AF606315

RYANODINE RECEPTORS

Structure, function and dysfunction in clinical disease

Developments in Cardiovascular Medicine

232. A. Bayés de Luna, F. Furlanello, B.J. Maron and D.P. Zipes (eds.): *Arrhythmias and Sudden Death in Athletes.* 2000 ISBN: 0-7923-6337-X
233. J-C. Tardif and M.G. Bourassa (eds): *Antioxidants and Cardiovascular Disease.* 2000. ISBN: 0-7923-7829-6
234. J. Candell-Riera, J. Castell-Conesa, S. Aguadé Bruiz (eds): *Myocardium at Risk and Viable Myocardium Evaluation by SPET.* 2000.ISBN: 0-7923-6724-3
235. M.H. Ellestad and E. Amsterdam (eds): Exercise Testing: New Concepts for the New Century. 2001. ISBN: 0-7923-7378-2
236. Douglas L. Mann (ed.): The Role of Inflammatory Mediators in the Failing Heart. 2001 ISBN: 0-7923-7381-2
237. Donald M. Bers (ed.): Excitation-Contraction Coupling and Cardiac Contractile Force, Second Edition. 2001 ISBN: 0-7923-7157-7
238. Brian D. Hoit, Richard A. Walsh (eds.): Cardiovascular Physiology in the Genetically Engineered Mouse, Second Edition. 2001 ISBN 0-7923-7536-X
239. Pieter A. Doevendans, A.A.M. Wilde (eds.): Cardiovascular Genetics for Clinicians 2001 ISBN 1-4020-0097-9
240. Stephen M. Factor, Maria A.Lamberti-Abadi, Jacobo Abadi (eds.): Handbook of Pathology and Pathophysiology of Cardiovascular Disease. 2001 ISBN 0-7923-7542-4
241. Liong Bing Liem, Eugene Downar (eds): Progress in Catheter Ablation. 2001 ISBN 1-4020-0147-9
242. Pieter A. Doevendans, Stefan Kääb (eds): Cardiovascular Genomics: New Pathophysiological Concepts. 2002 ISBN 1-4020-7022-5
243. Daan Kromhout, Alessandro Menotti, Henry Blackburn (eds.): Prevention of Coronary Heart Disease: Diet, Lifestyle and Risk Factors in the Seven Countries Study. 2002 ISBN 1-4020-7123-X
244. Antonio Pacifico (ed.), Philip D. Henry, Gust H. Bardy, Martin Borggrefe, Francis E. Marchlinski, Andrea Natale, Bruce L. Wilkoff (assoc. eds): Implantable Defibrillator Therapy: A Clinical Guide. 2002 ISBN 1-4020-7143-4
245. Hein J.J. Wellens, Anton P.M. Gorgels, Pieter A. Doevendans (eds.): The ECG in Acute Myocardial Infarction and Unstable Angina: Diagnosis and Risk Stratification. 2002 ISBN 1-4020-7214-7
246. Jack Rychik, Gil Wernovsky (eds.): Hypoplastic Left Heart Syndrome. 2003 ISBN 1-4020-7319-4
247. Thomas H. Marwick: Stress Echocardiography. Its Role in the Diagnosis and Evaluation of Coronary Artery Disease 2nd Edition. ISBN 1-4020-7369-0
248. Akira Matsumori: Cardiomyopathies and Heart Failure: Biomolecular, Infectious and Immune Mechanisms. 2003 ISBN 1-4020-7438-7
249. Ralph Shabetai: The Pericardium. 2003 ISBN 1-4020-7639-8
250. Irene D. Turpie; George A. Heckman (eds.): Aging Issues in Cardiology. 2004 ISBN 1-40207674-6
251. C.H. Peels; L.H.B. Baur (eds.): Valve Surgery at the Turn of the Millennium. 2004 ISBN 1-4020-7834-X
252. Jason X.-J. Yuan (ed.): Hypoxic Pulmonary Vasoconstriction: Cellular and Molecular Mechanisms. 2004 ISBN 1-4020-7857-9
253. Francisco J. Villarreal (ed.): Interstitial Fibrosis In Heart Failure 2004 ISBN 0-387-22824-1
254. Xander H.T. Wehrens; Andrew R. Marks (eds.): Ryanodine Receptors: Structure, function and dysfunction in clinical disease. 2005 ISBN 0-387-23187-0

Previous volumes are still available

RYANODINE RECEPTORS
Structure, function and dysfunction in clinical disease

Edited by

Xander H.T. Wehrens and Andrew R. Marks

Dept. of Physiology and Cellular Biophysics, Center for Molecular Cardiology, College of Physicians and Surgeons of Columbia University, 630 West 168th Street, P&S 9-401, New York, NY 10032, U.S.A.

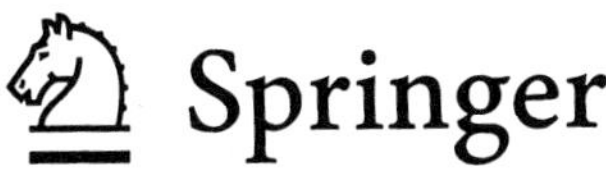

Xander H.T. Wehrens and Andrew R. Marks
Department of Physiology and Cellular Biophysics
Center for Molecular Cardiology
College of Physicians and Surgeons of Columbia University
630 West 168th Street, P&S 9-401
New York, NY 10032, U.S.A.
xw80@columbia.edu
arm42@columbia.edu

Cover illustration: Leaky ryanodine receptors in the failing heart may provide a trigger for cardiac arrhythmias (left). The drug JTV519 stabilizes the ryanodine receptor channel, thereby preventing lethal ventricular arrhythmias (right). Illustration by Nancy Heim.

Library of Congress Cataloging-in-Publication Data

Ryanodine receptors : structure, function and dysfunction in clinical disease / edited by Xander H.T. Wehrens and Andrew R. Marks.
p. ; cm. – (Developments in cardiovascular medicine ; 254)
Includes bibliographical references and index.
ISBN 0-387-23187-0 (alk paper) e-ISBN 0-387-23188-9
1. Ryanodine receptors. I. Wehrens, Xander H.T. II. Marks, Andrew R., 1955-III. Series.
[DNLM: 1. Ryanodine Receptor Calcium Release Channel—physiology. 2. Ryanodine Receptor Calcium Release Channel—chemistry. QH 603.I54 R989 2005]
QP535.C2R883 2005
612.3'924—dc22 2004058942

Printed in the United States of America.

9 8 7 6 5 4 3 2 1 SPIN 11053712

springeronline.com

Publication of this book was generously supported by:

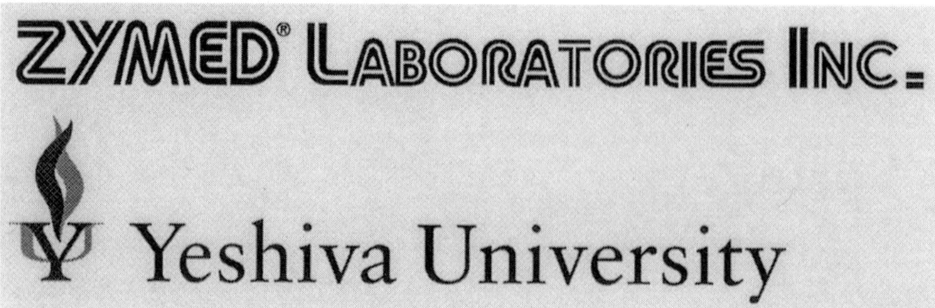

Dedication

This book is dedicated to Eve;
Marnie, Joshua, Daniel & Sarah

Contents

Contributing Authors

Donald M. Bers (Chapter 10)
Dept. of Physiology, Loyola University Chicago, Stritch School of Medicine, 2160 South First Avenue, Maywood, IL 60153 (dbers@lumc.edu)
Co-author: Kenneth S. Ginsburg

Henry R. Besch Jr. (Chapter 18)
Dept. of Pharmacology and Toxicology, Indiana University School of Medicine, 635 Barnhill Drive, Indianapolis, IN 46202 (besch@iupui.edu)
Co-authors: Keshore R. Bidasee, Chun Hong Shao

Keshore R. Bidasee (Chapter 21)
Dept. of Pharmacology, University of Nebraska Medical Center, 985800 Nebraska Medical Center, DRC 3047, Omaha, NE 6819 (kbidasee@unmc.edu)
Co-authors: Sarah Ingersoll, Chun Hong Shao

Robert T. Dirksen (Chapter 23)
Dept. of Pharmacology and Physiology, University of Rochester Medical Center, 601 Elmwood Avenue, Rochester, NY 14642 (robert_dirksen@urmc.rochester.edu)
Co-author: Guillermo Avila

Ehrlich, Barbara E. (Chapter 17)
Depts. of Pharmacology, and Cellular & Molecular Physiology, Yale School of Medicine, 333 Cedar Street, New Haven, CT 06510 (barbara.ehrlich@yale.edu)
Co-author: Edmond D. Buck

David A. Eisner (Chapter 11)
Unit of Cardiac Physiology, University of Manchester, 1.524 Stopford Building, Oxford Rd, Manchester M13 9PT, United Kingdom (eisner@man.ac.uk)
Co-authors: Mary E. Díaz, Stephen C. O'Neill, Andrew W. Trafford

Fill, Michael (Chapter 8)
Dept. of Physiology, Loyola University Chicago, 2160 South First Avenue, Maywood, IL 60153 (mfill@lumc.edu)
Co-author: Josefina Ramos-Franco

Franzini-Armstrong, Clara (Chapter 4)
Dept. of Cell Developmental Biology, University of Pennsylvania School of Medicine, Anatomy/Chemistry Building B42, Philadelphia, PA 19104 (armstroc@mail.med.upenn.edu)

Györke, Sandor (Chapter 7)
Dept. of Physiology, Texas Tech University HSC, 3601 4th Street, Lubbock, TX 79430 (sandor.gyorke@ttuhsc.edu)
Co-authors: Dmitry Terentyev, Serge Viatchenko-Karpinski

Susan L. Hamilton (Chapter 16)
Dept. of Molecular Physiology and Biophysics, Baylor College of Medicine, One Baylor Plaza, Room 400B, Houston, TX 77030 (susanh@bcm.tmc.edu)
Co-authors: Paula Aracena, Cecilia Hidalgo

Ikemoto, Noriaki (Chapter 6)
Boston Biomedical Research Institute, 64 Grove Street, Watertown, MA 02472, and Harvard Medical School, Boston, MA (ikemoto@bbri.org)

Lederer, W.J. (Chapter 9)
Medical Biotechnology Center, University of Maryland Biotechnology Institute, 725 W. Lombard Street, Baltimore, MD 21201
Co-authors: Silvia Guatimosim, Eric A. Sobie, Long-Sheng Song

Lehnart, Stephan E. (Chapter 25)
Dept. of Physiology and Cellular Biophysics, College of Physicians and Surgeons of Columbia University, New York, 630 West 168th Street, P&S 9-401, New York, NY 10032 (sel2004@columbia.edu)
Co-authors: Andrew R. Marks, Xander H.T. Wehrens

MacLennan, David H. (Chapter 2)
Banting and Best Department of Medical Research, University of Toronto, Charles H. Best Institute, 112 College St., Toronto, Ontario M5G 1L6, Canada (david.maclennan@utoronto.ca)
Co-author: Guo Guang Du

Marks, Andrew R. (15)
Depts. of Physiology and Cellular Biophysics, and Medicine, Center for Molecular Cardiology, College of Physicians and Surgeons of Columbia University, 630 West 168th Street, P&S 9-401, New York, NY 10032 (arm42@columbia.edu)
Co-authors: Stephan E. Lehnart, Xander H.T. Wehrens

Marx, Steven O. (Chapter 12)
Division of Cardiology and Center for Molecular Cardiology; Depts. of Medicine and Pharmacology, Columbia University College of Physicians and Surgeons, 630 W 168th Street, P&S 9-401, New York, NY 10032 (sm460@columbia.edu)

McCarthy, Tommie V. (Chapter 22)
Dept. of Biochemistry, University College Cork, Cork, Ireland (t.mccarthy@ucc.ie)
Co-authors: James J.A. Heffron, John Mackrill

Meissner, Gerhard (Chapter 20)
Depts. of Biochemistry and Biophysics, and Cell and Molecular Physiology, University of North Carolina, Chapel Hill, NC 27599 (meissner@med.unc.edu)
Co-author: Jonathan S. Stamler

Ogawa, Yasuo (Chapter 13)
Dept. of Pharmacology, Juntendo University School of Medicine, Tokyo 113-8421, Japan (ysogawa@med.juntendo.ac.jp)
Co-authors: Nagomi Kurebayashi, Takashi Murayama

Parness, Jerome (Chapter 24)
Dept. of Anesthesia, UMDNJ-Robert Wood Johnson Medical School, Staged Research Annex II, Rm 117, 661 Hoes Lane, Piscatway, NJ 08854 (parness@umdnj.edu)

Romi, Frederik (Chapter 27)
Dept. of Neurology, Haukeland University Hospital, N-5021 Bergen, Norway (fredrik.romi@haukeland.no)

Takeshima, Hiroshi (Chapter 14)
Dept. of Biochemistry, Tohoku University Graduate School of Medicine, Sendai, Miyagi 980-8575, Japan (takeshim@mail.tains.tohoku.ac.jp)

Valdivia, Héctor H. (Chapter 19)
Dept. of Physiology, University of Wisconsin Medical School, Madison, WI 53706 (valdivia@physiology.wisc.edu)
Co-authors: Georgina B. Gurrola, Xinsheng Zhu

Wagenknecht, Terence (Chapter 3)
Wadsworth Center, New York State Department of Health, Albany, New York 12201, and Dept. of Biomedical Sciences, School of Public Health, State University of New York at Albany, Albany, New York 12201 (tcw02@health.state.ny.us)
Co-author: Zheng Liu

Wehrens, Xander H.T. (Chapter 1)
Dept. of Physiology and Cellular Biophysics, Center for Molecular Cardiology, College of Physicians and Surgeons of Columbia University, 630 West 168th Street, P&S 9-401, New York, NY 10032 (xw80@columbia.edu)
Co-authors: Alexander Kushnir, A.K.M.M. Mollah

Williams, Alan J. (Chapter 5)
Cardiac Medicine, National Heart & Lung Institute, Imperial College London, London SW3 6LY, U.K. (a.j.Williams @imperial.ac.uk)
Co-authors: S.R. Wayne Chen, William Welch

Yano, Masafumi (Chapter 26)
Dept. of Medical Bioregulation, Division of Cardiovascular Medicine, Yamaguchi University School of Medicine, 1-1-1 Minamikogushi, Ube, Yamaguchi, 755-8505, Japan (yanoma@yamaguchi-u.ac.jp)
Co-authors: Masunori Matsuzaki, Takeshi Yamamoto

Preface

It has been 15 years since the ryanodine receptor/calcium release channel (RyR) cDNA was cloned, ushering in a new age of understanding for the largest known ion channel. Prior to the cloning of its cDNA, RyR was known to be a calcium release channel in the terminal cisternae of the sarcoplasmic reticulum (SR). However, it was shrouded in mystery, as even its molecular mass and subunit composition were not known.

From the deduced amino acid sequence, provided by cDNA cloning, the molecular mass of the channel became known and it was shown to be a homotetramer comprised of four RyR monomers each ~565,000 daltons. The availability of the cDNA, which ultimately enabled functional expression of the channel and site-directed mutagenesis to identify functional domains, revolutionized the study of RyR. What has emerged in the last decade of RyR research is a remarkable story that is still rapidly changing, almost on a daily basis. This ion channel, which is known to be required for such fundamental processes as muscle contraction, continues to challenge investigators by virtue of its massive size and complexity.

Despite many hurdles we have come a long way towards gaining insight about RyR structure-function relationships. While these studies continue, equally exciting and perhaps somewhat surprising has been the emergence of RyRs as central molecules in a number of major human diseases including heart failure and cardiac arrhythmias. The role of RyR in these diseases would not have been predicted a decade ago. Thus, RyR is emerging as a potentially important therapeutic target for the diseases that are the leading causes of mortality in the developed world.

It seemed fitting, on the 15 anniversary of the cloning of the RyR cDNA, to put together the first truly comprehensive book telling the story of this remarkable channel from many diverse perspectives. The scope of the book is from basic structure-function studies, to physiology to disease relevance. A central theme throughout many of the chapters is the role of the RyR macromolecular complex. Little did we know 15 years ago, when several laboratories were cloning the enormous 15 kb cDNA encoding RyR, that this was going to be just the beginning of the story! Indeed, multiple other proteins are integral components of the RyR complex. The first such component to be assigned a key function in the complex was the FK506 binding protein (FKBP12) now also known as calstabin1 (calcium channel stabilizing protein) which is required for normal gating of RyR1 in skeletal muscle by virtue of the fact that it stabilizes the closed (and the open) state of the channel. A similar function for calstabin2 (FKBP12.6) has been demonstrated for RyR2 in cardiac muscles. Subsequently, many other proteins have been assigned functional roles in the RyR channel complex and shown to bind to and/or interact with either the large cytoplasmic domain of the channel or the SR luminal domain of the channel.

It is important to note that stringent criteria must been used to define components of the RyR complex, and while several proteins have been proposed as candidates for inclusion in this macromolecular complex only those that meet the following criteria are bona fide members: 1) co-immunoprecipitation and co-sedimentation with solubilized RyR; 2) identification of binding site(s) on the RyR channel and targeting proteins with binding sites on the channel; 3) co-localization in relevant cells; 4) identification of physiologically important functional roles in the channel complex. Proteins that fail to qualify in all four of these aspects are not included in the RyR macromolecular complex. Doubtless future studies will identify new components of the complex that meet all four criteria and will be important for enhancing our understanding or RyRs. Truly, unless we understand the composition of the RyR complex it will be impossible to fully elucidate the regulation of this channel.

Looking to the next 15 years of RyR research, perhaps the most important advance will be solving the atomic structure of the channel. There are clear indications that the channel is regulated by long distance (allosteric) modulation of its structure through binding to molecules that regulate it. Solving the structure will be required to gain the next level of insight with regard to mechanisms of gating of the channel and modulation by such things as phosphorylation and drugs that are being developed as potential therapeutics.

Of course there are many, many unanswered questions about RyRs. Each of the following chapters provides a concise review of a specific aspect of the channel and includes thoughtful consideration of what is known, and what is not known. In instances where controversies exist in the field all sides have been presented in a fair and balanced manner so that the reader can understand that questions that remain and that the work is ongoing.

It is quite clear that RyRs are important molecules in virtually every organ system and we are just beginning to appreciate their central role in human diseases. No pharmacology currently exists for RyRs, so the opportunities for developing novel therapeutics that target RyRs are vast and this will be a most exciting avenue for investigation over the next 15 years.

Andrew R. Marks and Xander H.T. Wehrens
Editors

Acknowledgments: Publication of this book was generously supported by Zymed Laboratories Inc. and an educational grant from Yeshiva University, New York. Additional support was granted by Medtronic Inc., Pacer Scientific, and Tech Air Inc. We are indebted to Alexander Kushnir for his editorial assistance in preparing the book.

Foreword

Calcium is vital to life on earth. Its significance is preserved in the ocean beds and mountains of limestone, the remnants of countless organisms that used it to define their shapes. Only in the last couple hundred years did humans realize that the shells of organisms found at the tops of mountains were once at the bottoms of oceans. Without calcium to imprint the fossil and shell history of life, prehistoric life would have gone unrecorded. This record revolutionized the understanding of the earth's age, its restless, slow movement, and the billions of years span of life.

Particularly significant in light of the chapters that follow, cardiac muscle lies at the heart of our first understanding of calcium's significance in all living cells. In 1882, Sidney Ringer found that London's "hard" tap water sustained cardiac muscle contraction, which slowly came to a stop in distilled water. The significance of extracellular calcium in sustaining normal cell function, published in 1883 in *J Physiol.*, did not immediately draw the attention it deserved. Not until the 1950's did calcium begin to come into focus as the trigger molecule for muscle contraction and since then, the trigger or regulator of practically every cellular process ranging from cell division to cell death.

Both magnesium and calcium divalent cations are abundant in seawater. Calcium precipitates phosphate, while magnesium binds tightly to water. Apparently the roles of these two ions in biology were formed by the cell's need for preservation of free phosphate as the energy currency of cells. Calcium is actively excluded from the cytoplasm where phosphates are exchanged. Specialized proteins bind and extrude calcium to preserve a 20,000 fold gradient from the extracellular environment to the cytoplasm. In addition, the endo- or sarcoplasmic reticulum greatly expands the surface area for removal of cytoplasmic calcium, but preserving it as "stored" calcium. Calcium is a highly localized messenger. It diffuses much more slowly than calcium in water because it is bound by negative charges, particularly by the glutamates and aspartates of amino acids in proteins. Thus it diffuses no more than 0.1-0.5 μm before encountering a binding site, with the result that calcium stutters around the cell in roughly 50 ns steps.

The reticulum does not function as a simple storage reservoir from which calcium is released uniformly. Instead, calcium taken into the reticulum can be released in a highly localized manner. It appears that via the reticulum, calcium can be shunted across polarized cells, released near mitochondria to boost energy production, and used to trigger spatially localized subcellular events. The highest form of this organization is in muscle sarcoplasmic reticulum, where stored calcium can be electrically triggered for rapid, more uniform spatial synchrony. The ion channels that release the stored calcium are huge (>2.2 megadaltons) tetrameric proteins that span the sarcoplasmic reticulum. They are known as *ryanodine receptors*, based on their binding by the insecticidal alkaloid isolated from the ground stems of *Ryania speciosa*, a native plant of tropical America. At low concentrations ryanodine binds the open channel and locks the channel open in a subconducting state, but at higher concentrations it causes the channel to close. Caffeine also is an effective activator, but calcium itself is the presumed native activator of RyRs, resulting in amplified calcium-induced calcium release. Ryanodine receptors are encoded by three genes: *RyR1* (skeletal muscle), *RyR2* (heart, neurons), and *RyR3* (widespread expression).

The ryanodine receptor, and its smaller sibling, the inositol triphosphate receptor (IP_3R), have similar roles in releasing calcium from the reticulum, but the ryanodine receptor has evolved such that its gating is tightly linked to that of voltage-gated calcium channels in the plasma membrane, either by calcium entering through the voltage-gated channels or by conformational coupling (in the case of skeletal muscle). Its highly organized relation to the voltage-gated calcium channel makes it an integrated fast switch. The IP_3R in contrast, appears to be gated by comparatively slow generation of second messengers, although direct links with plasma membrane channels have been proposed. Both large calcium release channels appear to make many links to other proteins and are highly regulated in protein complexes. So far, both have been refractory to high-resolution structural determinations. Our understanding of intracellular channels lags understandably far behind the more accessible and smaller plasma membrane channels. There is much yet to do on this mega-channel, and there will be many surprises to come.

Drs. Xander Wehrens and Andrew Marks have gathered the collected wisdom of scientists who have devoted their working lives to the study of ryanodine receptors. In this series of brief but informative chapters, the contributions progress from the basic gene family and primary structure, through its 3D structure so far, to its regulation and physiology. The book ends with several chapters on mutations in the receptor that cause disease, and their role in adaptation to disease. There are interesting new developments in the control of ryanodine receptors by accessory proteins, the latest of which is the proposed role of leaky RyR channels in causing delayed afterdepolarizations, a cause of lethal ventricular arrhythmias. The series of reviews in this book will bring anyone rapidly up to speed in current progress in the field, as well as highlight remaining questions.

David E. Clapham

Boston, Massachusetts

Chapter 1

EVOLUTION OF THE RYANODINE RECEPTOR GENE FAMILY

Alexander Kushnir[1,2], A.K.M.M. Mollah[1], and Xander H.T. Wehrens[2]
[1]Dept. of Biology, Yeshiva College, New York, NY; [2]Dept. of Physiology and Cellular Biophysics, Center for Molecular Cardiology, College of Physicians and Surgeons, Columbia University, New York, NY

INTRODUCTION

Fluctuations in cytosolic calcium (Ca^{2+}) concentrations act to modulate a vast array of second messenger signaling pathways in living organisms. This control mechanism results in delicate regulation due to low cytosolic Ca^{2+} levels under resting conditions alternating with rapid and transient increases in Ca^{2+} upon stimulation. Key components of this pathway were initially evolved in primordial Ca^{2+} transport systems and then rapidly developed into more specialized Ca^{2+} pumps and Ca^{2+} channels on the plasma membrane. Following the evolution of the sarcoplasmic reticulum (or in some organ systems endoplasmic reticulum) as intracellular Ca^{2+} stores, intracellular calcium-release channels evolved.

Intracellular calcium-release channels are required for many cellular processes, such as excitation-contraction coupling in skeletal and cardiac muscle and signal transduction in the nervous system.[1] The system of endomembranes that forms the sarco(endo)plasmic reticulum plays a vital role in Ca^{2+} handling in most eukaryots.[2] Two families of intracellular calcium-release channels are found in this compartment: ryanodine receptors (RyRs) and inositol 1,4,5-trisphosphate receptors (IP_3Rs). The RyRs (560 kDa) and IP_3Rs (260 kDa) are similar in structure, both having large N-terminal and small C-terminal domains protruding into the cytoplasm, and several transmembrane regions near the C-terminus (Fig. 1-1).[3,4]

Ryanodine receptors consist of four monomers that assemble to form a functional calcium-release channel. The large N-terminal domain contains binding sites for channel modulators that regulate the channel pore including FK506-binding proteins FKBP12 (calstabin1) and FKBP12.6 (calstabin2), which are bound to RyR1 and RyR2, respectively (Fig. 1-1).[5] FKBP12/12.6 binding to RyR stabilizes the channel in the closed-state confirmation. Three leucine/ isoleucine zipper (LIZ) motifs on RyR2 allow binding of the adaptor proteins spinophilin, PR130, and mAKAP, which target the protein phosphatases PP1 and PP2A, and protein kinase A (PKA) to the channel complex, respectively (see Chapter 15).[6]

In the original topological model for RyR1 proposed by Numa and colleagues,[3] four transmembrane (TM) segments were proposed near the C-terminus. Subsequently, Zorzato *et al.*[7] proposed 12 hydrophobic sequences in the C-terminal region of RyR (see Chapter 2 for a more extensive review). The first two TM sequences (M' and M'') were considered to be very tentative, and the others were called M1-M10.[7] Based on an experimental study, MacLennan *et al.*[8] proposed a slightly different model (Fig. 1.1), in which the C-terminus contains six to eight TM segments. In addition, the pore segment (M9) is thought to line the pore of the channel as a selectivity filter described for voltage-gated ion channels,[9] allowing Ca^{2+} ions to transverse the membrane. This chapter will focus on the genetic characteristics and phylogenetic relationships among different RyR isoforms that have been identified thus far.

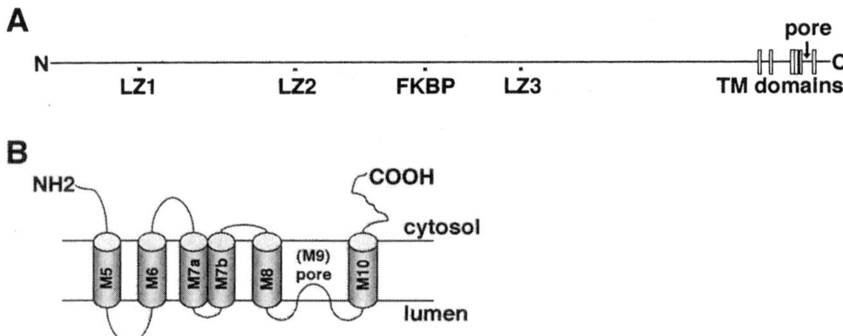

Figure 1-1. **Schematic diagram of the RyR protein. A**. Line diagram showing the RyR protein with the transmembrane (TM) domains and pore. Also shown are the leucine/isoleucine zippers (LIZ) and binding-site of FKBP12/FKBP12.6. **B**. Proposed organization of the transmembrane domains, according to MacLennan *et al.*[8] TM domains are numbered according to the Zorzato model.[7]

RYANODINE RECEPTOR GENES

Ryanodine receptors were first cloned from mammalian skeletal and cardiac muscle.[3,4,10] Analysis of the nucleotide sequences revealed that these two subtypes are about 66% homologous.[3,4] A third mammalian RyR isoform was cloned from rabbit brain and a mink lung epithelial cell line.[11,12] Similar RyR isoforms have been cloned from non-mammalian vertebrates (e.g., chicken, bullfrog, and blue marlin),[13-15] although they seem to express only two distinct isoforms. The non-mammalian vertebrate RyRα isoforms appear to be homologs of the mammalian skeletal muscle isoform RyR1, while the RyRβ isoforms are related to the mammalian RyR3.[13,15] Although RyRs were originally discovered in vertebrates, more recently they have been identified in invertebrates, including *Caenorhabditis elegans* and *Drosophila melanogaster* (Table 1-1).[16,17]

Table 1-1. **GenBank accession numbers and number of amino acids of the RyR isoforms**

Isoform	Species	Common name	Accession number	Amino acids	References
RyR2	*H. sapiens*	Human	Q92736	4967	Tunwell *et al.*[18]
RyR2	*O. cuniculus*	Rabbit	P30957	4969	Otsu *et al.*[4]
RyR2	*M. musculus*	Mouse	NP_076357	4967	Zorzato *et al.*[7]
RyR3	*H. sapiens*	Human	Q15413	4870	Leeb *et al.*[19]
RyR3	*O. cuniculus*	Rabbit	S27272	4872	Hakamata *et al.*[12]
RyR3	*Mustela sp.*	Mink	S74173	4859	Marziali *et al.*[20]
RyRβ	*G. gallus*	Chicken	CAA64563	4869	Ottini *et al.*[13]
RyRβ	*R. catesbeiana*	Bullfrog	BAA04647	4868	Oyamada *et al.*[15]
RyR1	*H. sapiens*	Human	P21817	5038	Zorzato *et al.*[7]
RyR1	*S. scrofa*	Pig	I46646	5035	Fujii *et al.*[21]
RyR1	*O. cuniculus*	Rabbit	P11716	5037	Takeshima *et al.*[3]
RyR1	*M. nigricans*	Fish	AAB58117	5081	Franck *et al.*[14]
RyRα	*R. catesbeiana*	Bullfrog	BAA04646	5037	Oyamada *et al.*[15]
RyR	*A. gambiae*	Mosquito	EAA13701	4872	Ensembl.org[22]
RyR	*D. melanogaster*	Fruit fly	AAB29457	5126	Takeshima *et al.*[23]
RyR	*H. pulcherrimus*	Sea urchin	BAB84714	5317	Shiwa *et al.*[24]

The gene for RyR1 is located on chromosome 19q13.2 in humans, and spans 104 exons. The RyR2 gene with 102 exons is located on chromosome 1q43, and the RyR3 gene with 103 exons on chromosome 15q13.3-14. Although the RyR genes are located on different chromosomes in mice (chromosomes 7A3, 13A2, and 2E4, for RyR1, RyR2, and RyR3, respectively),[25] the neighboring genes on these chromosomes are similar to those found on the corresponding human chromosomes. The organization in the phylogenetic tree supports the model that an expansion of the vertebrate gene family was associated with an initial duplication of the RyR1 gene, since only one RyR gene is found in invertebrates (Fig. 1-2). Indeed, non-mammalian vertebrates express two RyR genes.[15] It appears that a second duplication occurred in mammals, which distinguishes them from other vertebrates. This model is consistent with the theory that gene duplication is important in adaptive evolution because it allows the new proteins to have distinct functional characteristics.[26]

An additional means of generating diversity in RyR channels is through alternative splicing. Alternative splicing has been demonstrated for several vertebrate[18,27,28] and invertebrate RyR isoforms.[29] Although some data suggest that alternatively spliced variants of RyR3 exhibit reduced caffeine sensitivities, relatively little is known about the electrophysiological properties of alternatively spliced RyR channels.[30] Considering that invertebrate species appear to have only 1 RyR gene, in contrast to the three mammalian RyR genes, it is likely that invertebrates and vertebrates use fundamentally different means of generating diversity in RyR function. Indeed, there is evidence for alternative splicing of the insect *H. virescens RyR* gene, resulting in potentially different channels.[31] Thus, the major means of generating diversity in invertebrate RyR channels may involve alternative splicing, whereas vertebrate RyR diversity may result primarily from the presence of multiple genes.

PHYLOGENY OF RYANODINE RECEPTORS

Based on phylogenetic analysis, it is likely that all RyR isoforms evolved from a single ancestor (Fig. 1-2), and possibly that RyR and IP_3R evolved from a common ancestral channel.[32] It is thought that IP_3R have 6 and RyR have 6-8 transmembrane domains, although definitive structural evidence is currently lacking.[8,33] Sequence homology comparison has revealed a high degree of homology between the pore region and TM domains lining the pore region comparing RyRs and IP_3R.[32] Ryanodine receptors have not been detected in protozoa or algae. Although there seems to be some functional evidence for calcium-release channels in higher plants, primordial RyR seems to occur in *C. elegans*.[34]

No data are available yet on the origin and time of appearance of intracellular calcium-release channels.[35] However, an overall structural homology is present between the pore-forming region of ryanodine receptors and the superfamily of ion channels that encompasses most of the voltage-gated ion channels, the cyclic-nucleotide-gated channels and the transient receptor potential (TRP) channels.[36] There is ~35-40% homology at the amino acid level between *C. elegans* and vertebrates. The homology is higher in certain functionally important domains that are conserved among all RyR isoforms, including the leucine/isoleucine zipper domains, the pore region, and the transmembrane domains. The most similarity between the different isoforms is observed in the pore region, and the adjacent two TM regions (M8 and M10), in which many residues are conserved from *C. elegans* to the human RyR isoforms (Fig. 1-3). Mutations of many of the highly conserved amino acids in the ion-conducting pore region have diverse effects on channel functions such as caffeine-induced Ca^{2+} release, ryanodine binding, single channel conductance and modulation, and cation selectivity.[37,38]

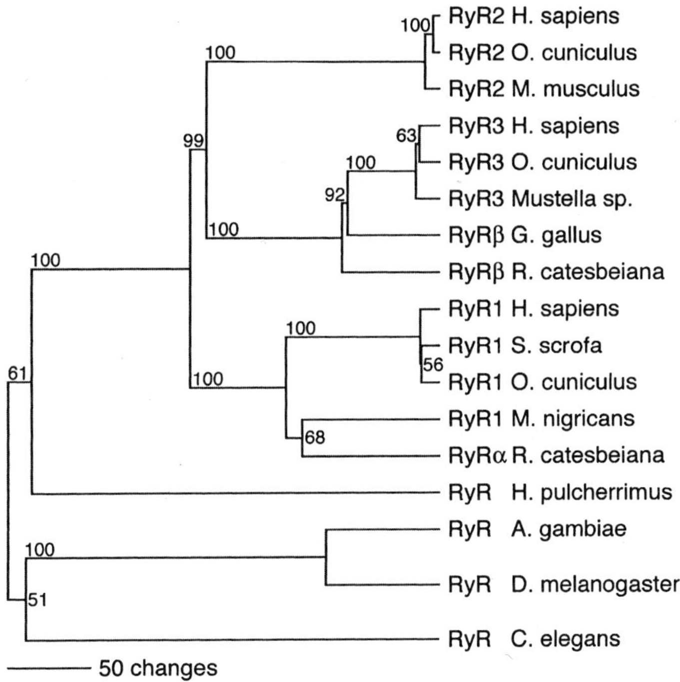

Figure 1-2. **Phylogenetic tree of the RyR gene family.** RyR protein sequences were aligned using ClustalW, and gaps were removed according to the method of Chiu *et al.*[39] Shown is the most-parsimonious tree using PAUP software. Numbers at each node represent bootstrap values (the probabilities that two lineages are joined together at the node to form a single cluster). Lengths of horizontal lines of the tree are proportional to the estimated number of amino acids substitutions. Abbreviations for the RyR isoforms are described in Table 1-1.

DIFFERENTIAL EXPRESSION OF RYR ISOFORMS

Expression of RyR1 is relatively abundant in skeletal muscle, although it is also expressed at lower levels in cardiac and smooth muscle, cerebellum, testis, adrenal gland, and ovaries.[3,10,13,40,41] Whereas RyR1 is predominantly expressed in Purkinje cells in the brain, RyR2 is localized mainly in the somata of most neurons.[40] RyR2 is expressed robustly in the heart and brain, and at lower levels in the stomach, lung, thymus, adrenal gland, and ovaries.[27,41] The RyR3 isoform is expressed in the brain, diaphragm, slow twitch skeletal muscle, as well as several abdominal organs.[11-13,41] The non-mammalian RyRα isoform is expressed strongly in skeletal muscle and weakly in brain, whereas the RyRβ isoform is expressed in a variety of tissues, including skeletal and cardiac muscle, lung, stomach, and brain.[15] There is some evidence that alternative splicing of RyR genes may underlie the tissue-specific expression of certain isoforms.[28]

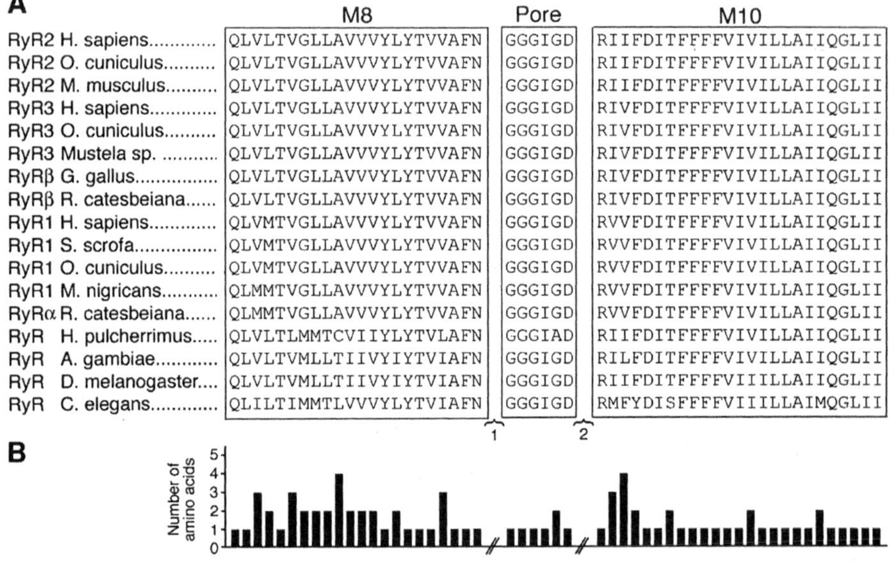

Figure 1-3. **The ryanodine receptor pore-forming region**. **A**. Alignment of 17 RyR isoforms showing the pore region and transmembrane regions 8 and 10 (M8, M10). Numbers 1 and 2 indicate regions not shown in alignment. **B**. The bar graph indicates the number of different amino acids among the different isoforms at the indicated residues.

RYANODINE RECEPTOR FUNCTION

In *C. elegans*, RyRs are found in vesicles of the body wall musculature that resemble the vertebrate junctional sarcoplasmic reticulum.[23] Expression of RyR has been reported in the body wall, pharyngeal, vulval, anal, and sex muscle of adult worms, as well as in embryonic muscle, but not in non-muscle cells.[42] Compared to RyR channels from mammalian cells, *C. elegans* RyR channel exhibit different conduction properties, although the functional significance of these findings remain to be elucidated.[29,43]

Wild-type *C. elegans* move by coordinated contraction and relaxation of the opposing dorsal and ventral muscle strips attached to the cuticle along the body length, producing sinusoidal waves that propel the animal forward or backward.[44] Mutant *C. elegans* defective in the RyR gene (unc68) propagate more slowly than wild-type, and exhibit an incomplete flaccid paralysis, despite normal muscle ultrastructure.[16] Although it appears that RyR plays a role in *C. elegans* pharyngeal and body-wall muscle contraction by amplifying depolarization-induced Ca^{2+} transients, intracellular Ca^{2+} release via RyR is not essential for EC coupling in *C. elegans*.[16,45] In nematodes, RyR-induced Ca^{2+} release also mediates periodic muscle contraction in the male sexual organ which is necessary during mating,[46] and in egg laying and embryogenesis.[47]

Similar to *C. elegans*, *D. melanogaster* only expresses one RyR isoform,[17] which is expressed in the mesoderm of early embryos, and in somatic, hypodermal and visceral muscle of larvae.[29] *D. melanogaster* larvae with a hypomorphic allele (ryr^{16}) display a reduced heart rate relative to wild-type larvae.[48] In adult *Drosophila*, RyR is expressed in nearly all tissues, most notably in the digestive tract and the nervous system.[32] Antibody staining for RyR is cytoplasmic, consistent with labeling of the endoplasmic reticulum. Therefore, it is believed that RyRs play an important role in intracellular Ca^{2+} cycling in *D. melanogaster*.

In non-mammalian vertebrates such as birds and fish, many organs express both the RyRα and the RyRβ isoforms.[49] In contrast, certain functionally specialized muscles, such as the extraocular muscles and the swimbladder muscle, express only the RyRα isoform.[49] The appearance of the RyRα isoform alone in these muscles in fish provides evidence that this isoform is selectively expressed when rapid contraction is required. The evolutionary development of three RyR isoforms in mammals possibly allowed for even further differentiation of intracellular calcium-release characteristics according to the needs of individual muscles or other cell types.

RYANODINE RECEPTOR MUTATIONS AND INHERITED DISEASE

Allelic variants of some RyR genes have been associated with phenotypic effects including genetic abnormalities. The *unc-68* mutation in the *ryr* gene of *C. elegans* has been linked to abnormal ketamine response, convulsions, and paralysis. Unc-68 null mutant worms move poorly as a result of defects in contraction and relaxation of body wall musculature. The unc-68 mutation occurs at a splice-acceptor sequence of intron 21, and acts like a null mutation.[16] Body contraction is attenuated in *Drosophila* unc-68 mutants, which often display tremors. In addition, severe defects in ingestion and passage of food into the gut and excretion have also been observed. Thus, in invertebrates the single RyR gene is functionally involved in a multitude of Ca^{2+} release mechanisms responsible for contraction in skeletal, cardiac, and visceral muscles.

Since vertebrates express more than one *ryr* gene, the regulation of Ca^{2+} release is more complex. Mutations that specifically eliminate RyR1 channels in mice ($skrr^{m1}$) or RyRα in 'crooked neck dwarf' chicken (*cn*) have recessive lethal phenotypes, resulting in perinatal death.[23,50] In contrast, mice deficient of the *RyR3* gene are viable and exhibit functional excitation-contraction coupling in skeletal muscle (Chapter 14).[51] Missense mutations in the porcine and human *ryr1* gene have been linked to malignant hyperthermia and central core disease, inherited myopathies in which skeletal muscle contracture with attendant hypermetabolism and elevation of body temperature are triggered by stress or anesthetics (see Chapters 22-24).[52] In humans, two distinct clinical syndromes causing exercise-induced sudden cardiac death, catecholaminergic polymorphic ventricular tachycardia (CPVT) and arrhythmogenic right ventricular cardiomyopathy/dysplasia (ARVC/D), have been linked to mutations in the human *ryr2* gene (see Chapter 25).[53,54]

CONCLUDING REMARKS

Ryanodine receptor calcium-release channels play an important role in many cellular processes, such as excitation-contraction coupling in skeletal and cardiac muscle. In evolution, functionally different RyR isoforms have evolved by gene duplication or alternative splicing. Several domains have been highly conserved from *C. elegans* to human RyR isoforms, and are now increasingly being recognized to mediate critical calcium-release channel functions.

Chapter 2

TOPOLOGY AND TRANSMEMBRANE ORGANIZATION OF RYANODINE RECEPTORS

Guo Guang Du and David H. MacLennan
Banting and Best Department of Medical Research, University of Toronto, Toronto, Ontario, Canada

INTRODUCTION

The transient elevation of Ca^{2+} in the myoplasm is a key element in excitation-contraction (EC) coupling. In muscle, Ca^{2+} is released from a store located in the lumen of the sarcoplasmic reticulum (SR) by a class of Ca^{2+} release channels referred to as ryanodine receptors or RyR. They are located in the junctional terminal cisternae of the sarcoplasmic reticulum, where they form a cluster of tetrameric molecules, each with a transmembrane (TM) component and a much larger cytosolic component. The cytosolic structure is often referred to as the "foot" component, since it appears to be the foot on which the sarcoplasmic reticulum stands as it extends away from the transverse tubular membrane.[55] The foot component bridges the 140 Å gap that exists between transverse tubular and sarcoplasmic reticulum membranes.

Three-dimensional reconstruction of RyR1 at 25-30 Å has been carried out using averaged electron microscopic images of large numbers of individual molecules.[56-58] Isolated RyR1, viewed from above, is roughly 290 x 290 Å with four equal subunits resembling a quatrefoil. These structures are observed in the junctional terminal cisternae of the sarcoplasmic reticulum and in corbular sarcoplasmic reticulum in cardiac muscle, but are absent from *RYR1* null mice.[59] At 30 Å resolution, the cytoplasmic quatrefoils are seen to be about 120 Å high and to be highly hydrated, with numerous canals lying among at least 10 loosely assembled protein domains (see Chapter 3). The architecture is that of a scaffold that provides a mechanical linkage between the SR and the transverse tubule, while facilitating flow of Ca^{2+} from a central channel to the periphery. The open channel has a visible, solvent-filled opening on the luminal side, which disappears in the closed configuration. The intramembrane domain, seen from below or from the side, is about 70 Å tall and could accommodate multiple TM amino acid sequences. Estimates have been made of the mass of the protein contained in the TM domains, based on the total volume of the transmembrane domain and the volume occupied by a TM helix. The TM domain could accommodate 24 to 32 TM helices,[60,61] suggesting that the most likely number of TM helices per monomer is between 6 and 8.

The close apposition between the transverse tubular and junctional terminal cisternae membranes has led to speculation concerning the identity of the proteins in these two membranes that must interact. Block *et al.*[62] demonstrated that, in skeletal muscle, every other foot protein is directly apposed to a cluster of four L-type Ca^{2+} channel complexes referred to as dihydropyridine receptors or DHPR, located in the transverse tubules. Each of the four DHPR complexes is associated with one subunit of the huge tetrameric RyR molecule. These observations led to the proposal that there is a direct interaction in skeletal muscle between RyR and DHPR molecules. Further support for the interaction between RyR and DHPR comes from physiological evidence which shows that inward Ca^{2+} currents through the DHPR are a late event in skeletal muscle EC-coupling and are not essential.[63] An essential component of EC coupling is the "charge movement", which represents the translocation of a voltage-sensing helix across the membrane, with consequences for the conformation of other physically associated TM helices.[64,65] These physical movements in the DHPR are believed to be transmitted physically to closely apposed RyR molecules to alter the conformation of RyR1 and bring about the activation of Ca^{2+} release channels that triggers muscle contraction.[63]

The random apposition of RyR and DHPR molecules that is observed in cardiac muscle shows that cardiac isoforms of RyR and DHPR do not interact directly. Moreover, in cardiac muscle, inward Ca^{2+} through the DHPR is an early and essential event[63]. These results suggest that Ca^{2+}-induced Ca^{2+} release accounts for virtually all EC coupling in cardiac muscle, but for only 50% of EC coupling in skeletal muscle.

A second protein that helps to bring the transverse tubule into apposition with the terminal cisternae is mitsugumin 29.[66] This protein has a single TM component and a cytosolic domain which also bridges the gap between the transverse tubule and the terminal cisternae. This protein does not appear to be involved directly with the interaction between RyR and DHPR.

It has been of great interest to understand which parts of RyR and DHPR interact. These segments occur in the part of RyR which is most distal from the TM segments of the four subunits which make up the RyR molecule. The identity of these segments is covered in Chapter 4 of this book. The focus of this chapter is the question of which parts of the ryanodine receptor form the TM domain. We conclude that there are six essential TM segments which lie between amino acids (aa) 4557 and 4935. They include three TM hairpin loops and a selectivity filter which is located within the final hairpin loop between aa 4854 and 4911. We also conclude that RyR contains an additional upstream TM hairpin loop which is contained within a single contiguous hydrophobic sequence between aa 4323 and 4363 and is preceded by a very basic sequence of about 19 aa which lies in the cytosol. This TM sequence has some regulatory properties, but is not essential to channel function, since recombinant RyR1 molecules in which aa 4274-4535 are deleted retains Ca^{2+} release channel function.[67] Thus the entire molecule contains 8 TM sequences in 4 TM hairpin loops, but only 3 of these TM hairpins are required for Ca^{2+} release channel function.

IDENTITY OF TM SEQUENCES

RyR Ca^{2+} release channel molecules are homotetramers of 2,350,000 Da, formed from four monomers, each of 565 kDa. TM sequences from each of the four monomers interact to form the ion-conducting pore.[68] When the sequences of the ~5000 aa that constitute rabbit and human skeletal muscle RyR1[3,7] were first deduced from cDNAs, they were subjected to analysis using hydropathy plots that were based on criteria defined by Kyte and Doolittle.[69] The data obtained were interpreted in minimalist fashion by Takeshima *et al.*[3] Among the predicted TM sequences, four potential TM sequences are clearly more hydrophobic than others, with hydropathy indices between 2.0 and 2.9. These four sequences: aa Phe^{4564}-Tyr^{4580}; Pro^{4641}-Leu^{4664}; Gln^{4836}-Phe^{4859}; and Ile^{4918}-Ile^{4937}, were designated M1 to M4 and were proposed to form two hairpin loops in the topological model proposed by Takeshima *et al.* (the Takeshima model).[3]

In the studies of Zorzato *et al.*[7] a more complex interpretation was attempted, based on previous experience in the prediction of TM sequences in the sarco(end)plasmic reticulum Ca^{2+} ATPase or SERCA.[70] With the view that TM sequences in pumps and channels might require charged residues in TM sequences, the criteria for prediction of a TM sequence were made less stringent. Nevertheless, the view that each TM sequence would exist in partnership to form a hairpin loop was adhered to. In the topological model proposed by Zorzato *et al.*[7] (the Zorzato model), eight additional hydrophobic sequences were identified in the C-terminal fifth of the molecule, with hydropathy indices ranging from 0.8 to 1.6, and proposed to form four additional hairpin loops. The first two sequences in the Zorzato model, M' (Gly^{3124}-Phe^{3144}) and M" (Pro^{3188}-Leu^{3206}), were considered to be very tentative; the others were: M1 (Leu^{3985}-Ala^{4004}); M2 (Met^{4023}-Ala^{4041}); M3 (Gly^{4277}-Ala^{4300}); M4 (Ala^{4342}-Phe^{4362}); M5 (Phe^{4559}-Tyr^{4580}); M6 (Leu^{4648}-Phe^{4671}); M7 (Phe^{4789}-Val^{4820}); M8 (Leu^{4837}-Phe^{4856}); M9 (Met^{4879}-Gly^{4898}); and M10 (Val^{4914}-Ile^{4937}). M1, M2, M3 and M4 in the Takeshima model correspond to M5, M6, M8 and M10 in the Zorzato model. In further discussion, we will identify the predicted TM sequences through use of the numbering system of Zorzato *et al.*[7]

Subsequent analysis of the aa sequences of RyR2, deduced from cDNAs, confirmed the pattern of hydrophobicity first seen in RyR1.[4] However, the sequences of M3 and M4 were not well conserved and the hydrophobicity of M4 could clearly be extended to over 40 aa. The sequencing of RyR3,[12] however, led to a different pattern. In RyR3, the sequence corresponding to M3 was not hydrophobic and could not be TM, but the possibility now existed that M4 alone might be long enough to form a hairpin helix.

Brandt *et al.*[71] proposed that as many as four additional TM segments might be located in the first 3000 aa of RyR1: at aa 599-614; 1514-1530; 1838-1855; and 2555-2570. This prediction was based in part on evidence that a 70-kDa fragment, which was deduced to contain the hydrophobic sequences, 1514-1530 and 1838-1855, and a 360 kDa C-terminal fragment containing previously predicted TM sequences, were both labeled with a hydrophobic probe, 3-(trifluoromethyl) 3-(*m*)[^{125}I]iodophenyl diazarine.

The first functional evidence for the location of the TM sequences at the C-terminus of the molecule came from investigations by Takeshima *et al.*[72] which showed that a second RyR1 transcript can be found in brain. This transcript encoded only 656 aa, which would begin just before M^{4382} and extend to the end of the molecule. When a recombinant RyR1 protein with a deletion of aa 183-4006 was expressed in CHO cells, it could be shown to encode a channel, which, when measured in planar bilayers, had a huge conductance, corresponding to that of intact RyR1, and a probability of opening close to 1. Thus, it appeared to contain the channel forming segment, but to be missing key regulatory sequences.[73]

Studies of a K^+ channel containing only two TM sequences and a pore[9] showed that the selectivity filter is located between two C-terminal TM sequences. These findings focused attention on M9 in RyR1 and RyR2 as a candidate for the selectivity filter and M8 and M10 as candidate outer and inner pore helices. Alanine-scanning mutagenesis and analysis of the mutant products in a variety of assay systems[37,38,74] showed that amino acids in M9 had properties associated with a selectivity filter sequence. These properties included alterations in conductivity, ryanodine binding and channel regulation. If M9 is assigned as the selectivity filter and M8 and M10 as outer and inner pore helices, then a significant revision is required in the topological predictions of the Zorzato model, but not of the Takeshima model.

The location of other mutation-sensitive aa in TM segments has been investigated in a number of experiment. In a study of the mutation-sensitivity of conserved polar aa in TM sequences,[75] mutations in Glu^{4032} in M2, Asn^{4086} and Asp^{4815} in M7 and Asp^{4917} and Gln^{4933} in M10 had functional consequences that suggested that they might be involved in channel function and regulation. Indeed, the properties assigned to the mutation Glu^{3895} in RyR3, which corresponds to Glu^{4032} in RyR1, were those of a Ca^{2+} sensor.[76] These results do not provide direct evidence, however, that the sequences in which these critical residues lie are, in fact, TM sequences.

M10 has been proposed to be the inner pore inner helix of RyR and to play a role in channel activation and gating that is similar to the role of the inner helix in bacterial K^+ channels.[9,77] When systematic mutagenesis of M10 was carried out, mutants D4847A, F4850A, F4851A, L4858A, L4859A and I4866A had curtailed caffeine-induced Ca^{2+} release when expressed in HEK-293 cells and [^{3}H]ryanodine binding was diminished in cell lysates.[78] Mutants F4846A, T4849A, I4855A, V4856A, and Q4863A lost or had markedly reduced [^{3}H]ryanodine binding, but retained caffeine-induced Ca^{2+} release.[79] These two groups of mutants are largely located on opposite sides of the M10 helix. Single channel measurements showed that mutant Q4863A had altered kinetics and apparent affinity for ryanodine and was insensitive to ryanodol, an analogue of ryanodine. The single channel conductance of the Q4863A mutant and its responses to caffeine, ATP, and Mg^{2+}, however, were comparable to wild type. The effect of ryanodine on single Q4863A channels was influenced by the transmembrane holding potential. These results suggest that the M10, and Gln^{4863} in particular, play an important role in ryanodine binding. Single I4862A mutant channels exhibited considerable channel openings and altered gating at very low Ca^{2+} concentrations. All of these data indicate that M10 constitutes an essential determinant of channel activation and gating, in keeping with its proposed role as an inner helix of the pore region of RyR.

In the absence of a high-resolution structure for RyR, attempts have been made to elucidate the structure and topology of RyR using biochemical approaches. Proteolytic digestion of RyR1 yielded several major fragments,[80-82] identified by sequencing[80,82] or by immunoblotting with a series of seven antibodies[81]. Five major fragments were estimated to span the molecule. They had masses and deduced aa sequence boundaries as follows: 135 kDa (aa 1-1397 or 1508), 100 kDa (1398 or 1509-2401), 50 kDa (2402-2840), 160 kDa (3119-4475) and 76 kDa (4476-5037). The more N-terminal

150, 50 and 100 kDa tryptic fragments and their subfragments could be extracted by Na_2CO_3, indicating that they did not contain TM sequences.[81] The more C-terminal 160 kDa fragment reacted with an antibody against an epitope contained within aa 4382-4417 and was resistant to Na_2CO_3 extraction,[81] implying that TM sequences exist in the sequence between aa 3119 and 4476. This sequence would include M', M'', M1, M2, M3 and M4 from the Zorzato model. The 76 kDa C-terminal fragment (4476-5037) could not be extracted into Na_2CO_3, indicating that it was membrane-associated[81]. This fragment would include M5 to M10 from the Zorzato model and M1 to M4 from the Takeshima model.

In a thorough analysis of RyR1,[82] similar major fragments were generated, which spanned the whole molecule. Sequence analysis clarified which aa were located at the beginning and the end of each of these fragments. The masses and approximate aa sequence of these fragments, beginning at the N-terminus are: 40 kDa (aa 1-426); 110 kDa (aa 426-1508); 100 kDa (aa 1508-2401); 50 kDa (aa 2401-2840); 33 kDa (aa 2840-3119); 150 kDa (aa 3119-4475); and 76 kDa (4475-5037).

According to the hydropathy analysis and evidence obtained from other studies, the N- and C-termini of RyR1 are both located in the cytoplasm,[83-85] indicating that an even number of sequences traverse the membrane. Antibodies against synthetic peptides corresponding to N-terminal aa 2-15[84] and C-terminal aa 5027-5037[84] or 4941-5037[83] in rabbit skeletal muscle RyR1 bound to intact SR, confirming that both ends of the membrane-embedded RyR1 are exposed to the cytoplasm. Degradation of the C-terminal end of RyR1 in the intact SR, using carboxypeptidase A, caused a loss of reactivity with anti-C-terminus antibodies.[84] Denaturation of RyR1 in SR vesicles by transient incubation at alkaline pH under condition where few of the vesicles were permeabilized increased its sensitivity to antibodies.[83]

A useful approach to the topology and localization of specific regions of RyR has involved the insertion of glutathione-S-transferase (GST) or green fluorescent protein (GFP or EGFP) tags into various regions of the molecule. The mutant protein is expressed, purified, and subjected to cryoelectron microscopy and single particle image analysis, and reconstruction of the three-dimensional structure of the tagged protein.[85] Comparison of the three-dimensional reconstructions of wild type and mutant RyR3 with GST attached to the N-terminus showed that GST was located at the corners of the square-shaped cytoplasmic region of homotetrameric RyR3. This finding proves that the N-terminus of RyR3 lies in the cytoplasm.[85] Insertion of GFP after Thr^{1874} in the middle of the highly divergent region 3 (DR3) between aa 1872 and 1923 did not alter the function of the channel.[86] The tag, representing the DR3 region, was located in domain 9, in the clamp-shaped structure adjacent to the binding sites for FKBP12 and FKBP12.6. A similar analysis was carried out with RyR2 in which GFP was inserted into divergent region 1 after Asp^{4365}.[87] Again, channel function was not impaired. The inserted GFP, and consequently, DR1, was mapped to RyR domain 3, referred to as the "handle" domain. These studies provide evidence that the N-terminus and divergent regions 1 and 3 are all located in the cytosol.

Confocal microscopy of EGFP fused to a variety of RyR1 sequences indicated that the ER retention signal is present within the C-terminal portion of RyR1 containing the TM sequences [88]. Evidence showed that aa 4918-4943 of RyR1 may be responsible for ER retention of the Ca^{2+} release channel.[89]

Further studies[83] have shown that antibodies against aa 2804-2930 of RyR1, lying upstream of M', bound to either intact or permeabilized SR vesicles, confirming the cytoplasmic location of this sequence. Antibodies against aa 4581-4640, between M5 and M6, did not bind to intact SR vesicles but bound well to permeabilized vesicles, supporting a lumenal location for this peptide sequence. Antibodies against aa 4860-4886 between M8 and M9 did not bind to intact vesicles, but exhibited weak binding to the permeabilized vesicles, suggesting that this epitope is exposed to the lumen. In a study of human RyR2,[18] an antibody against aa 4594-4718 between M6 and M7 bound to intact or permeabilized SR vesicles, indicating that this epitope is located in the cytoplasm.

These epitope location results are largely consistent with the predictions inherent in both the Takeshima and Zorzato models for membrane topology of RyR1. However, there is a very informative discrepancy for the location of the epitope against aa 4860 and 4886, lying between M7 and M8. In the Zorzato model aa 4860-4886 are predicted to lie in the cytoplasm. In the most recently revised topological model,[8,90] described in the next section and Fig. 2-1, the value of this antibody is evident: it is consistent with the revised view that M7 (M7a/M7b) forms a hairpin loop, that M8 is oriented cytosol to lumen; that M9 is a selectivity filter located between M9 and M10; and that M10 is oriented lumen to cytosol.

Thus after more than a decade of investigation using a variety of tests, it was still not possible to distinguish clearly between the Takeshima and Zorzato models. Progress had been made, however, since M9 was transferred from TM status to selectivity filter status, allowing M8 and M10 to form a hairpin loop, and M3 was no longer considered to be a TM sequence. Moreover, there was clear recognition that both M4 and M7 are long helical sequences, which might, themselves, form TM hairpin loops. Clearly a systematic investigation of the TM sequences was required and new technologies, such as the fusion of EGFP to various sites in RyR1, was a new technology suited to this type of investigation.

SYSTEMATIC ANALYSIS OF RYR TOPOLOGY

Membrane protein synthesis is initiated at the N-terminus and nascent proteins are translocated into membranes cotranslationally using machinery shared with secretory proteins only to the point where membrane proteins become integrated into the ER membrane.[91] On the basis of these principles, it was possible to design strategies to analyze predicted membrane sequences in RyR1 through the insertion of EGFP, with a stop codon at its C-terminus, into virtually any site in RyR1 where membrane association and orientation was to be interrogated. Nascent proteins could then be truncated sequentially from the C-terminus and tagged with EGFP. Through investigation of the location of EGFP fluorescence in the cell using confocal microscopy, it was possible to determine whether the truncated protein was uniformly distributed in the cell or membrane bound. By examining the fate of the fluorescence after saponin permeabilization of the cell, it was possible to determine solubility – soluble proteins were leached out of the cell; membrane bound proteins were retained within a reticular network.

Other studies could be carried out at the biochemical level following isolation of microsomal fractions from these cells. If EGFP in the fusion protein was soluble, it would be detected in the soluble fraction, but if membrane bound, it would be detected in the microsomal fraction following Western blotting with an EGFP antibody. If loosely bound to membrane fractions, it would be extracted with sodium carbonate, which dissociates peripheral proteins from membranes (but has limited capacity to extract aggregated proteins from membrane fractions). Finally, it was possible to determine whether EGFP was located in the cytoplasm or in the lumen of microsomal vesicles following tryptic digestion. EGFP is intrinsically resistant to digestion by common proteases due to its tight folding. If EGFP were folded appropriately in the cytosol, it would be freed into solution as a trypsin-resistant, 27 kDa product. If it were folded appropriately in the lumen, it would remain in the membrane pellet, but its mass would be increased in proportion to the length of the trypsin-protected TM sequence to which it was attached. Problems that arise using this strategy are that it is difficult to interpret experiments in which EGFP does not fold properly and it is not always possible to insert EGFP into the exact site desired because of technical problems involving the cDNA sequence of RyR1.

The basis for insertional site selection was analysis of the rabbit skeletal muscle RyR1 amino acid sequence using the Argos algorithm[92,93] for prediction of TM domains (Fig. 2-1 A). Stretches of hydrophobicity, compatible with TM sequences, were found mainly in the last 1000 aa. Those stretches in which the average index for each amino acid is over 1 include: Glu^{4275}-Ala^{4300} (average index 1.137); Thr^{4323}-Gly^{4363} (1.197);

Arg^{4557}-Ile^{4576} (1.241); Gly^{4637}-Asn^{4662} (1.170); Gln^{4776}-Thr^{4825} (1.092); Gly^{4834}-Val^{4854} (1.201); Leu^{4911} - Leu^{4935} (1.253). These sequences correspond closely to M3, M4, M5, M6, M7, M8 and M10 in the Zorzato model. With the Argos algorithm, M1, M2 and M9 are only weakly hydrophobic, but the hydrophobic region of M4 is over 40 aa long and, of M7, about 50 aa long. Thus both M4 and M7 sequences are long enough to form a TM hairpin. Prediction of TM domains for RyR2 and RyR3 using the same program gave results similar to that for RyR1, except that M3 is not predicted as a hydrophobic TM sequence in RyR3.

In the C-terminal-truncated RyR1-EGFP fusion constructs that were designed to analyze membrane sequences in RyR1, EGFP was attached: PreM1 at aa 3224, which lies after the proposed M'/M" hairpin loop sequence and just before M1 (designated PreM1); PostM2 (aa 4186); PostM3 (aa 4302); PostM4 (4556); PostM5 (aa 4628); PostM6 (aa 4771); PostM7b (aa 4836); PostM8 (aa 4888); and PostM10 (aa 5037). The possibility that M7 (aa Gln^{4776}-Thr^{4825}) forms an independent hairpin loop was also examined by placing EGFP after aa 4806 in the middle of M7 (PostM7a).

It was anticipated that any EGFP fusion protein in which EGFP lies before the first TM sequence would be translated in the cytosol, would not enter the secretory protein pathway, would not be translocated into the ER lumen and would not associate with the membrane. As a corollary, any EGFP fusion protein in which EGFP lies after a TM sequence with cytosol to lumenal orientation would be translated in the cytosol, would enter the secretory protein pathway, would be translocated into the ER lumen and would associate with the membrane. Finally, any EGFP fusion protein in which EGFP lies after a TM sequence with lumen to cytosol orientation would be translated in the cytosol, where it would remain in association with the membrane. On the basis of these principles, it was possible to determine the boundary between the cytosolic portion of RyR1 and the first membrane-associated sequence. It was expected that EGFP located after TM helices would be translated and translocated to the side of the membrane corresponding to the native orientation of the TM sequence. However, a caveat exists in this reasoning in that a lone signal anchor sequence may not be sufficiently strong to cause translocation into the lumen; in some cases, this occur only in the presence of a combined signal anchor sequence and a stop-transfer sequence.[94] The fusion-truncation proteins were expressed in mammalian MEF or HEK-293 cells and confocal microscopy was used to visualize the fluorescent proteins in the cell in the absence or presence of saponin, which permeabilizes the cells. Alkali was also used to extract peripheral proteins, leaving behind integral membrane proteins, which formed a reticular network, but also insoluble recombinant protein aggregates, which were distinguished by their amorphous nature.

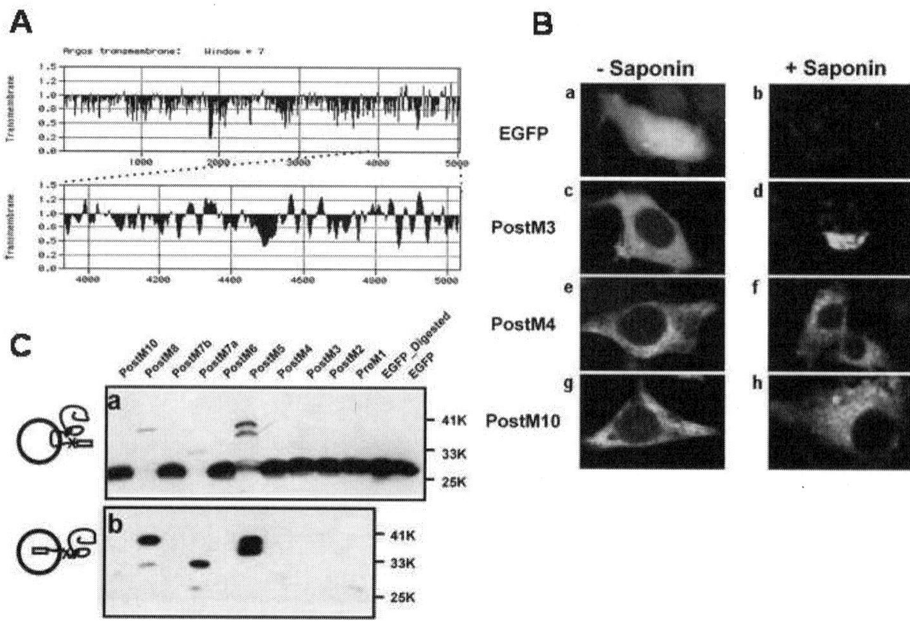

Figure 2-1. **Evidence for a model of RyR1 topology. A**. Prediction of transmembrane sequences in rabbit skeletal muscle RyR1with the Argos transmembrane algorithm.[92] The top panel shows the analysis of the full length RyR1 sequence and the lower panel shows the expanded C-terminal region. Ten potential TM sequences are apparent,but M4 and M7 are very long. **B**. Confocal microscopy of MEF cells expressing EGFP and RyR-EGFP fusion proteins. The left panel shows transfected MEF cells prior to treatment with saponin and the right panel shows cells after treatment with saponin, which releases soluble proteins (eg. **b** and **d**), leaving aggregated (**d**) and membrane proteins in situ (**f** & **h**). The designation for each construct is on the left side of the image. **C**. Localisation of EGFP in HEK-293 cells transfected with RyR1 fusion protein constructs. Microsomes from transfected HEK-293 cells were digested with trypsin and centrifuged. Proteins in the supernatant (**C**, **a**) and microsomes (**C**, **b**) were immunoblotted with anti-EGFP antibody. The cartoon on the left of **C**, **a** shows that EGFP will be released to the cytosol with a normal mass, following tryptic digestion, if it lies on the cytosolic side. The cartoon on the left of **C**, **b** indicates that EGFP will remain membrane-bound with an increased mass, following tryptic digestion, if it lies at the lumenal side. In PostM8, PostM7a and PostM5, EGFP remained in membranes with an increased mass. EGFP from other fusion proteins was exclusively in the supernatant.

RyR1 fusion proteins truncated PreM1, PostM2 and PostM3 (aa 4302) gave off a uniform fluorescence throughout the cell, indicating that they were located in the cytosol and were not membrane-bound (Fig. 2-1 B). Since they were released from cells treated with saponin and were extracted by Na_2CO_3 it was clear that they were soluble. These studies effectively eliminated M', M", M1, M2 and M3 as TM helices. Although M2 is not a TM sequence, it contains at least one residue that is critical to channel function and is possibly the Ca^{2+} sensor,[75,76] indicating that this sequence must form part of an important regulatory domain.

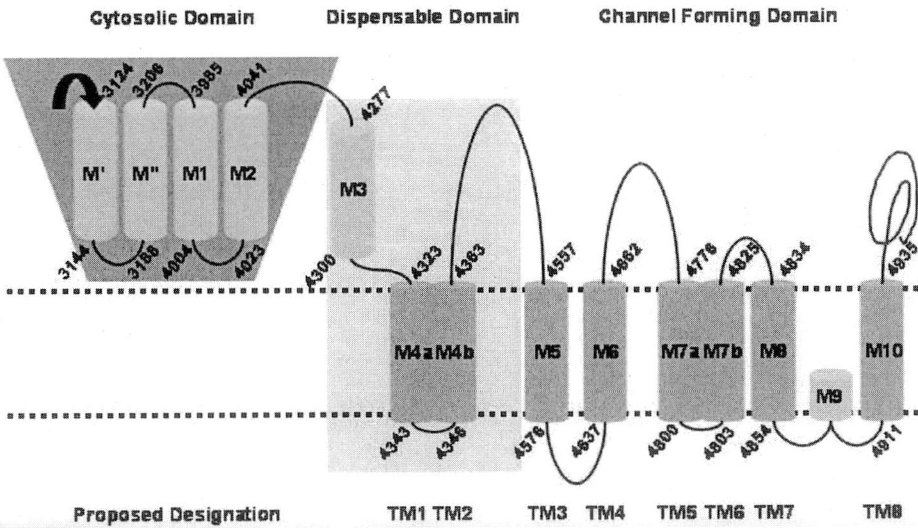

Figure 2-2. **Proposal for a model of RyR1 topology.** Dark grey cylinders inserted into the membrane represent the eight proposed TM sequences. Numbers inside the cylinders preceded by M are those in the Zorzato model. However, sequences M4 and M7 are now divided into M4a/M4b and M7a/M7b. New designations for these eight TM sequences are proposed at the bottom of the figure, in which the number of the TM sequence is preceded by TM. Light grey cylinders in the cytosol represent those sequences proposed as TM sequences in the Zorzato model, but which are now known to be located in the cytoplasm. They are identified by numbers preceded by M. Cytosolic and lumenal boundaries of predicted and confirmed TM segment are indicated by numbers that represent amino acids in RyR1. M9 is now proposed to be the selectivity filter between M8 and M10. The cytosolic domain of RyR is believed to extend to ~aa 4323 at the beginning of the M4 sequence and to include M3. A region which includes aa 4274-4535 is referred to as a dispensable domain, since its removal in the Δ4274-4535 deletion mutant does not affect structural stability, Ca^{2+} release channel function or ryanodine binding (see Fig. 2-3) and a corresponding sequence is not present in functional IP_3R Ca^{2+} release channels. The last six TM sequences form the Ca^{2+} release channel, but the first two TM sequences may interact with them in a regulatory fashion, thus forming a part of the channel domain.

The RyR1 fusion protein PostM4, truncated at aa 4556 so that it included M4 and the M4/M5 loop, was membrane-associated, as indicated by the reticular nature of its fluorescence, its indifference to saponin permeabilization and its resistance to extraction by Na_2CO_3. All fusion proteins that were truncated downstream of M4 had similar properties. These results indicate that the region containing the M4 sequence is the first sequence in RyR1 to associate the ~4,300 aa cytosolic portion of the molecule with the membrane.

Further evidence concerning the number of TM sequences and their orientation was derived from proteolytic digestion of microsomal fractions (Fig. 2-1 C). EGFP was recovered after tryptic digestion of SR vesicles as a 28 kDa protein. EGFP from PostM4, PostM5, PostM7a and PostM8 remained largely in the membrane after trypsin digestion and with molecular masses increased in proportion to the mass calculated for each TM domain and/or linker (7-8 kDa for PostM5 and PostM8 and 2-3 kDa for PostM7a). These results show that EGFP in these three proteins was located on the lumenal side of the membrane, demonstrating that the orientation for M5, M7a, and M8 is from cytoplasm to lumen. EGFP from all of the other fusion proteins was present in the supernatant and had a molecular mass similar to that of wild type EGFP. These results show that EGFP from PreM1, PostM2 and PostM3 is located in the cytosol because it forms part of a long soluble sequence, while EGFP fused to PostM4, PostM6, PostM7b, and PostM10 lies in the cytosol because it is located at the C-terminus of a hairpin loop. Thus the orientation of M6, M7b and M10 is from lumen to cytoplasm and this must also be true of the second half of M4 (M4b if M4 alone forms a hairpin loop).

These data confirm the view that M5/M6 and M8/M10 form helical hairpin loops and provide new evidence that the long M7 sequence forms a helical hairpin loop. In PostM7a, a construct only 35 aa longer than PostM6, EGFP was translocated to the lumen, preventing its proteolysis by trypsin. In PostM7b, only 30 aa longer than PostM7a, EGFP was dissociated from the membrane after digestion by trypsin, indicating that it was located on the cytoplasmic side. These data provide conclusive evidence that the 50 aa Gln^{4776}-Thr^{4825} sequence forms two TM helices with a relatively short lumenal loop confirming the prediction of the Argos algorithm (Fig. 2-1 A).

Since M5 is a membrane sequence with an N-cytoplasmic to C-lumenal orientation, any TM sequences upstream of M5 must exist as hairpin loops. The PostM3 fusion truncation protein is soluble and PostM4, truncated just before PreM5, is ER associated and located on the cytosolic surface. Thus it is possible that the 40 aa M4 sequence forms a hairpin loop. Indeed, the TMHMM2.0[95] predicts that M4 in both RyR1 and RyR2 is a TM sequence formed by two helices with a loop in the middle.

In unpublished work, it has been possible to show that fusion truncation proteins immediately PostM4 are insoluble, that fusion truncation proteins immediately PreM4 are soluble and that an RyR2 fusion truncation protein with an epitope in the middle of M4 is soluble. These data are consistent with the view that M4 forms a TM hairpin loop in which the first half (M4a) forms a signal transfer sequence which is not strong enough to anchor the protein, but which can interact with the second half (M4b) to form a signal anchor-stop transfer hairpin sequence, which is the first site of anchorage of RyR1 to the membrane (Fig. 2-2).

Ironically, since so much effort has been spent on investigation of the topology of the M3/M4 region, it is possibly of little functional concern whether M4 does or does not form a hairpin loop in RyR1 (Fig. 2-3). Alignments of the sequence of ryanodine receptors with their homologues, the IP_3 receptors, show that a large gap exists in the IP_3R family, which encompasses the M3/M4 region in RyR1. Thus three C-terminal hairpin loops in IP_3R[94] are all that are required for Ca^{2+} release channel function. Of more immediate significance is the fact that the RyR1 deletion mutant, Δ4274-4535, is expressed in HEK-293 cells at a level that is enhanced up to four-fold over that of wild-type recombinant RyR1 (Fig. 2-3). Thus, the 4274-4535 sequence appears to be inhibitory to expression of RyR1 in HEK-293 cells. The corresponding sequence in RyR2 is not inhibitory, so that expression of RyR2 in HEK-293 cells is also up to four-fold higher than expression of RyR1. These results show that deletion of aa 4274-4535 does not disrupt RyR1 structure – if the protein were misfolded during synthesis, it would have been degraded. The Δ4274-4535 deletion mutant also forms a functional Ca^{2+} release channel, which is activated by caffeine (Fig. 2-3 B). Caffeine affinity is intermediate between the high affinity of RyR1 and the lower affinity of RyR2. The deletion mutant also binds ryanodine with the same affinity as RyR1 and RyR2 (Fig. 2-3 C). These results indicate that the aa 4274-4535 region, which encompasses both M3 and M4, is not required for function. In Fig. 2-2, we have delineated the approximate range of this sequence and have labelled it as a dispensable domain. It is probable, however, that the sequence is retained in RyR molecules because it has a unique regulatory function.

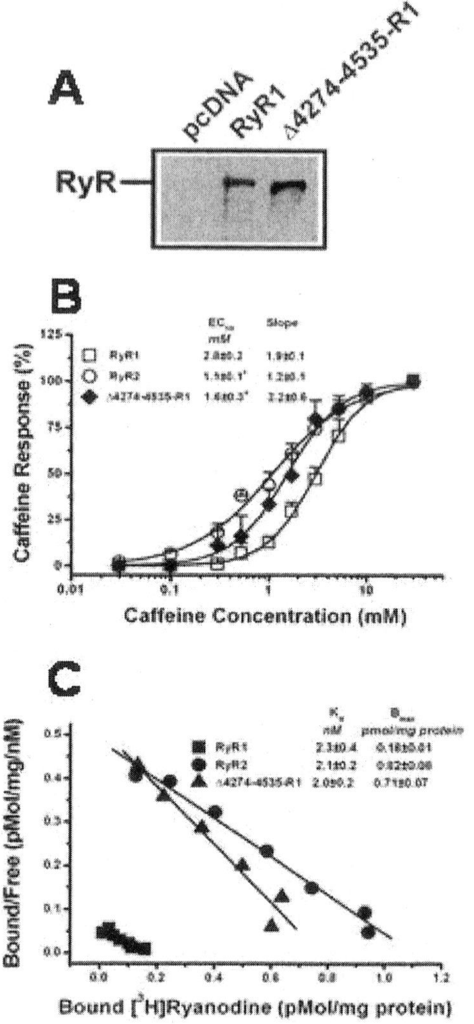

Figure 2-3. **Evidence that the region surrounding M3/M4 is dispensable in RyR1. A.** Expression of RyR1 and the Δ4274-4535 deletion mutant in HEK-293 cells. CHAPS lysates from HEK-293 cells were harvested 48 h after transfection with cDNas encoding RyR1 and the Δ4274-4535 deletion mutant and subjected to Western blotting.[67] The expression of the Δ4274-4535 deletion mutant is enhanced over that of RyR1. **B**. Dose-response curves obtained from fluorescence measurements of *in vivo* Ca^{2+} release induced by incremental concentrations of caffeine in HEK-293 cells expressing RyR1, RyR2 and the Δ4274-4535 deletion mutant. Dose-response curves were used to obtain the EC_{50} values and Hill coefficients for caffeine-induced Ca^{2+} release that are presented as an inset.[67] **C**. Scatchard analysis of $[^3H]$ryanodine binding to solubilized RyR1 RyR2 and the Δ4274-4535 deletion mutant expressed in transfected HEK-293 cells. K_d and B_{max} values are inserted.[67] On the basis of ryanodine binding, presented as an inset, the expression of the Δ4274-4535 deletion mutant is enhanced four-fold over that of RyR1.

CONCLUDING REMARKS

In summary, it is now clear that M', M", M1, M2 and M3 do not exist as TM sequences. It is also clear that three hairpin loops do exist: they are formed from M5-M6, M7a-M7b and M8-M10, with M9 inserted between M8 and M10 to form a selectivity filter, as depicted in Fig. 2-2. Results with the M4 sequence show that about 40 aa comprising M4 create the first site of association of RyR1 with the membrane. The precise nature of this association is not yet established, but it is likely to be a TM hairpin loop from M4a/M4b. The cytosolic domain of RyR is believed to extend to ~aa 4323 at the beginning of the M4 sequence and to include M3. A region which includes aa 4274-4535 is referred to as a dispensable domain, since its removal in the Δ4274-4535 deletion mutant does not affect structural stability, Ca^{2+} release channel function or ryanodine binding, as shown in Fig. 2-3, and a corresponding sequence is not present in functional IP_3R Ca^{2+} release channels. The sequence may, however, be retained in RyR1 because it has important regulatory functions. The last six TM sequences are believed to form the Ca^{2+} release channel, but the first two TM sequences may well interact with them in a physical and regulatory fashion, thus forming a part of the channel domain.

ACKNOWLEDGEMENTS

Original work from our laboratory, described in this review, was supported by grant MT-3399 to D. H. M. from the Canadian Institutes of Health Research.

Chapter 3

THREE-DIMENSIONAL RECONSTRUCTION OF RYANODINE RECEPTORS

Zheng Liu[1] and Terence Wagenknecht[1,2]
[1]Wadsworth Center, New York State Dept. of Health, Albany, New York; [2]Dept. of Biomedical Sciences, School of Public Health, State University of New York at Albany, Albany, NY

INTRODUCTION

Calcium ions function as second messengers in all types of cells and regulate many fundamental cellular processes, including muscle contraction and relaxation, secretion, synaptic transmission, fertilization, nuclear pore function, transcription, and apoptosis.[96,97] One of the major calcium channels responsible for Ca^{2+} release from intracellular stores is the ryanodine receptor (RyR).

RyRs are highly enriched in skeletal and cardiac muscle, or more precisely, in those regions of the sarcoplasmic reticulum (SR) membrane that interact with the plasma membrane/transverse tubule system (see Chapter 4). The SR is the major storage site for the bulk of cellular calcium. RyRs play a central role in excitation-contraction coupling, a process in which neuron-induced depolarization of the plasma membrane causes RyRs to release Ca^{2+} from the SR, and the resulting increase in cytoplasmic $[Ca^{2+}]$ activates the myofilaments to generate muscle contraction.

Three genetic isoforms of RyR have been identified. In mammals, these isoforms are encoded on separate chromosomes. Type 1 RyR (RyR1) is predominant in skeletal muscle, while the type 2 isoform (RyR2) is most abundant in cardiac muscle, and the type 3 RyR isoform (RyR3) is also expressed in mammalian striated muscle, but at relatively low levels. Because the RyR isoforms share a high degree (~70%) of sequence homology, their three-dimensional (3D) structures are expected to be nearly identical. RyRs are homo-tetramers of molecular mass ~2.3MDa, making them the largest and the most structurally complex ion channels known.

CRYO-ELECTRON MICROSCOPY, SINGLE PARTICLE IMAGE PROCESSING, AND THREE-DIMENSIONAL RECONSTRUCTION OF RYRS

3D structural information is essential to an understanding of the functional properties of RyRs. However, because RyRs are both very large and integral membrane proteins, it seems problematic that an atomic structure of the intact receptor will be determined in the near future by X-ray crystallography, although efforts are being made to accomplish this goal.

Cryo-electron microscopy (cryo-EM) has thus far been the only feasible technique by which to obtain reliable information about the 3D structure of RyRs. In the past decade, cryo-EM of isolated macromolecules, in conjunction with computerized single particle image processing, has emerged as a powerful methodology for determining the 3D structures of macromolecules and macromolecular assemblies[57,98-102] In this conceptually simple technique, a few microliters of aqueous solution containing the macromolecule of interest (0.02 - several mg/ml) is applied to a standard EM grid on which a carbon support was placed. Following extensive blotting of excess solution, the grid is rapidly plunged into liquid ethane. The rapid rate of freezing (from 4°C to -180°C in less than a millisecond) prevents the aqueous solution from forming cubic ice, and consequently the macromolecules become preserved in a thin layer of vitreous ice in their native and fully hydrated state. The cryo-grids can be stored in liquid nitrogen and subsequently transferred into a special cryo-transfer holder for insertion into a transmission electron microscope as they are needed. The temperature of the grid inside the microscope is maintained well below the devitrification temperature, which is ~-140°C.

Cryo-EM has eliminated the artifacts associated with chemical fixation, dehydration, and contrast enhancement by heavy metals that have plagued EM in the past, and it permits resolution of the "true" structure of the specimen. However, to compensate for the low signal-to-noise ratio inherent in micrographs of ice-embedded macromolecules, it is necessary to average in the computer large numbers (thousands) of images of individual macromolecules to achieve even moderate (~20Å) resolution. Unlike other structural techniques for which "smaller is better", this approach is best suited to large assemblies of macromolecules. Probably the technique's most appreciated advantages are that crystallization of the specimen is unnecessary and that rather small quantities of specimen are required (e.g., less than a microgram of protein is required to make a single grid, which can provide sufficient data to determine a 3D structure to moderate resolution).

The first 3D reconstructions from micrographs of frozen-hydrated, detergent-solubilized RyRs were reported in the mid 1990s by two research groups.[57,58] The main limitation of the approach is that atomic resolution, although possible in principle, has proven difficult to attain, and for studies of RyRs, the best resolution reported to date is 22 Å.[103]

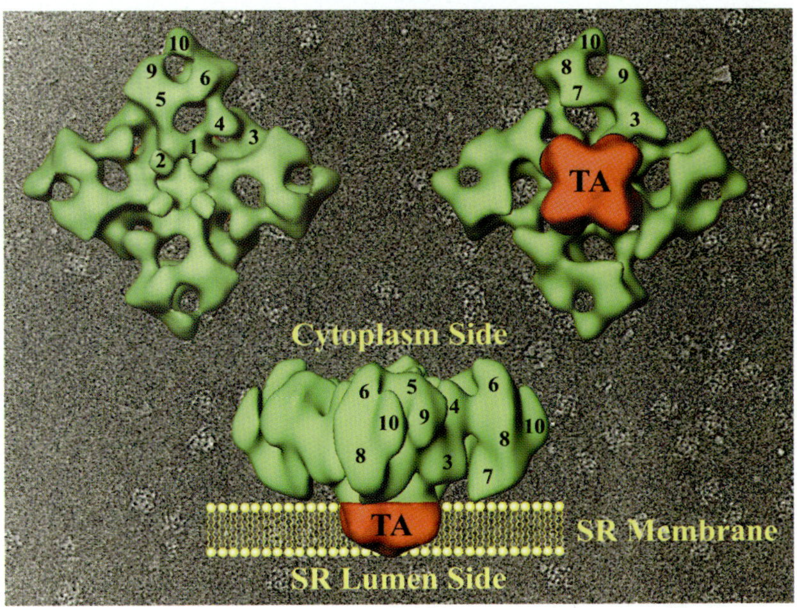

Figure 3-1. **Cryo-electron microscopy and three-dimensional reconstruction of skeletal muscle ryanodine receptor.** The background shows a typical cryo-electron micrograph of RyRs. Numerous individual RyR molecules that are embedded in a thin layer of vitreous ice are visible. For computation of a 3D reconstruction by single-particle image processing methods,[104] over ten thousand such particles are typically selected from a data set comprising up to hundreds of micrographs. In the foreground, a solid body representation of RyR is shown in three views: **upper left**, top view of the cytoplasmic region that *in situ* would face the transverse tubule membrane; **upper right**, bottom view, which would face the SR; **bottom**, side view. The side view shows that RyR comprises two main components, a transmembrane assembly (TA, shown in red) and a larger cytoplasmic assembly (in green).

As expected, 3D reconstructions of the three RyR isoforms reveal a highly conserved structure, having the overall shape of a mushroom and consisting of two major components (Fig. 3.1): a large, square prism-shaped cytoplasmic assembly (290×290×130Å) composed of at least 10 distinct domains (the "cap"), and a differentiated small transmembrane assembly (the "stem") of dimensions 120×120×70Å. As discussed in Chapter 2, sequence analysis[3,18] and biochemical studies[8,83] indicate that the amino-terminal ~4,000-4,500 amino acid residues form the large cytoplasmic assembly, while the remaining ~500-1,000 carboxy-terminal residues comprise the transmembrane regions. Still controversial is the precise number of transmembrane segments per protein monomer: four-, six-, and ten-segment models have been proposed. The most recent report[8] supported the six-transmembrane model, with two intervening membrane associated loops (see Chapter 2, and the schematic representation of RyR's sequence in Fig. 3-3 C). A more detailed correlation of RyR's amino acid sequence with its 3D architecture will require either much higher resolution 3D reconstructions or the use of sequence-specific labels of sufficient size to be resolved in the currently achievable reconstructions. The latter approach is discussed further below.

In retrospect, it is apparent that the cytoplasmic assembly was first visualized several decades ago as darkly staining, rectangular-shaped so-called "feet" in conventional thin-section electron micrographs of skeletal muscle triad junctions,[55] but the biochemical identity of the feet was unknown until RyRs were purified and characterized in the late 1980s. The cytoplasmic assembly appears to consist of 10 or more discrete globular domains per subunit that are clearly resolvable, due to their separation by solvent-accessible regions. Reassuringly, the arrangement of the various domains, as illustrated in Fig. 3.1 (where each domain has been assigned arbitrarily a numeral), is essentially identical in all of the reconstructions that have been reported thus far. The four "3" domains, which form the sides of the square-shaped cytoplasmic assembly, are the largest of the domains, and have been referred to as "handles".[58] A cluster of domains ("5" through "10") form the corners of the cytoplasmic assembly, and have been named "clamps".[58] The four "2" domains surround a central 40-50 Å-diameter solvent-filled pocket that appears to extend to the cytoplasmic end of the transmembrane region. Domain 1 appears to connect the cytoplasmic and transmembrane structures.

3D reconstructions have now been determined for RyRs under conditions that favor both closed and open states for all three isoforms of the receptor.[105-108] Functional studies have established that open conformations of RyR1 are favored by the presence of Ca^{2+} (optimal at about 0.1 mM) and millimolar levels of ATP. Channel closing is favored by the absence of nucleotide and by submicromolar levels of Ca^{2+}. Also, the plant alkaloid ryanodine, binding to its high (nanomolar) affinity site, locks the receptor in a state whose conductance is about 40% that of the open state achieved with Ca^{2+} and nucleotide (see Chapter 18 and Sutko *et al.*[109]). Through exposing of purified, solubilized receptors to these conditions and application of 3D cryo-EM, structures of putatively open and closed states of RyR were determined. A caveat to all these studies is that functional studies must be done on receptors in their native bilayer environment, and the results may not be directly applied to the solubilized receptors used for cryo-EM. Remarkably, despite the limited resolution attained, several reproducible differences appear to distinguish the closed and open states of all three RyR isoforms, as is illustrated in Fig. 3-2 for RyR3.

STRUCTURE OF OPEN AND CLOSED STATES

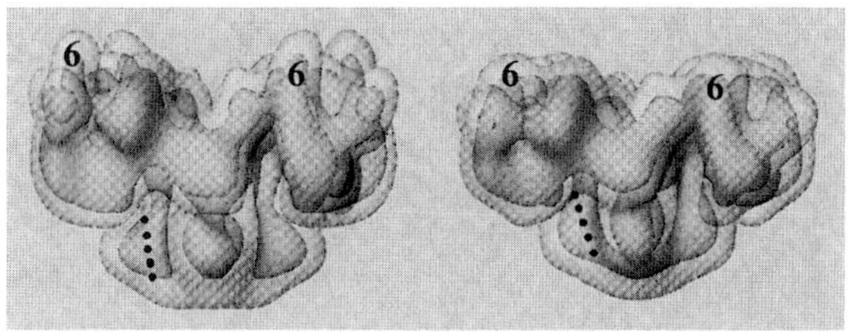

Figure 3-2. **Comparison of putatively open and closed states of RyR3.** Open RyR3 (left) and closed RyR3 (right) are displayed at two density thresholds. The higher threshold (solid, darker grey) illustrates how the mass density shifts between the open and closed forms, particularly in the transmembrane region. Dotted line indicates an elongate region of density that splays outward in the open, relative to the closed, state. Scale bar, 100 Å. Adapted from Sharma *et al.*[105]

Fig. 3-2 shows the open (left) and closed (right) structures at two density threshold levels: a semitransparent grey defines the molecular boundaries, and a higher threshold in a darker shade of grey is used to better reveal the nature of the structural differences between the two states, particularly in the transmembrane region. Differences in both the transmembrane and cytoplasmic regions are apparent between the open and closed states: the transmembrane assembly appears more expanded in the open as compared to the closed state, apparently due to a radial movement outward of four columns of protein mass (two of which are indicated by the dotted lines in Fig. 3-2). When viewed along the 4-fold rotation axis (not shown), the transmembrane assembly appears to rotate by a few degrees when the conformation switches between the two states. Intriguingly, structural differences between the two states are also present in the clamps of the cytoplasmic assembly. Perhaps the most striking of these is the increase in height of the cytoplasmic region due mainly to a change in configuration of clamp domain 6, which appears to flip upward in transitioning from the closed to the open state (Fig. 3-2). The structural changes that occur in the clamps are separated by well over 100 Å from changes that occur in the transmembrane region - an indication that long-range conformational communication between the clamps and the transmembrane pore-containing region are important to receptor functioning. Further evidence for long-range allosteric interactions comes from ligand binding studies, described below.

MAPPING OF LIGAND BINDING SITES

RyRs are regulated by numerous natural and pharmacological ligands, and by covalent modifications such as phosphorylation, nitrosylation, and oxidation/reduction of cysteine sulfhydryl moieties (see Meissner[110]; see also Chapters 7, 15, 16, 18-20). Most of these ligands bind or modify specific sites on the cytoplasmic assembly, a fact which perhaps offers one explanation for the unusually large size of the cytoplasmic region. 3D cryo-EM has been utilized to determine the physical locations of some of these modulatory sites. Among the macromolecular modulators of RyRs are calmodulin (CaM), a 12-kDa or 12.6-kDa FK506-binding protein (FKBP12, FKBP12.6), and, for skeletal RyR1, the dihydropyridine receptor (DHPR), which localizes in the transverse tubule membrane at triad junctions (see Chapter 4). Many of the RyR protein ligands are likely to be resident components of the excitation-contraction coupling apparatus. For example, the role of FKBP may be to mediate interactions between RyRs, enabling them to form arrays at triad junctions.

Fig. 3-3 A illustrates results that have been obtained for RyR-FKBP (see Chapter 15), RyR-calmodulin (Chapter 16), and RyR-imperatoxin complexes (Chapter 19).[111-113] The concept of the experiments is straightforward: RyR and ligand are mixed *in vitro* under conditions favoring complex formation, and then applied to specimen grids and quickly frozen for cryo-EM. If necessary, a control reconstruction is done of RyR lacking the ligand but otherwise identical. Finally, the reconstructions of the RyR with and without ligand are quantitatively compared, by subtracting the corresponding voxels of the control from the experimental reconstruction, to generate a 3D difference map.

Skeletal and cardiac RyRs are somewhat unusual, in that they bind both apo- and Ca^{2+}-calmodulin, unlike most calmodulin-regulated proteins, which bind only the Ca^{2+}-form. As can be appreciated from Fig. 3-3 (middle panel), the two forms of calmodulin bind to distinct sites that appear to be spatially separated by about 35 Å.[113] Imperatoxin is a peptide that is thought to mimic the region of the DHPR that interacts with skeletal (and perhaps cardiac) RyR (for additional details see Chapter 19). It binds at a location near that of

Ca^{2+}-calmodulin. FKBP, in contrast, binds on the side of domain 3 opposite to that where apo- and Ca^{2+}-calmodulin bind.

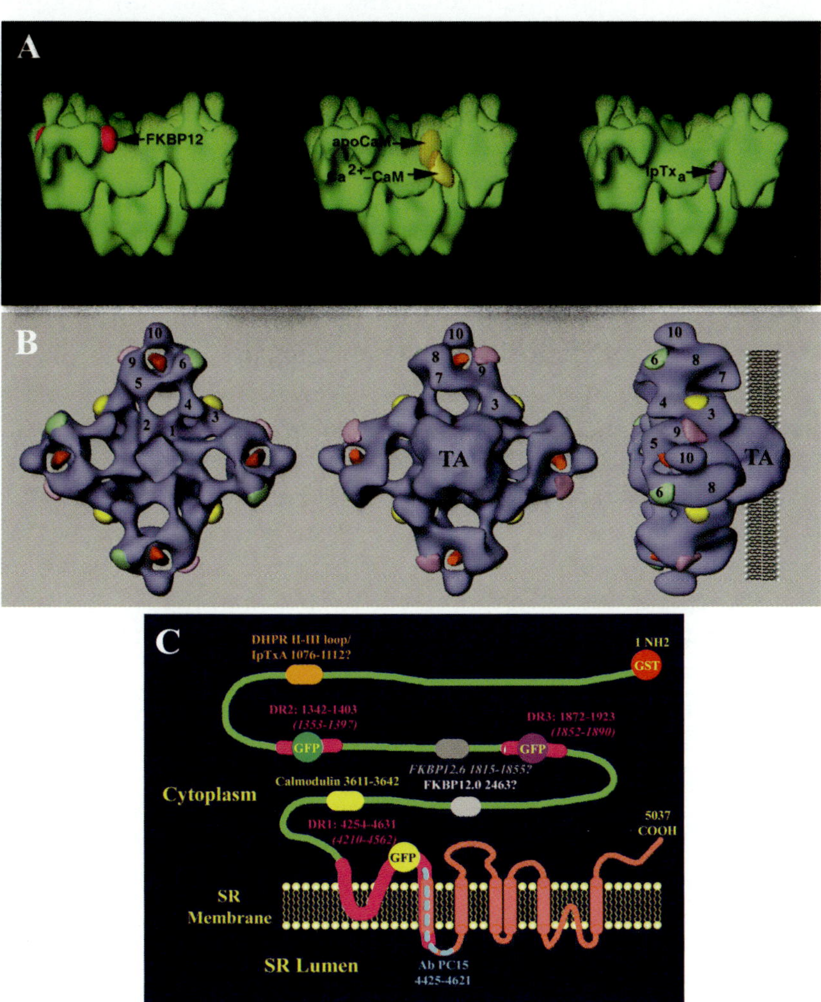

Figure 3-3. **Correlation of amino acid sequence of RyR to its 3D structure. A**. Ligand binding locations on RyR. Left, location of FKBP12 (fuchsia). Middle, location of both forms of CaM: apoCaM (transparent orange) and Ca^{2+}-CaM (solid yellow). Right, location of imperatoxin A (purple). The differences attributed to the ligands are superposed onto a common 3D reconstruction of RyR1 in absence of any ligand. **B**. Mapping of the amino terminus and the three divergent regions on RyR. 3D structure of RyR2 is shown in blue. Red, location of GST fused to amino terminus; divergent regions (DR1-D4365, DR2-T1366, and DR3-T1874) are shown in yellow, green, and purple, respectively. **C**. Schematic representation of RyR sequence. Six transmembrane segments are shown as previously proposed.[8] The ligand binding sites, amino terminus fused GST, and GFP in the three divergent regions that have been localized by 3D cryo-EM are highlighted.

The observation that all three of the RyR-modulating ligands depicted in Fig. 3-3 bind to sites on the cytoplasmic assembly that are quite remote (100 Å or more) from the transmembrane pore argues for long-range conformational changes in the functioning of RyRs.

CORRELATING THE LINEAR SEQUENCE TO THE 3D STRUCTURE USING RECOMBINANT RYR

Recently, the feasibility of expressing cloned RyRs in mammalian cell lines for structural analysis by cryo-EM has been demonstrated.[87] 3D cryo-EM of RyRs obtained from cells expressing genetically modified RyRs that contain insertions of autonomously folding peptides at specific sites in the amino acid sequence is illustrative of a general, efficient experimental approach for mapping the locations of surface-exposed amino-acid residues onto the 3D architecture of the receptor.[85-87,114] Gene fusions of RyRs and glutathione S-transferase (GST) or green fluorescent protein (GFP) have been shown to be useful for 3D cryo-EM. In this approach, since the GST or GFP labels are covalently attached to the RyR, every receptor image contains the label within each of the four RyR subunits, unlike the situation for noncovalently linked ligand:RyR complexes in which ligand dissociation often complicates the analysis.

Thus far, the amino terminus has been localized on the 3D structure of RyR3 using a GST fusion protein, and amino acids Asp-4365, Thr-1366, and Thr-1874, which lie within DR1, DR2, and DR3, respectively, have been located on the 3D structure of RyR2 using appropriate RyR2-GFP fusion proteins (Fig. 3-3 B). DR1-3 refer to three divergent regions where the amino acid sequences of the three isoforms are highly variable relative to the average sequence identity among the isoforms, which is nearly 70%.[115] These divergent regions have been the focus of a number of structural and functional studies, as they are thought to be largely responsible for the differing properties of the isoforms. For example, sequence variations in the DR1 region, between RyR1 and RyR2, have been shown to account for these isoforms' differing sensitivities to Ca^{2+} inactivation.[67]

CONCLUDING REMARKS

An atomic structure for RyR is unlikely to be determined in the near future, and, unfortunately, information on the distribution of amino acid residues within the 3D architecture of the RyR is not revealed at the resolutions currently being attained by cryo-EM (20-30 Å). It is not entirely clear why higher resolution has not been attained by cryo-EM, which can attain resolutions of 10 Å or better for some macromolecular complexes of comparable size to RyR.[98] Recent results suggest that higher resolutions should be achievable,[116] and that at least part of the difficulty is due to heterogeneity in RyR's structure following detergent solubilization and purification, a process which removes the receptor from its natural membrane environment.[117] Thus, improved methods of purification and/or specimen preparation for cryo-EM could be the key to attaining high resolution RyR structures. Also, RyRs from only a few taxonomic species have been characterized by cryo-EM. Based upon findings for other membrane proteins, it is quite possible a receptor that is more amenable to structural studies will be isolated from some as-yet unexamined organism. A receptor that is amenable to crystallization would of course greatly facilitate structural analyses by electron crystallography (two-dimensional crystals) or X-ray crystallography (3D crystals).

In the meantime, even at the moderate resolutions currently achieved routinely, the locations of surface-exposed amino acids can be determined, if these residues can be appropriately labeled with probes of sufficient mass, as we have shown in the previous section (Fig. 3-3 B). A comprehensive study by cryo-EM of RyR-GFP fusion proteins, with the GFP inserted at various surface-exposed residues of the RyR, should allow determination of those regions of RyR's amino acid sequence that comprise each of the 10 or more domains that form the cytoplasmic assembly. Such studies will also allow us to decipher the organization of the transmembrane segments. Even at current resolution levels, it should in some cases be feasible to propose functions for particular regions of the sequence, and to evaluate the plausibility of hypothesized functions for particular amino acids derived from biochemistry experiments. For instance, RyR amino-acid residues that are hypothesized to interact directly with a ligand, such as FKBP or calmodulin, should map to a spatially restricted region on the surface of the receptor that coincides with the location where the ligand itself is found to bind.

For so large a structure as RyR, a piecemeal approach to solving its atomic structure may well prove the most practical. In this, the multiple domains that appear to compose RyR would be expressed individually (or as clusters of adjacent, interacting domains) and solved to high resolution by X-ray or electron crystallography. Then, the high resolution structures of the domains would be fitted ("docked") into the lower resolution cryo-EM reconstructions ("envelops") of the intact RyR using algorithms such as those already employed in studies of other macromolecular complexes.[118,119] The docking would be greatly facilitated by knowledge of one or a few of the domain's amino acid residues on the receptor's surface as determined from RyR-GFP fusion protein complexes (described in the previous section). As an illustration of this strategy, an X-ray derived structure of an oxidoreductase domain, whose sequence bears homology to a region of RyR's sequence, has recently been modeled and docked into a cryo-EM reconstruction of RyR.[103]

Chapter 4

RYR-DHPR RELATIONSHIPS IN SKELETAL AND CARDIAC MUSCLES

Clara Franzini-Armstrong
Dept. of Cell Developmental Biology, University of Pennsylvania School of Medicine, Anatomy/Chemistry Building B42, Philadelphia, PA

INTRODUCTION

The functional link between depolarization of the plasmalemma and the release of calcium from the sarcoplasmic reticulum (SR) in all types of muscle cells involves two calcium channels. The L-type calcium channels of the plasmalemma and transverse (T) tubule, also called dihydropyridine receptors (DHPRs), act as voltage sensors and initiate the cascade of events linking excitation to contraction (EC coupling). The calcium release channels of the sarcoplasmic reticulum, also called ryanodine receptors (RyRs), have a high permeability to calcium and allow a rapid efflux of calcium from the SR lumen to the myofibrils, driven by the large lumenal-cytoplasmic concentration gradient.

The two channels can be detected by immunolabeling with specific antibodies and more directly by various electron microscopy techniques. These approaches have established the fact that DHPRs and RyRs are components of stable macromolecular complexes within calcium release units (CRUs)[120] at sites where one or two SR cisternae dock on the plasmalemma/T tubules forming intracellular junctions named triads, dyads and peripheral couplings (Fig. 4-1). Regardless of their shape, CRUs of skeletal and cardiac muscle *in vivo* and *in vitro* contain a common complement of major components. These include the SR docking protein junctophilin;[121] the two calcium channels defined above; the internal calcium binding protein calsequestrin (CSQ);[122] the two proteins that mediate CSQ-

RyR link, triadin and junctin;[123,124] and a large number of proteins associated with and regulating the cytoplasmic domains of RyRs (Fig. 4-1).

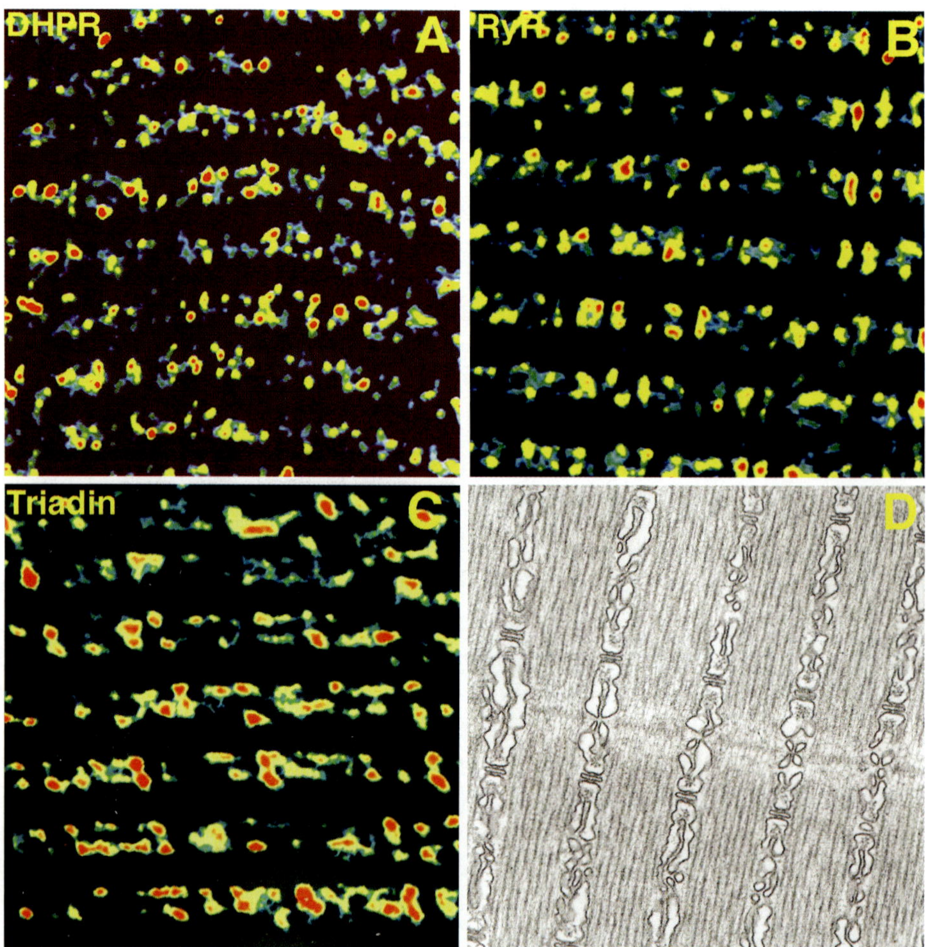

Figure 4-1. **Calcium release units** (usually in the form of triads in skeletal muscle) contain L-type calcium channels (DHPRs), the sarcoplasmic reticulum calcium release channels (RyRs) and other SR proteins. In these false-color confocal images, the position of hot spots of DHPRs (**A**), RyRs (**B**) and triadin (**C**), labeled by the correspondent antibodies, mark the positions of the triads at the A-I junction. In the electron microscope (**D**) triads are composed of a central transverse tubule flanked by two SR cisternae.

RYR DISPOSITION

The structure, location and disposition of RyRs *in situ* is detected by electron microscopy of thin sections (Fig. 4-1), of freeze-fracture replicas and of replicas from shadowed isolated SR vesicles. In thin sections, the large cytoplasmic domains of RyRs appear as electron dense masses that bridge the gap between apposed SR and plasmalemma/ T tubule membranes, called feet. In grazing views of the gap, each cytoplasmic domain (or foot) has an approximately square shape and is closely associated with those of the neighboring channels to form extensive arrays. Feet arrays have a handedness, that is they appear different when viewed from the cytoplasmic or from the lumenal side of the SR membrane. The cytoplasmic domains of RyRs are mirror symmetric and also they do not abut at the corners within the arrays, but they overlap with each other by about a third of their sides. Thus in the array, RyR profiles are skewed relative to the lines connecting the centers of the tetrameric RyR feet, which is parallel to the long axis of the T tubules (Fig. 4-2). RyRs have an inherent ability to organize themselves into arrays even in the absence of all other proteins of the sarcoplasmic reticulum[125,126] and they are also targeted to CRUs in the absence of DHPRs.[127]

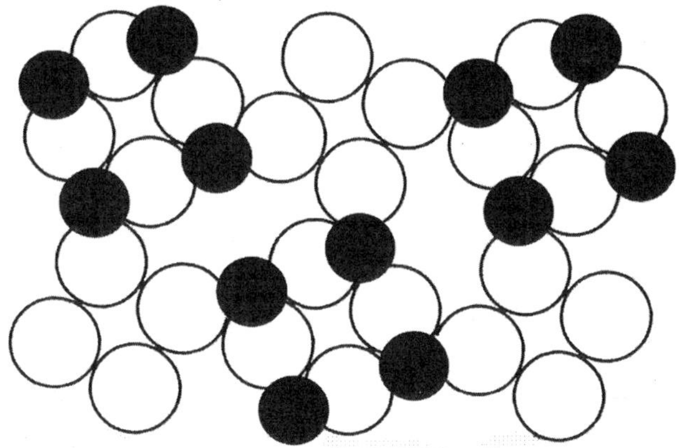

Figure 4-2. **RyRs (shown as four white circles) form precise arrays within the junctional SR membrane.** This is due to the fact that their cytoplasmic domains interlock with each other. In skeletal muscles of all vertebrates, DHPRs (each shown as a black sphere), are located in precise apposition to the four identical subunits of RyRs, thus forming a group called a tetrad. Tetrads are located opposite alternate feet in the array, probably due to steric hindrance that does not allow DHPRs to be associated with subunits of adjacent RyRs.

RYR-DHPR RELATIONSHIP

DHPRs are detected in freeze-fracture replicas of the plasmalemma/T tubule membranes. Each DHPR appears as a large intramembranous particle mostly associated with the cytoplasmic leaflet. In skeletal muscle, the DHPRs are arranged into arrays that are closely related to the arrays of RyRs. In particular, four DHPRs, constituting a tetrad, are associated with the four equal subunits of the RyR (or feet), but are positioned over alternate feet (Fig. 4-2).[62] Dysfunctional CRUs containing RyR, but not DHPRs are formed in skeletal muscle in the absence of the $\alpha 1$ subunit of DHPRs[128,129] and units containing DHPRs are formed in the absence of RyRs.[127,130] This indicates that the two proteins are independently targeted to and retained within CRUs. However, DHPRs require an association with skeletal type RyRs (RyR1) in order to form tetrads and tetrad arrays.[131] The alpha 2 subunit of DHPR also needs the alpha1 for appropriate targeting.[129]

The recent availability of 3-D reconstructions of both RyR and DHPR is bringing us close to a final understanding of the structural interaction between these two molecules.[57,107,116,132] We have recently reexamined the relative positions of DHPR and RyRs arrays relative to each other by superimposing arrays of DHPR tetrads as seen in freeze-fracture and arrays of feet as seen in rotary shadowed replicas of isolated heavy SR vesicles. Both images contain orientation clues, and if care is taken with mounting the grids in the electron microscope, images that have the same orientation can be obtained. Superimposition of an oriented array of tetrads over a similarly oriented array of feet shows that each of the four DHPR freeze-fracture particles is in the same relationship with the four RyR subunits and that each is close to, but not quite halfway, along the side of the square outline defining the foot (Fig. 4-2). In addition it is clear that overall the DHPR tetrad is larger than the outline of the foot and this in part explains why tetrads are associated with alternate feet. These images define specific restrictions on the location of DHPRs, which will acquire importance in the near future, once higher resolution images will be available. The specific positioning of skeletal type DHPRs in relation to RyR1 molecules is at the basis of the proposed bidirectional interaction that allows the two channels to control each other's function during excitation contraction coupling.[133] More on this below.

RYR3 LOCATION

Many skeletal muscles contain type 3 ryanodine receptors (or beta in the lower vertebrates) in addition to type one (or alpha), some at equal molar concentrations.[134,135] RyR3 fails to sustain EC-coupling *in vitro* and *in vivo*[23,50,136,137] and to induce tetrad formation by DHPRs when expressed in dyspedic (RyR1 null) cells that have skeletal DHPR.[131] Structural observations give some clues to the possible role of RyR3. Comparison of muscles that contain, alternatively, none, few or a relatively high proportion of RyR3, show that presence of RyR3 correlates well with the presence of parajunctional feet, located not within the area of SR membrane that associate with T tubules, but immediately adjacent to it.[138] Identification of these parajunctional feet with RyR3 (Fig. 4-3) suggests that activation of RyR3 is not directly via an interaction with DHPRs, but indirectly, perhaps by calcium released from the RyR1, as also indicated by the known properties of the RyR3 channels.

Comparison of RyR and DHPR dispositions in skeletal and cardiac muscles also yields results that are significant in functional terms. Differently from those in skeletal muscle, the cardiac isoforms of the two channels (RyR2 and α1c DHPR) do not interact directly. As a result, while in skeletal muscle EC-coupling is independent of extracellular calcium, and thus it does not require calcium permeation through the DHPR channel, cardiac EC-coupling depends on extracellular calcium.[139-141] In cardiac muscles, DHPRs and RyRs are colocalized at CRUs,[142-144] but the DHPRs are not organized into tetrads, an indication that they are not specifically linked to the RyR subunits. One may infer from this that like in the case of RyR3 in skeletal muscle, the cardiac RyR is not directly activated by a molecular interaction with DHPRs, in keeping with the physiology. Expression of RyR2 in dyspedic (RyR null, or lacking feet) cells fails to restore EC-coupling (either of the skeletal or cardiac type) and DHPR tetrads.

EXPERIMENTAL APPROACHES

The availability of null mutations for RyR1 in mouse skeletal muscle where RyR3 plays a minor role[23] and of a cell line carrying the RyR1 mutation[137] opened the possibility of exploring the functional and structural requirement for the skeletal type, or direct, DHPR-RyR interaction. The functional experiments performed in K.G. Beam's laboratory[133] clearly led the way. Nakai *et al.*[133] showed that the talk between skeletal type DHPR and RyR goes in both directions: DHPR activity directly affects the open probability of the RyR channel, but interaction with RyR is also necessary for effective calcium permeation through the DHPR. RyR1-RyR2 chimerae and an effective virus based infection mechanism were engineered in P. D. Allen's laboratory, allowing the following structural observations. An initial result is that DHPRs are targeted to CRUs in the absence of RyR, but they require an interaction with RyR1 in order to assemble into tetrads. Thus the presence of tetrads is indicative of a specific link between α1s-DHPR and RyR1.[59] Regions of RyR1 necessary for these interactions have been identified. The immediate question is whether there is a relationship between the requirements for a functional talk and those for the formation of DHPR tetrads, indicative of a specific molecular link with the RyR subunits. Interestingly, while the general answer is that indeed those RyR1-RyR2 chimerae that restore skeletal type EC-coupling also restore the presence of tetrads, the effectiveness of specific chimerae to restore tetrads is not exactly the same as that in restoring the functional link.[145] It appears that several regions of the RyR sequence may be involved in both the functional and structural interaction, but the regions that are required for holding the two molecules in the appropriate relative position are not exactly the same as those required for the functional interaction during EC-coupling. An interesting, if not unexpected, result.

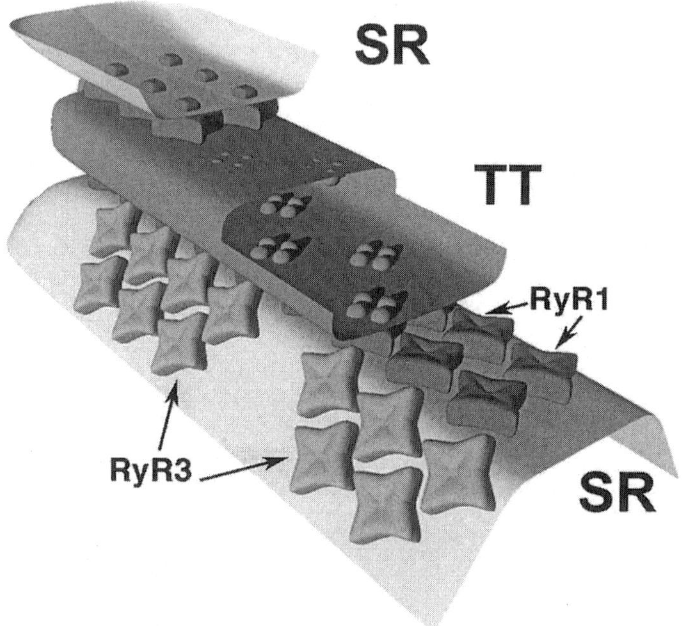

Figure 4-3. **Diagrammatic view of the relationship between type 1 and type 3 RyRs in the triads of skeletal muscles** (e.g., from the frog, the tail of some fish and some birds) that contain a 1:1 ratio of RyR1 and RyR3. RyR1 are positioned in the junctional gap between SR and T tubules, so that they can associate directly with DHPRs. RyR3 are located in a parajunctional region, where they are in proximity of RyR1, but cannot interact with DHPRs. It is assumed that they are activated independently. Courtesy of E. Felder.[138]

Thus in skeletal muscle DHPRs and RyRs are held in close physical proximity by a molecular connection that may be direct, and this proximity is a requirement for their functional interaction.

Further interesting confirmation of the specificity of the DHPR-RyR link in skeletal muscle comes from recent experiments exploring the possibility that conformational changes in the RyR may be revealed by an alteration of DHPR tetrads.[146] Ryanodine induces substantial and persistent conformational changes in RyR. At relatively high concentrations (above ~100 μM) ryanodine locks the channel in a closed state by binding to low affinity sites. Two cells lines (BC3H1 and RyR1-infected 1B5) that have extensive clusters of associated α_{1s}-DHPR and RyR1 at the cell surface were treated with 500 μM ryanodine for 24 hrs, freeze-fractured and rotary shadowed. The center-to-center distances between individual DHPR within tetrads decreased by ~2 nm in the ryanodine-treated cells relative to the control cells. These results indicate that the DHPR-RyR complex acts as a single unit, confirming a specific interaction between the channels, and further suggest that ryanodine induces large conformational changes in the cytoplasmic RyR domain responsible for linking to DHPR.

CONCLUDING REMARKS

The specificity of the RyR-DHPR interaction in skeletal muscle is revealed by electron microscopy studies that define the special relationship between the two channels.

ACKNOWLEDGEMENTS

The work presented in this chapter was performed in collaboration with Drs. P.D. Allen; Kurt Beam and Isaac Pessah and is due to the contributions of Drs. Edward Felder, Feliciano Protasi, Cecilia Paolini, and Hiroaki Takekura.

Chapter 5

THE PORE OF THE RYANODINE RECEPTOR CHANNEL

Alan J. Williams[1], S.R. Wayne Chen[2], and William Welch[3]
[1]*Cardiac Medicine, National Heart & Lung Institute, Imperial College London;* [2]*Cardiovascular Research Group, Dept. of Physiology and Biophysics, and Dept. of Biochemistry and Molecular Biology, University of Calgary, Calgary, Alberta, Canada;* [3]*Dept. of Biochemistry, University of Nevada School of Medicine, Reno, NV*

THE PHYSIOLOGICAL ROLE OF THE RYANODINE RECEPTOR CHANNEL

As is highlighted in various other chapters of this book, the ryanodine receptor functions as an intracellular membrane Ca^{2+}-release channel; providing a regulated pathway for the movement of Ca^{2+} from a storage organelle, such as the sarcoplasmic reticulum in muscle, down an electrochemical gradient to initiate a wide variety of cellular processes.[96]

The efficiency of the ryanodine receptor as a Ca^{2+}-release channel in a process such as excitation-contraction coupling is underpinned by both its ability to open and close in response to appropriate stimuli and its ability to allow the movement of very large numbers of Ca^{2+} ions per unit time. This second component of RyR channel function reflects both the capability of the channel to discriminate between ions present in the lumen of the sarcoplasmic reticulum and to maximize rates of ion throughput.

In this chapter we will discuss the mechanisms and structural features of the pore region employed by the RyR channel to select and then to translocate Ca^{2+} across the sarco(endo)plasmic reticulum membrane. We will also consider the emerging proposition that the RyR pore contains a high-affinity binding site for ryanodine.

WHAT AND WHERE IS THE RYR PORE?

An individual RyR channel is composed of four identical monomers, each of which contains approximately 5000 amino acid residues (variations between isoforms are described in Williams *et al.*[147]). It has been proposed that each RyR monomer could contain a viable pore and that the function of an individual RyR channel reflects coordinated gating of these four pores.[148] However, a growing body of evidence, arising from the investigation of the function of heteromeric channels containing wild type and mutant monomers,[37] and studies of the influence of chemical modifiers of channel function,[149] indicates that each tetrameric RyR channel contains a single pore.

The pore of any membrane ion channel is the region of the molecule that provides a pathway for the movement of ions across the dielectric barrier of a phospholipid membrane. As a consequence, this region of the RyR channel will inevitably be formed by membrane spanning regions of the molecule. Potential membrane-spanning regions of the RyR monomer have been identified in the C-terminal 1000 residues with the number of transmembrane sequences present in each monomer estimated at between 4[3] and 10.[7,8] Experiments involving tryptic cleavage[150] or truncation of RyR channels[29,73] indicate that the region of the molecule encompassing the probable transmembrane domains can, in isolation, provide a pathway for cation translocation.

Balshaw *et al.*[77] have proposed a role for a specific sequence of residues in the formation of the RyR pore. These authors noted that a mutation in the human RyR1 that underlies an unusually severe form of central core disease (I4898T)[151] occurred in a sequence of residues that shared a degree of homology with the consensus selectivity sequence of K^+ channels (Fig. 5-1). Balshaw *et al.*[77] also noted that this sequence of residues was found in a loop, equivalent to the pore forming or P-loop in K^+ channels, which links the probable penultimate and last transmembrane domains of all topology models of RyR. This potential RyR P-loop occurs within the lumen of the SR and Balshaw *et al.* proposed that, as is the case for K^+ channels, the loop could fold back into the membrane to contribute to the formation of the RyR pore.

Evidence in support of the involvement of residues, analogous to the K^+ channel selectivity filter and within a RyR P-loop, in ion translocation has been provided by investigations of the properties of individual channels in which specific residues have been mutated; an approach that has proved to be invaluable in the identification of selectivity sequences in other ion channels. Residue substitutions in and around the putative selectivity filter sequences in both RyR1[38] and RyR2[37,74] decrease, to a greater or lesser extent, unitary conductance of both Ca^{2+} and K^+.

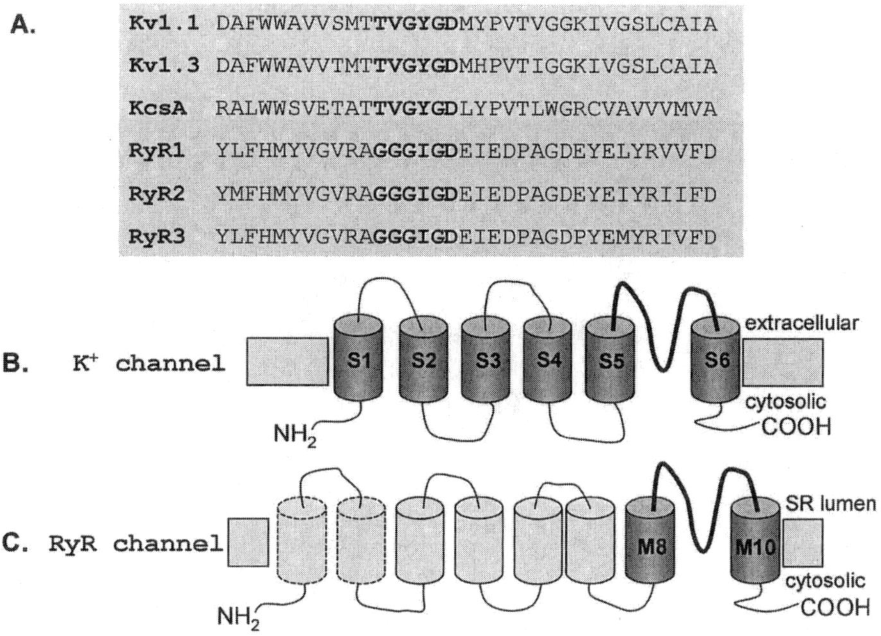

Figure 5-1. **Signature selectivity sequences of representative K^+ channels (bold) and analogous motifs of three rabbit RyR isoforms are shown in A.** In K^+ channels these motifs occur in an extracellular pore forming or P loop linking S5 and S6 in voltage-activated channels (as shown in **B**) and M1 and M2 in KcsA. The putative RyR selectivity sequence occurs in an analogous position in this species of channel between the penultimate and last transmembrane segments (M8 and M10 in the topology model described in Du *et al.*[8] and shown in **C**). In both **B.** and **C.** the P-loop (bold) is shown folding back into the membrane to contribute to the formation of the pore.

Analogies between the pore regions of RyR and K channels

The foregoing discussion indicates certain analogies between the pore regions of RyR and K^+ channels. Both species of channel are homotetramers; in both cases the pore of the channel appears to be formed by elements of an equivalent extracellular/luminal loop linking the last two transmembrane domains and within this loop RyR contains a sequence of residues analogous to the selectivity sequence of the K^+ channels. Whilst we have no direct information concerning the structure of the RyR pore, a wealth of structural information has been made available for the pore of K^+

channels as the result of the crystallization of simple bacterial K^+ channels.[9,152] The essential features of these structures are as follows. The pore is formed at the long axis of four identical subunits. Each subunit contributes two transmembrane helices (in KcsA the outer helix (M1) and the inner helix (M2)). The extracellular loop linking these helices folds into the membrane and itself contains two elements of differing secondary structure, a short helix referred to as the pore helix and an extended chain of residues including the identified selectivity sequence. When the channel is closed, a gate is formed at the crossing of the four inner helices at the cytosolic entrance to the structure.[9] The transition to an open conformation involves a flexing of the inner helices at a glycine hinge located somewhere near the middle of each helix.[153] A K^+ ion entering the pore from the bulk solution at the cytosolic side of the open channel is stabilized in a water-filled cavity by dipoles of the four pore helices.[9] On entering the selectivity filter of the channel the K^+ is dehydrated and coordinated by backbone carbonyl oxygens of the signature selectivity residues.[154,155] The cation is re-hydrated as it leaves the filter and re-enters the extracellular bulk solution.[155]

The extraordinary powers of discrimination of K^+ channels arise from the very precise coordination of this ion within the fairly rigid selectivity filter; Na^+ ions are not coordinated and are hence excluded, as the filter is a poor solvent for Na^+ relative to water. In these channels, rates of translocation are maximized by electrostatic repulsion between ions occupying multiple sites within the selectivity filter.

Examinations of predictions of the secondary structure of elements of the putative RyR P-loop have identified a helical region in the RyR P-loop that occurs in a location equivalent to the pore helix in K^+ channels (Fig. 5-2).[147,156] The sequence of structural elements in KcsA is M1 (outer helix); pore helix; selectivity filter; M2 (inner helix). In RyR the elements occur in an equivalent order (using the topology profile recently described by Du *et al.*[8]) M8 (transmembrane helix); M9 (putative pore helix); loop containing residues analogous to K^+ channel selectivity sequence; M10 (transmembrane helix). These observations have led to the suggestion that the putative RyR P-loop may adopt a tertiary configuration equivalent to that determined for the P-loop of KcsA and that the pore of the RyR channel could, as a consequence, adopt a broadly similar structure to that determined for KcsA (Fig. 5-3).[147,156]

In such an arrangement an ion entering the pore from the SR luminal bulk solution would encounter a region formed by the apposition of the four chains containing residues analogous with the K^+ channel selectivity sequence. Having passed through this region the ion would enter a water-filled cavity lined with residues of the M10 helices before leaving the pore into the cytosolic bulk solution. A general structure of this form would provide the RyR pore with a means to accomplish the fundamental requirement of a membrane ion channel. As in KcsA the presence of a water-filled cytosolic cavity, into which are orientated four helix dipoles, would effectively bring the cytosolic bulk solution into the membrane and provide a means of overcoming the potential electrostatic destabilisation of a cation within the membrane.

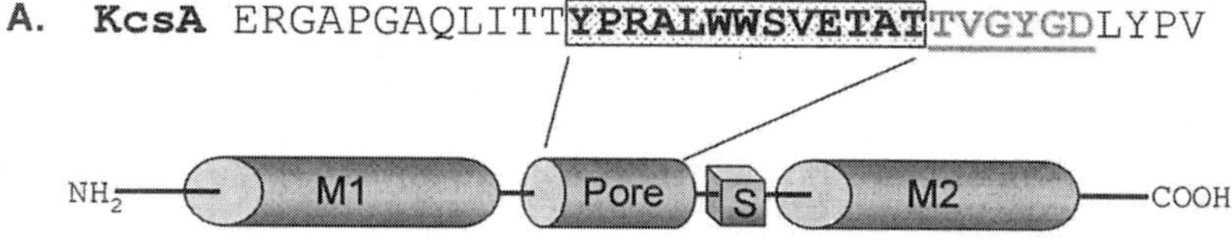

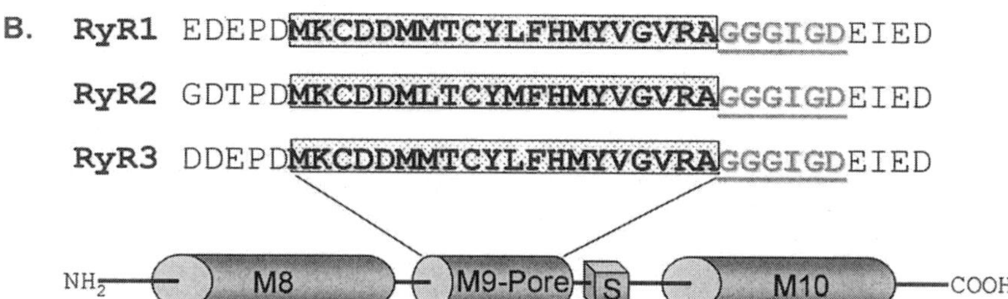

Figure 5-2. **Pore forming loops of KcsA and RyR. A**. The P loop of KcsA contains a short helical element referred to as the pore helix (pore) and a signature selectivity sequence (S). Secondary structure predictions for the putative RyR P loop have identified motifs equivalent to the K^+ channel pore helix in all isoforms of the channel. The residues contributing to the putative pore helices of three rabbit isoforms of RyR and their location within the P loop are shown in panel **B**. In both panels residues of the selectivity sequence are underlined.

Evidence in support of this putative structure

Whilst there are very significant fundamental differences in the characteristics of ion discrimination and translocation in RyR and K^+ channels (see later), there are some similarities that could support the suggestion that the channels share a basically similar pore structure. Permeant cation movement is blocked in both species of channel by a range of tetra alkyl ammonium cations.[147] The demonstration of block of RyR by large polycations[157] and K^+ channel N-type inactivation peptides from the bulk solution at the cytosolic face of RyR[158] would be consistent with the proposal that access to the site of block in a putative selectivity filter is via a large water-filled cavity at this entrance to the structure.

We have already indicated that residue substitution in the selectivity filter of the putative RyR pore modifies rates of monovalent and divalent cation translocation. It should also be noted that expression of heteromeric mouse RyR2 channels comprising different combinations of wild type monomers and monomers in which an alanine residue has been substituted for glycine 4824 (a substitution that reduces K^+ conductance to 3% of wild type conductance when expressed as a homotetramer) gives rise to channels with a range of conductance values intermediate between wild type and homomeric G4824A.[37] These observations indicate that each monomer contributes to ion handling and would suggest that a single pore is formed at the axis of the tetramer.

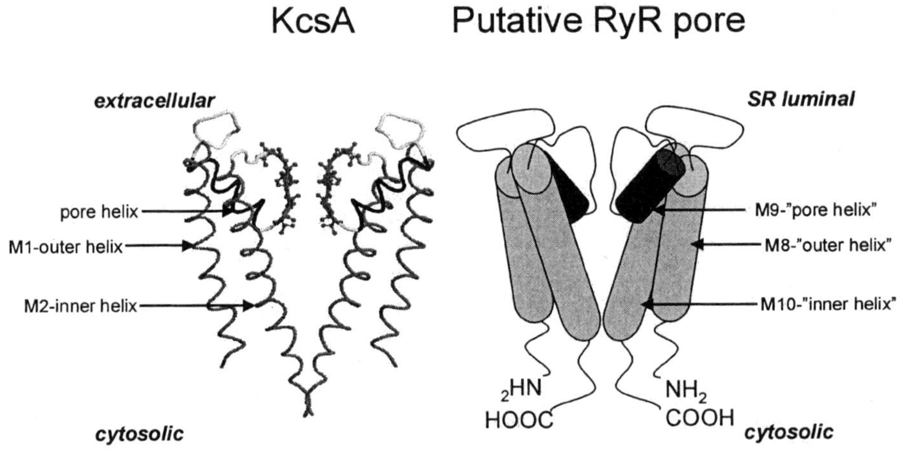

Figure 5-3. **The KcsA pore** (pdb 1BL8 from Doyle *et al.*[9]) is shown in the left-hand panel; two diagonally apposed monomers have been removed for clarity. The two transmembrane helices of each monomer are shown in grey, the pore helices in black and the residues of the selectivity filter in ball and stick representation. The equivalent arrangement of structural elements identified in the RyR putative P loop, are shown in the right-hand panel.

Further support for this putative pore structure comes from the recent identification of residues of RyR1 that are involved in interactions with the sarcoplasmic reticulum luminal accessory protein, triadin. Lee *et al.*[159] identified three acidic residues in the luminal loop linking M8 and M10 that appear to be critical for this interaction. As noted by these authors all three residues would be located at the luminal face of the putative RyR pore described in this chapter, with one located towards the N-terminus of the putative pore helix and two others in the loop containing the selectivity sequence residues linking the putative pore helix and M10.

Finally, models of the proposed pore region of RyR, incorporating a putative pore helix, have been produced by extrapolating from the crystal structure of KcsA.[156,160]

ION SELECTION AND TRANSLOCATION IN RYR

The various observations outlined above have led us to conclude that it is reasonable to hypothesize that the pore of the RyR channel shares a broadly common architecture with the equivalent region of K^+ channels. However, a comparison of the discrimination and translocation properties of these two species of channel suggests that the mechanisms underlying these processes must be very different. K^+ channel function is characterized by high rates of translocation coupled with extremely high specificity and these intuitively contradictory properties are made possible by a pore and selectivity filter structure that permits very precise coordination of K^+ and electrostatic interactions between adjacent cations in the filter.[161]

The ion handling properties of RyR have been reviewed in detail in Williams *et al.*[147] and are summarized here. The first observation to emerge from these investigations is that RyR is not a particularly selective channel. While it does completely exclude anions, RyR discriminates only relatively poorly between cations. Unlike K^+ channels, RyR is permeable to a very wide range of divalent and monovalent inorganic cations and some organic monovalent cations. Calculations of relative permeability from reversal potentials monitored for single RyR channels under bi-ionic conditions reveal that, as a group, the alkaline earth divalents are essentially equally permeant in RyR. Similarly, RyR is equally permeable to the group 1a monovalent cations. However RyR is able to discriminate to some extent between divalent and monovalent inorganic cations with divalents 6 to 7 fold more permeant than monovalents.

Another striking feature to emerge from these studies is the rate of both monovalent and divalent cation translocation achieved in RyR. Unitary conductance for K^+ increases with increasing activity and plateaus at approximately 1nS. Equivalent experiments with Ba^{2+} demonstrate a maximal unitary conductance of approximately 200pS. Despite these very high rates of cation translocation and very limited discrimination, permeant cations interact with the RyR pore with high affinity. Values obtained from conductance-activity relationships and from rate theory modelling indicate that 50% maximal conductance is achieved at activities of 100-400 μM for alkaline earth divalents and activities of 10-20 mM for group 1a monovalents. While rates of cation translocation in RyR are significantly greater than those in K^+ channels all available evidence indicates that this does not reflect multi-ion occupancy in a RyR selectivity filter; rather RyR behaves as a single-ion channel. Theoretical considerations indicate that to achieve the measured rates of cation translocation with single ion occupancy, RyR is likely to possess a short, wide, selectivity filter. In agreement with this suggestion, investigations involving a range of permeant and impermeant monovalent and divalent organic cations have produced estimates of approximately 3.5 Å for the minimum pore radius and approximately 10 Å for the length of the voltage drop across the channel.

Even this very brief comparison of the ion handling properties of RyR and K^+ channels indicates that the mechanisms underlying discrimination and translocation are likely to be very different in the two channels. If, as we have proposed, the channels share a broadly comparable pore structure to overcome the dielectric barrier of the membrane, it is clear that the arrangement of structural elements and hence the processes governing interactions of cations with the pore must be very different in the two structures.

DOES THE RYR PORE CONTAIN A RYANODINE-BINDING SITE?

The RyR channel is so named because each functional channel contains a high-affinity binding site for the plant alkaloid ryanodine and, as described elsewhere in this book, the binding of ryanodine to this site has dramatic consequences for both channel gating and rates of cation translocation.

Initial attempts to identify the ryanodine binding site within RyR1 involved proteolysis and photoaffinity labelling.[82,162] These approaches localised the site to a 76 kD portion at the C-terminus of the molecule which encompasses the putative pore region discussed in this chapter. The suggestion that a ryanodine-binding site is located within the pore of RyR has arisen as the result of several observations. It is well established that high affinity ryanodine binding involves interaction of the ligand with an open conformation of the channel.[163,164] This could mean that the binding site is located within the pore and is only accessible when the channel is open or that a site outside the pore is made available by a conformational alteration associated with channel opening. Single channel investigations of the interactions of derivatives of ryanodine (ryanoids) have demonstrated that these events are influenced by transmembrane holding potential[164,165] and, whilst it has been established that the vast majority of this voltage dependence arises from a potential-driven alteration in receptor affinity,[166] the possibility remains that ryanoids might bind at a site at the extremity of the voltage drop across the channel; such a site is likely to be within the pore.

Also contributing to a proposed pore location for a ryanodine-binding site is the observation that the mutation of several residues located within the putative RyR P-loop alters the interaction of ryanodine with the channel. Substitution of residues in and around those equivalent to the K^+ channel selectivity sequence has been shown to prevent the binding of [^{3}H]-ryanodine to populations of channels or to either increase or decrease the affinity of the interaction.[37,38,74,167]

Investigations in which the interactions of charged ryanoids with individual RyR channels have been monitored have revealed that the high-affinity ryanodine binding site is only accessible from the cytosolic side of the channel.[164] We have investigated the possible involvement of the putative cytosolic cavity in ryanodine binding by investigating the interactions of the ligand with mouse RyR2 channels in which residues of M10, the helix that lines the cavity of the proposed RyR pore, have been mutated. Alanine substitution of several of these residues results in alterations in the response of channels to Ca^{2+} and caffeine[78] and reduced levels of [^{3}H]-ryanodine binding.[79] One substitution has been studied in detail by monitoring ryanodine interactions with individual, voltage-clamped, channels. Although we were unable to detect binding of [^{3}H]-ryanodine to populations of Q4863A channels, single channel investigations revealed that ryanodine does interact with the channel. On the timescale of a single channel experiment the interaction of ryanodine with wild type RyR channels is irreversible; observations with Q4863A revealed that this mutation produced a dramatic increase in the rate of dissociation of bound ryanodine from the channel so that, in the continued presence of ryanodine, we observed reversible interactions of the ligand with the channel. Interestingly the consequences of the Q4863A substitution appear to be very specific.[79] These channels respond to physiological and pharmacological regulators of gating in a manner equivalent to wild type channels. Similarly, unitary conductance and the fractional conductance of the Q4863A RyR-ryanodine complex have the same values as these parameters in wild type channels. Finally, rates of ryanodine association with, and dissociation from, Q4863A channels are sensitive to changes in transmembrane holding potential and these parameters vary in a manner analogous to those of reversible ryanoids such as ryanodol and 21-amino-9α-hydroxyryanodine with wild-type sheep RyR2 channels. Taken together, the effects of residue substitution in both the putative selectivity filter and M10 indicate that residues of the proposed pore are likely to make an important contribution to the high affinity binding site for ryanodine in RyR.

CONCLUDING REMARKS

In this chapter we have given a very brief overview of the evidence for the involvement of residues of a C-terminal luminal loop in the formation and function of the RyR channel pore. Further investigations will be aimed at elucidating the relationships between pore structure and the mechanisms that a) give rise to the very unusual characteristics of ion discrimination and translocation displayed by RyR, and b) contribute to the binding of ryanodine to the channel.

ACKNOWLEDGMENTS

The work in the authors' laboratories is supported by research grants from the British Heart Foundation to A.J.W., the Canadian Institutes of Health Research and the Heart and Stroke Foundation of Alberta, Northwestern Territories, and Nunavut to S.R.W.C, and the National Science Foundation (MCB 9817605) to W.W.

Chapter 6

INTRA-MOLECULAR DOMAIN-DOMAIN INTERACTION

A KEY MECHANISM FOR CALCIUM CHANNEL REGULATION OF RYANODINE RECEPTORS

Noriaki Ikemoto
Boston Biomedical Research Institute, 64 Grove Street, Watertown, MA; and Harvard Medical School, Boston, MA

DOMAIN-DOMAIN INTERACTION FOR Ca^{2+} CHANNEL REGULATION

Introduction

E-C coupling in both skeletal muscle and cardiac muscle is mediated by a common mechanism as well as by tissue-specific mechanisms.[168] The most important common feature is that the ryanodine receptor plays a central role in this process.[169] Some tissue-specific differences may be ascribable to the fact that the RyR is expressed by different tissue-specific genes and that its structural arrangements with another important component DHPR are quite different (see Chapter 1).[170]

The skeletal RyR isoform (RyR1) and the cardiac RyR isoform (RyR2) show about 60% homology, and interestingly, homologous regions and non-homologous regions appear to be segregated along the RyR polypeptide chain. An early analysis identified the three major divergent (non-homologous) regions; the so-called D1, D2 and D3 regions as indicated in Fig. 6-1.[115] Fig. 6-1 also shows a heterogeneity map we constructed on the basis of the residue distance score of individual corresponding residues of the two isoforms. As seen (the peak height shows heterogeneity), there are several additional divergent regions in the RyR. It is quite reasonable to assume that some of the tissue-specific differences in the RyR function mentioned above are ascribable to these divergent regions, and some common features may be ascribable to the homologous regions as discussed in the following parts.

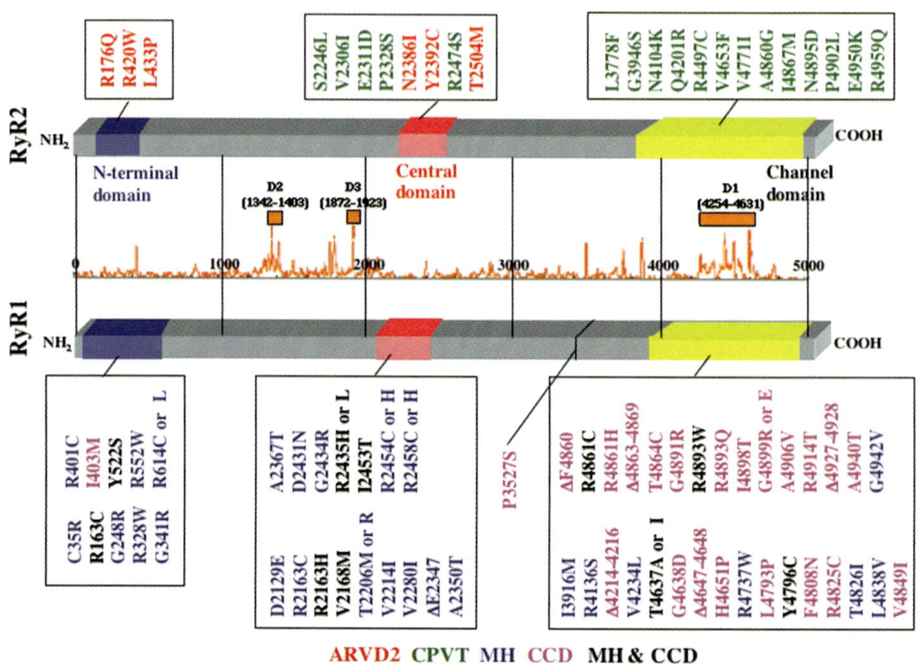

Figure 6-1. **The locations of MH/CCD mutation sites (RyR1) and cardiac disease mutation sites (RyR2).** Most of these mutations are located in the three well-definable regions, the N-terminal domain, central domain, and channel domain. As a reference, the heterogeneity map is indicated. Three highly divergent regions D1, D2 and D3 are shown. Note that the two hot-spot domains located in the cytoplasmic lobe of the RyR (i.e. N-terminal domain and central domain) are relatively homologous between RyR1 and RyR2. ARVD2, arrhythmogenic right ventricular dysplasia/cardiomyopathy type 2; CCD, central core disease; CPVT, catecholaminergic polymorphic ventricular tachycardia; MH, malignant hyperthermia.

THE CONCEPT OF 'DOMAIN SWITCH'

Critical regulatory domains

Presumably, a number of domains and sub-domains of RyR are working in a coordinated manner to perform the necessary conformational control of RyR Ca^{2+} channels. In searching for such regulatory domains, Ikemoto and his colleagues, as well as other investigators, have paid particular attention to the fact that the reported sites of MH/CCD mutations on RyR1 are not randomly distributed. As a matter of fact, they are localized to three rather restricted regions: the N-terminal, central, and the channel domains (Fig. 6-1). For further details of these mutations, the readers must refer to Chapters 22 and 23. The vast majority of MH mutations are located in the N-terminal and central domains. In contrast, most mutations conferring susceptibility to CCD, a rare myopathy linked to RyR1, are located in the C-terminal channel region.[171] These MH mutations cause aberrations in the RyR1 channel function, such as hyper-activation of the channel by, and hyper-sensitization to, various physiological and pharmacological agonists, resulting in a leaky Ca^{2+} channel and an elevated cytoplasmic Ca^{2+} level.[172-174] The studies on the Ca^{2+} release properties of heterologously[175] or homologously[176] expressed RyR1 channels containing randomly selected MH mutations from the N-terminal and central domains demonstrated that these channels in fact display MH-like hyper-activation and hyper-sensitization of RyR Ca^{2+} channels. However, the expressed RyR1 containing selected CCD mutations from the C-terminal channel domain displayed a different phenotype: that is, unlike RyR1 containing MH mutations, it showed normal response to pharmacological agonists, but it showed no response to the physiological stimulus ('EC uncoupling').[177] These facts suggest that mutations occurred in the N-terminal and central domains affect primarily upon the intra-molecular control of channel functions, while those in the C-terminal channel domain affect primarily upon the inter-molecular (DHPR-RyR1) signal transmission.

The primary structure of the RyR2 corresponding to both of the skeletal N-terminal and central domains are relatively well conserved (Fig. 6-1, heterogeneity map). This suggests that the cardiac domains corresponding to these N-terminal and central domains also play a key role. Recently several RyR2 mutations have been reported that are related to inheritable cardiac diseases[53,54,178]; for further details, see Chapters 25. Many of these mutations are located in either of the predicted N-terminal or central domain of the RyR2 (see blue and red coded regions, respectively, Fig. 6-1), although many more are located in the putative transmembrane channel region (yellow-coded). Of particular interest is that one of the cardiomyopathy (ARVD2) mutations in the N-terminal domain of the RyR2, Arg176Gln, corresponds exactly to the Arg163Cys human MH mutation of the RyR1. One must also note that the amino acid residues in RyR1 or RyR2 that are mutated in disease are usually ones that are identical in RyR1 and RyR2. Thus, it is very likely that the essentially identical sets of regulatory domains are operating for channel regulation in both RyR1 and RyR2.

Domain-domain interaction for Ca^{2+} channel regulation

Considering again the afore-mentioned properties of the expressed RyR1 channels containing randomly selected MH mutations[175,176], we notice a quite important feature. That is, wherever these mutations are, any of these mutations produces more or less identical MH-like effects (hyper-activation/hyper-sensitization) on Ca^{2+} channels, so far as those mutations were located in either N-terminal domain or central domain of RyR1. One of the most feasible explanations is that these hot domains (i.e. N-terminal and central domains) constitute the intra-molecular machinery that controls Ca^{2+} channel functions, hence mutations occurring in either domain will produce a global impact on the operation of the machinery, and in turn abnormal Ca^{2+} channel regulation.

Based on the above consideration, Ikemoto and his colleagues have proposed a 'domain-switch' model (Fig. 6-2) that involves inter-domain interactions between the N-terminal and central domains of RyR serving as a key mechanism for Ca^{2+} channel regulation.[179,180] The model assumes that in the resting or non-activated state, the N-terminal and central domains make close contact at several as yet undetermined sub-domains (e.g. sub-domains x/y). The conformational constraints imparted by the 'zipped' configuration of these two domains stabilize the closed state of Ca^{2+} channel (Fig. 6-2, the left state of row a). The model proposes this conformation as the 'off' configuration of the implicit 'on/off switch' constituted by these two domains. Under usual stimulating conditions (EC coupling or pharmacological agonists), the inter-domain contacts are weakened leading to an 'unzipped' or 'on' configuration. This leads to Ca^{2+} channel opening (Fig. 6-2, the right state of row a). According to this model, if a mutation should occur in critical sub-domain *x* of the central domain for example, the interaction of this sub-domain with its mating sub-domain located in the N-terminal domain would weaken or be lost, causing a partial 'unzipping', and resulting in a lowering of the energy barrier necessary for channel opening (Fig. 6-2, the middle state of row b). Such a partially 'unzipped' domain pair is readily turned to its fully opened configuration by weaker-than-normal stimuli, causing the hyper-activation/hyper-sensitization effects seen in channels containing disease-causing mutations in both cases of skeletal and cardiac muscles (Fig. 6-2, the right state of row b).

This model has been tested by examining the effects of a family of synthetic peptides corresponding to the putative critical domains of RyR (designated as domain peptides, DP) on several aspects of channel function. The underlying assumption in rationalizing the use of synthetic domain peptides as a functional probe is that they are capable of mimicking native conformations in the *in vitro* solution. The strategy of the domain peptide

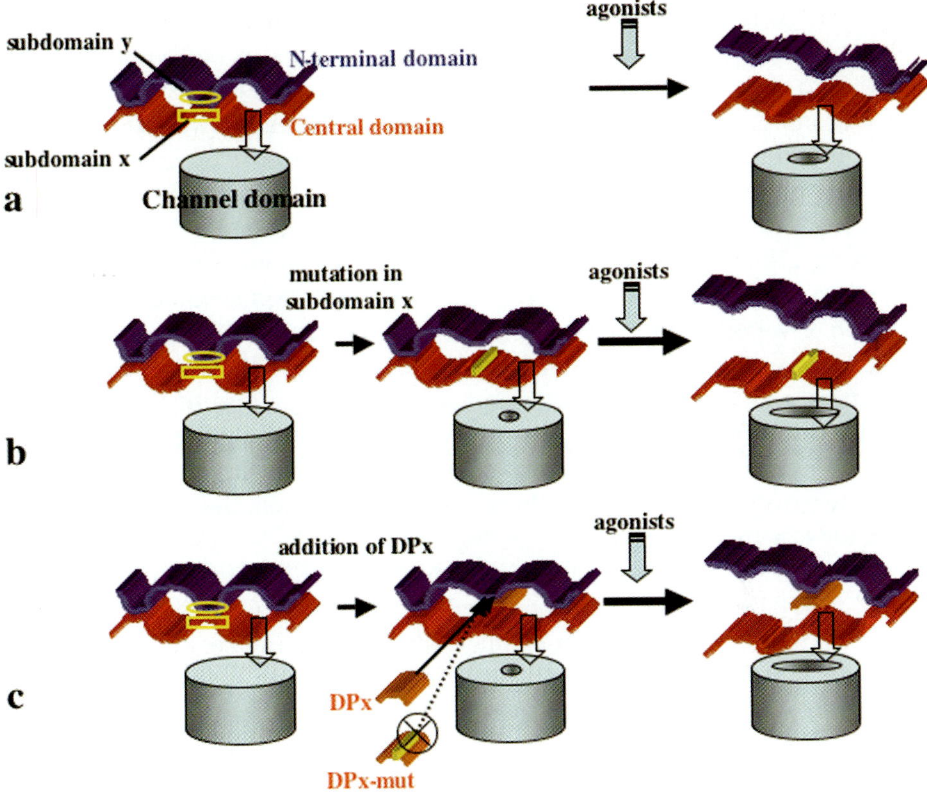

Figure 6-2. **Hypothetical model showing how the changes in the mode of interaction between the two key domains (N-terminal and central) control the state of the RyR Ca^{2+} channel. A**. Close contact between the N-terminal (blue) domain and the central domain (red, zipping) stabilizes the closed state of the Ca^{2+} channel. Upon activation of the RyR by adding the agonist, the close contact of the domain pair is removed (unzipping), then de-blocks the channel to open. **B**. Mutations in either of the N-terminal or the central domain (in this example, in sub-domain x of the central domain) weakens the interaction between sub-domain x and sub-domain y, causing a partial unzipping of the domain switch even before receiving the agonist signal. The activation by the agonist readily unzips domain switch even with lower than normal stimulus. This is manifested in the hyper-activation and hyper-sensitization effects seen in the channels of diseased muscle. **C**. Domain peptide (in this example, the peptide corresponding to sub-domain x of the central domain; namely domain peptide x or DPx) binds to its mating sub-domain: sub-domain y of the N-terminal domain. As a result of competition between DPx and sub-domain x for their binding to their mating sub-domain y, the interaction between sub-domains x and y (consequently, the interaction between the N-terminal and central domains) is weakened. This causes partial unzipping of the interacting domain pair and activation of the channel. Disease-causing mutation made in DPx (DPx-mut) abolishes its ability to bind to sub-domain y, resulting in the loss of the activating function of DPx. Thus, DPx-mut provides us with an excellent negative control.

approach is as shown in row c of Fig. 6-2. Addition of synthetic peptide DP*x*, corresponding to sub-domain *x*, to RyR results in the binding of the peptide to the N-terminal mating domain of sub-domain *x* (i.e sub-domain y), in competition with native sub-domain *x*. Resultant weakened native inter-domain interactions cause partial "unzipping" of RyR, thereby destabilizing the closed or 'off' conformation (Fig. 6-2, the middle state of row c).

An excellent negative control to test the physiological relevance of the observed activation effect of DP*x* is as follows. Since mutation in sub-domain *x* weakens the interaction between sub-domains *x* and *y* as mentioned above, the same mutation made in DP*x* (namely DP*x*-mut) will reduce the affinity of its binding to sub-domain *y*, causing a loss of the activating function that would have been present in the un-mutated peptide.

As an example of successful domain peptides, which worked exactly as predicted from the above hypothesis, Table 6-1 depicts the results obtained with DP4, which corresponds to the Leu^{2442}-Pro^{2477} region of the central domain of RyR1 (^{2442}LIQAGKGEALRIRAILRSLVPLDDLVGIISLPL-QIP^{2477}). DP4 enhanced ryanodine binding,[181] induced Ca^{2+} release from the SR,[181] induced contraction in skinned muscle fiber at an inhibitory Mg^{2+} concentration,[182] increased the sensitivity to caffeine,[181,182] increased the frequency of Ca^{2+} sparks in saponin-permeabilized fibers,[183] and increased the open probability of single channels.[183] DP4-mut, in which one mutation was made to mimic the Arg2458Cys or Arg2458His MH mutation, produced no appreciable effect on any of these parameters.

It has been shown that the central domain peptide DP4 binds to the N-terminal region of the RyR, as evidenced by the fact that the DP4-mediated site-directed probe labeling (see below) resulted in an exclusive fluorescence labeling of the ~150 kDa N-terminal segment of the RyR,[184] and according to more recent study in the 50 kDa segment starting from the N-terminus, that corresponds to the N-terminal domain.[185] This supports the view that the sub-domain of the central domain corresponding to DP4 interacts with the N-terminal domain. These data suggest that at least some of the synthetic domain peptides are capable of mimicking native conformations, and that experimental data obtained with them are physiologically relevant.

Several other domain peptides have also been used to test the domain switch hypothesis. For instance, DP1 corresponding to the Leu^{590}-Cys^{609} region of the N-terminal domain of RyR1 (^{590}LDKHGRNHKVLDVLCSLCVC^{609}) produced MH-like hyper-activation/hyper-sensitization effects on RyR1 channels.[186] Importantly, this peptide contains the binding site for dantrolene, the drug that is used to treat MH (see Chapter 24).[187] Moreover, DP1 was recognized by mAb anti-RyR1 raised to native rabbit RyR1, and this antibody inhibits dantrolene binding to

RyR1,[187] indicating that the drug-binding site is located within the Leu^{590}-Cys^{609} region of the N-terminal domain.

Table 6-1. **A central domain peptide DP4 produces MH-like hyper-activation effects on the RyR Ca^{2+} channel as seen in various systems**: from the level of the single channel to the level of the whole cell. Single mutation in the peptide abolishes its activating function. (+):increase, (-):no change.

System	Function	DP4	DP4-mut
Triad	Ryanodine binding	+	-
	SR Ca^{2+} release	+	-
	Apparent affinity to agonist	+	-
Skinned fiber	Force response to caffeine	+	-
	Force response to sub-max depolarization	+	n.d.
Permeabilized fiber	Frequency of Ca^{2+} sparks	+	-
Single channel	Po	+	-

N.d.: not determined.

As described above, many mutations related to the inheritable cardiac myopathies occur in the regions of the RyR2 corresponding to the N-terminal and central MH domains of the RyR1 (Fig. 6-1). This suggests that these domains and their inter-domain interactions also play an important role in cardiac Ca^{2+} channel regulation. To test this hypothesis, a cardiac RyR domain peptide DPc10 corresponding to the Gly^{2460}-Pro^{2495} region (a portion of the central domain of RyR2 (^{2460}GFCPDHKAAMVLFLDRV-YGIEVQDFLLHLLEVGFLP^{2495}) was used. This peptide was found to enhance the ryanodine binding activity and increased the sensitivity of the RyR2 to activating Ca^{2+}: the effects that resemble the typical phenotypes of cardiac diseases.[188] A single Arg-to-Ser mutation made in DPc10, mimicking the recently reported Arg2474Ser mutation in the patient with polymorphic ventricular tachycardia,[53] abolished all of these effects that would have been produced by non-mutated DPc10. Furthermore, both skeletal domain peptides DP4 and DP1 activated RyR2 as they activated RyR1, again supporting the concept that the cardiac Ca^{2+} channel is controlled by the basically identical mechanism as in the RyR1. However, the site of DPc10 binding has not yet been identified.

MONITORING THE OPERATION OF THE DOMAIN SWITCH

All of these findings described above are consistent with the hypothesis that zipped and unzipped states of the domain switch constituted by the two regulatory domains (viz. N-terminal and central domains) are directly involved in down-regulation and up-regulation of the RyR Ca^{2+} channel, respectively. The next important question is how one can monitor such actions of the domain switch. Fig. 6-3 illustrates two independent approaches that have been used favorably for this purpose. The important first step for both approaches is to label the conformation sensitive fluorescence probe, MCA, to the designated site of the RyR in a site-directed manner. Site-specific fluorescent labeling of the domain peptide binding site of RyR was performed using the cleavable heterobifunctional cross-linking reagent, sulfo-succinimidyl-3-((2-(7-azido-4-methylcoumarin-3-acetamido)-ethyl)dithio)propionate (SAED) in the following way. First, the selected domain peptide is incubated with SAED to form peptide-SAED conjugate. The peptide-SAED conjugate, after purification, is mixed with RyR and photolyzed to cross-link the conjugate *via* the azido group, followed by the treatment with reducing reagent to cleave the disulfide bond of SAED and the domain peptide used as a site-direction carrier is removed. As illustrated in row a of Fig. 6-3, the agonist-induced domain unzipping decreases the fluorescence intensity of the MCA probe attached to either the N-terminal domain or the central domain of the domain switch, because a more hydrophobic environment of the MCA attachment site, that has prevailed in the zipped configuration, becomes less hydrophobic upon domain unzipping. This method was suitable to follow a rapid process of domain unzipping. The other method involves the determination of the accessibility of the attached MCA probe to a bulky fluorescence quencher (QSY conjugated with BSA: QSY-BSA). As shown in row b of Fig. 6-3, the MCA that is attached to the designated sub-domain of the domain switch is relatively inaccessible to the fluorescence quencher QSY-BSA in the zipped configuration of the domain switch, because the QSY-BSA is excluded from the gap between the interacting domains. Upon unzipping of the interacting domains, the attached MCA becomes accessible to the QSY-BSA, causing an appreciable decrease in the fluorescence intensity of the attached MCA probe.

As described in above, DP4 binds to the N-terminal domain of RyR1. Hence, MCA is introduced to the N-terminal domain in a site-directed manner if DP4 is used as a carrier. Recent fluorescence quenching studies showed that all agents known to produce channel hyper-activation and hyper-sensitization, such as DP4 and DP1,[184] produced domain unzipping, as evidenced by a significant increase in the accessibility of the N-terminal domain-attached MCA to the QSY-BSA quencher. These findings indicate that MH-like Ca^{2+} channel dysfunction (hyper-activation and hyper-sensitization) is produced by domain unzipping as predicted from the domain switch concept (Fig. 6-2).

According to the recent fluorescence quenching study by Yano *et al.* (see also Chapter 26), it appears that the activation and sensitization of RyR2 channels by cardiac domain peptide DPc10 are produced also by domain unzipping, although it has not yet been confirmed that the DPc10-mediated MCA labeling takes place in the putative domain switch of RyR2.[189]

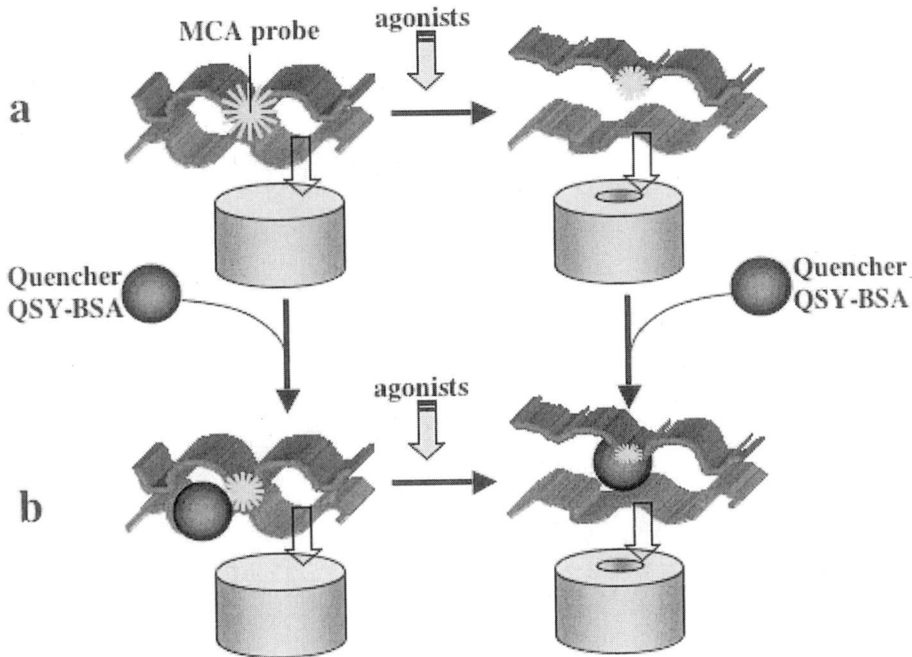

Figure 6-3. **Schematic illustration of the principle of the methods to monitor the process of domain unzipping. A**. In the zipped state, the fluorescence intensity of the attached MCA is high because of a more hydrophobic environment of the probe attachment site. Upon addition of agonists, the fluorescence intensity of the MCA decreases because the environment becomes less hydrophobic due to unzipping. **B**. A bulky fluorescence quencher, QSY-BSA, cannot enter the gap between the interacting domains in the zipped configuration, but can enter the widened inter-domain gap after the agonist has induced domain unzipping. Thus, in the zipped state, the quencher has only slight effect on the MCA fluorescence; after unzipping, the MCA fluorescence shows a considerable decrease because of the conferred access to the quencher.

Therapeutic drugs directed to the domain switch

Dantrolene is a hydantoin derivative that is widely used to treat malignant hyperthermia (MH) (see Chapter 24). One of dantrolene derivatives, azumolene, is also effective for the treatment of MH. However, virtually no other pharmacological reagents are known that are effective for the treatment of skeletal muscle disease. Since MH mutations in either N-terminal domain or central domain of RyR1 produce severe aberrations of channel function, one might expect that the pharmacological effect of dantrolene is directed to the domain switch and its operation. Most important in this context is the recent finding that dantrolene binds to the Leu^{590}-Cys^{609} region of RyR1, which is located in the C-terminal portion of the N-terminal domain (see Chapter 24).[187] Thus, the drug binds to a well-defined site located within the domain switch. According to the recent experiment in the author's laboratory (Kobayashi *et al.*, unpublished data), dantrolene decreased significantly the magnitude of agonist-induced domain unzipping, as determined by the fluorescence quenching technique described in above. This is particularly important because the increased tendency of domain unzipping causes MH-linked Ca^{2+} channelopathies. Thus, the evidence accumulated to this date suggests that the actual mechanism of drug action of dantrolene is to stabilize the zipped configuration of domain switch and prevent unwanted domain unzipping caused by mutations.

According to general consensus, dantrolene has no effect or much less effect (if any) on cardiac muscle and RyR2. Since RyR2 appears to have a potential drug binding region in the N-terminal domain as RyR1 does,[187] the site of drug binding may be occluded due to conformational constraint in the native RyR2, although it might become partially accessible in diseased conditions. Recently, Yano *et al.* have found that a new compound, the 1,4-benzothiazepine derivative JTV519, prevents heart failure by stabilizing RyR2 (see Chapter 26).[189] Although the binding site of JTV519 has not yet been identified, it is tempting to speculate that the pharmacological action of this drug may also be to stabilize the zipped state of domain switch of RyR2, as dantrolene does for RyR1.

DOMAIN-DOMAIN INTERACTION IN E-C COUPLING

Domains involved in the DHPR-to-RyR communication

Voltage-dependent activation of skeletal muscle-type E-C coupling is mediated by physical interaction between the DHPR and the RyR, presumably by mediation of the cytoplasmic loops of the DHPR $\alpha 1$

subunit[190] and β subunit.[191] Then, which portions of the RyR are involved in such a physical interaction in the case of the RyR1? Studies by several groups, yielding rather controversial results, have addressed this important question. There are many regions implicated in the coupling: e.g. residues 1635-2636,[192] a short 1076-1112 segment,[193] and the residues 1303-1406 D2 region.[194] Interestingly, according to the recent studies of immuno-localization of anti-D2 antibody in the 3D image, the site of antibody reaction is located in the so-called clamp region, which is regarded as the area for the interaction with the DHPR.[195] According to more recent information by Perez *et al.*, the residues 1-1,680 containing the D2 region is critical for RyR1-DHPR coupling.[196] Thus, the critical regions suggested in the literature are spread in a wide region of the primary structure encompassing residues 1-2636.

The fact that the DHPR-binding regions are distributed in widespread areas of the RyR polypeptide chain would indicate that the putative DHPR-interaction domain of RyR is constructed by a number of sub-domains derived from different regions of the RyR chain. Binding regions of some peptides corresponding to the DHPR II-III loop were localized within the RyR primary structure. Using the peptide-mediated site-directed probe-labeling technique, the conformation-sensitive fluorescence probe MCA was introduced into the binding sites of peptide A and peptide C (the peptides corresponding to the Thr^{671}-Leu^{690} and the Glu^{724}-Pro^{760} regions of the II-III loop, respectively) on the RyR. The A site and C site were localized at different sides of the major calpain cleavage site (residue #1400, which is located in the D2 region, which is regarded as the area for the interaction with the DHPR as described above).[197,198] Together with the accumulated information in the literature (see above), it is tentatively proposed that the putative DHPR-RyR signal transmission port of the RyR consists of several non-covalently but tightly associated domains flanking the D2 region.

Role of domain switch in E-C coupling

MH mutation causes hyper-activation and hyper-sensitization effects on depolarization-induced Ca^{2+} release.[199] This suggests that the domain switch unzipping mechanism is used also for the depolarization-induced activation of Ca^{2+} channels.[182] This idea was tested by monitoring the changes in the fluorescence intensity of the MCA probe attached to the N-terminal domain of the RyR moiety of the triad after depolarizing the T-tubule moiety.[184] It was found that T-tubule depolarization produces a rapid decrease of the MCA fluorescence at a rate significantly higher than the Ca^{2+} release rate. This suggests that the environment of the domain switch, to which the MCA probe is attached, has become less hydrophobic, indicative of domain unzipping produced by T-tubule depolarization (cf. row a of Fig. 6-3). Thus, it appears that the domain switch is used for the activation of RyR1 Ca^{2+} channels in the skeletal muscle-type E-C coupling.

CONCLUDING REMARKS

Recent structure-function studies of the ryanodine receptor (RyR) have led us to the concept that inter-domain interaction within the RyR serves as a key mechanism in the process of channel gating. Of such regulatory domains of the RyR known so far, three domains (designated as N-terminal domain, central domain and transmembrane channel domain) are particularly important when we consider their role in channel regulation, because disease-linked mutations that have occurred in these domains cause severe problems in Ca^{2+} channel regulation (e.g. malignant hyperthermia and central core disease in skeletal muscle, and inheritable cardiac diseases). Evidence accumulated to this date suggests the hypothesis that the N-terminal and central domains constitute, at least partly, the interacting domain pair, which serves as the implicit on/off switch for the channel operation (domain switch). Namely, unzipping and zipping of such domain pair cause opening and closing of Ca^{2+} channels, respectively. Several domains located in widely spread regions of the RyR polypeptide chain have been identified as the putative sites for RyR's interaction with the DHPR, suggesting that these domains come together to constitute the putative DHPR-to-RyR signal transmission port. Recent studies with an *in vitro* E-C coupling model indicated that the domain switch mediates the voltage-dependent activation of RyR Ca^{2+} release channels. The RyR Ca^{2+} channel can be regulated by a variety of pharmacological and immunological agents and proteins. Most important physiological regulators among these are the two satellite proteins of RyR: calmodulin and FKBP. Their binding domains on the RyR have been characterized, but the important question whether the domain switch is also involved in the satellite protein-mediated channel regulation is left as an important subject for future studies.

As shown in the mutation map (Fig. 6-1), disease-causing RyR mutations are located in three regions (Regions 1, 2 and 3) in both skeletal and cardiac muscle systems. The concept of domain switch described in this chapter was born out from the consideration of the fact that MH mutations are located chiefly in Region 1 (N-terminal domain) and Region 2 (central domain), while CCD mutations are located chiefly in Region 3 (channel domain). Since the phenotypes of MH and CCD are different, it is reasonable to assume that Region 3 may be involved in a mechanism other than the domain switch mechanism. However, it is anticipated that there is an intimate interaction between the domain switch (Region 1 plus Region 2) and Region 3. Furthermore, those mutations causing inheritable cardiac diseases are also located in the three regions of RyR2 corresponding to the three hot regions of RyR1. To elucidate the details of inter-domain interactions among these three regions in both RyR1 and RyR2 will be one of the most important tasks in the future study. Clear understanding of the channel regulation mechanism mediated by these key domains will immediately provide us a valuable clue for the understanding of the pathogenic mechanism of channel-linked skeletal and cardiac muscle diseases, because these domains are the very places where those problems are originated from. Some therapeutic drugs, such as dantrolene, are targeted to the domain switch, as described in this chapter. This finding has hinted us a new guideline for the development of therapeutic drugs for channel-linked skeletal and cardiac diseases; that is to screen a group of reagents that bind to the domain switch and stabilize the zipped configuration of the domain switch.

ACKNOWLEDGMENTS

The author wishes to thank Drs. Robert T. Dirksen, Xander H. Wehrens, and Andrew R. Marks for their help in updating the information concerning the mutation sites of RyR1 and RyR2, and Dr. Graham D. Lamb for his comments on the manuscript. National Institutes of Health Grants AR16922 and HL072841 supported this work.

Chapter 7

REGULATION OF SARCOPLASMIC RETICULUM CALCIUM RELEASE BY LUMINAL CALCIUM

Sandor Györke, Dmitry Terentyev, and Serge Viatchenko-Karpinski
Texas Tech University Health Sciences Center, Lubbock, TX

INTRODUCTION

Cardiac excitation-contraction (EC) coupling relies on transient efflux of Ca^{2+} from the sarcoplamic reticulum (SR), an intracellular Ca^{2+} storage and release organelle in muscle. While the events leading to initiation of Ca^{2+} release have been well established and are known to involve activation of the SR Ca^{2+} release channels/ ryanodine receptors (RyR2s) by Ca^{2+} that enters the cytosol from the extracellular milieu (i.e. Ca^{2+}-induced Ca^{2+} release, CICR),[63,200] the mechanisms responsible for SR Ca^{2+} release termination only begin to emerge. Yet, these restraining mechanisms are of particular importance in view of the inherent predisposition of CICR to self-activation. Because Ca^{2+} released to the cytosol has the tendency to feedback on the release channels to induce more release, it is expected that some sort of negative control mechanisms exist that account for termination of CICR in cardiac mytocytes. Growing evidence indicates that restraining and termination of CICR involves Ca^{2+} signaling processes inside the SR lumen.[201] In particular, the decline of *free* intra-SR Ca^{2+} concentration ($[Ca^{2+}]_{SR}$) during release provides a signal for RyR2 closure (i.e. luminal Ca^{2+}-dependent deactivation),[202] resulting in robust termination of CICR and in a refractory state that lasts till $[Ca^{2+}]_{SR}$ is restored by the SR Ca^{2+}-ATPase. Recently, genetic defects in the SR intraluminal Ca^{2+} binding protein calsequestrin (CASQ2) have been linked to inherited cardiac arrhythmia and sudden cardiac death underscoring the importance of the role of intra-SR Ca^{2+} signaling mechanisms to normal Ca^{2+} handling.[203-206]

Early indications that the functional state of the Ca^{2+} release mechanism might be modulated by intra- SR Ca^{2+} came from studies of the effects of SR Ca^{2+} load on contraction and SR Ca^{2+} release in intact and permeabilized myocytes.[207-209] However, clear demonstration of this mechanism and elucidation of its molecular basis became only possible through a combined use of tools of modern cellular physiology, molecular biology and biophysics. The purpose of this chapter is to review experimental evidence in support of such SR intraluminal Ca^{2+} signaling mechanisms and discuss their molecular determinants and functional implications for intracellular Ca^{2+} handling in normal and diseased heart.

EFFECTS OF LUMINAL Ca^{2+} ON RYR2s IN LIPID BILAYERS

The mechanisms of regulation of SR Ca^{2+} release by Ca^{2+} inside the SR have been challenging to study in cardiac cell- and isolated SR vesicle preparations because of technical difficulties associated with controlling and measuring Ca^{2+} levels inside this closed compartment. The planar lipid bilayer approach permits unrestricted access to both sides of the RyR2 release channel. Therefore, RyR2s reconstituted into planar lipid bilayers have been a preparation of choice for studying the effects of luminal Ca^{2+} on the SR Ca^{2+} release mechanism. The RyR2 activity in bilayers is controlled by high affinity Ca^{2+} activation and low-affinity inactivation sites accessible from the cytosolic side of the channel.[210,211] Changes in $[Ca^{2+}]$ at the luminal side of the RyR2 have been shown to positively affect RyR2 open probability in the range of 0.2 to 20 mM (EC_{50}~2 mM, Fig. 7-1 A).[212] Modulation of RyR2 by luminal Ca^{2+} seems to require the presence of such cytosolic agonists as caffeine, ATP or sulmazole and is usually not observed in channels exposed to cytosolic Ca^{2+} as the only activating ligand.[209,212,213] This observation supports the allosteric nature of the modulatory influences of luminal Ca^{2+} upon the RyR2 and is consistent with the existence of distinct luminal Ca^{2+} sensing sites that modulate RyR2 activity. An alternative possibility is that Ca^{2+} flowing through the open RyR2 channel activates the channel by interacting with its cytosolic Ca^{2+} activation sites (i.e. 'feed-through" regulation). Xu and Meissner[214] demonstrated such feed-through effects in purified RyR2s by correlating the impact of luminal Ca^{2+} upon RyR2 open probability with calculated luminal-to-cytosolic Ca^{2+} fluxes through the channel. However, Györke and Györke[212] found that the luminal Ca^{2+} dependence of native RyR2s from SR vesicles was similar regardless whether Ca^{2+} was flowing from the luminal-to-cytosolic or from the cytosolic-to-luminal directions, indicating that luminal Ca^{2+} must act on the luminal side of the RyR2 complex. Additionally, Ching *et al.*[215] reported that trypsin digestion of the luminal side of the RyR2 channel leads to the loss of luminal Ca^{2+} sensitivity of the channel.

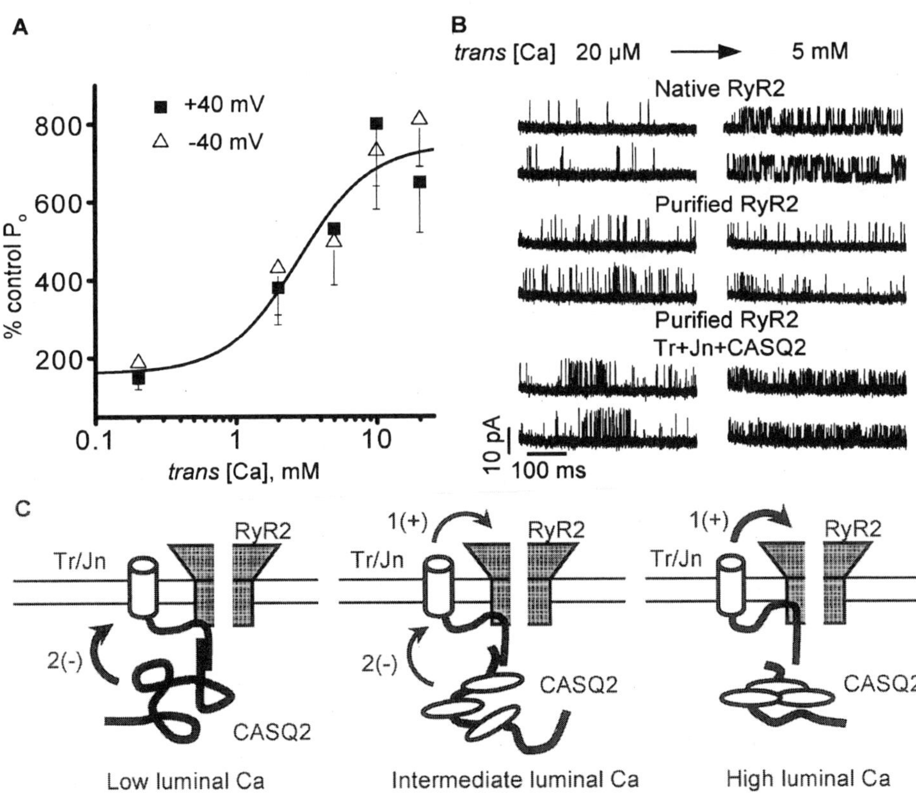

Figure 7-1. **Modulation of RyR2 by luminal Ca^{2+} and the auxiliary proteins CASQ2, triadin (Tr) and junctin (Jn). A**. Relative open probability (P_o) as a function of luminal [Ca^{2+}]. Single-channel currents were recorded at holding potential of +40 or -40. Data are from Györke *et al.*[212] **B**. Effects of increasing luminal (*trans*) [Ca^{2+}] from 20 μM to 5 mM on activity of native RyR2 from SR vesicles (upper panel), purified RyR2 (middle panel) and purified RyR2 re-associated with CASQ2, Tr and Jn. **C**. Hypothesized functional interactions between CASQ2, Tr, Jn and RyR2 in the cardiac SR membrane. Tr and Jn stabilize RyR2 in an increased activity mode (1 (+)). CASQ2 acts by removing the potentiatory influence of Tr and/or Jn on the RyR2 channel through Ca^{2+}-dependent interaction with Tr/Jn (2 (-)). Different RyR2 functional states, i.e. CASQ2-inhibited, -partially inhibited and -uninhibited, at low, intermediate and high luminal [Ca^{2+}], respectively. Data are from Györke *et al.*[216]

More recently Györke at al.[216] reported that purification of RyR2 by sucrose-gradient centrifugation also results in the loss of RyR2 responsiveness to luminal Ca^{2+}, implicating the potential role of auxiliary proteins such as calsequestrin, triadin and junctin in these effects (see below). Thus, the single RyR2 channel data accumulated to date indicate that luminal Ca^{2+} controls RyR2 functional activity by acting at distinct Ca^{2+} regulatory sites located at the luminal side of the RyR2 channel complex, although under certain conditions luminal Ca^{2+} can have access to the cytosolic Ca^{2+} regulatory sites of the channel as well.

CALCIUM IN THE SR

In what form and at what concentrations is Ca^{2+} present in the SR lumen? In general, the total amount of Ca^{2+} sequestered in the SR is determined by the balance between Ca^{2+} uptake by the SR Ca^{2+}-ATPase, binding of Ca^{2+} to luminal buffers, and Ca^{2+} leak from the SR through the RyR2s. It is believed that at rest most of the Ca^{2+} present in the SR is bound to luminal Ca^{2+} buffers such as calsequestrin.[1,201] During release, Ca^{2+} bound to luminal buffers dissociates from these binding sites and contributes to the Ca^{2+} efflux to the cytosol. Although the amount of bound Ca^{2+} is an important contributor to the functional size of the SR Ca^{2+} pool, however, it is the free rather than the total $[Ca^{2+}]$ in the SR governs RyR2 gating behavior. Additionally, it is the free Ca^{2+} that determines the concentration gradient and electrochemical driving force for Ca^{2+} across the SR membrane. Therefore, free $[Ca^{2+}]$ levels inside the SR are critical to the role of this organelle in intracellular Ca^{2+} signaling. Because, free intra-SR $[Ca^{2+}]$ measurements are difficult to perform, only few such determinations have been done to date.[217,218] According to these studies, $[Ca^{2+}]_{SR}$ is close to 1 mM in resting cardiac myocytes. Following electrical activation of myocytes, $[Ca^{2+}]_{SR}$ declines to levels of ~0.3-0.6 mM, indicating that the SR loses only a fraction of its free Ca^{2+} in the process of EC coupling. The partial depletion of $[Ca^{2+}]_{SR}$ is also an indication that CICR is terminated by an active extinguishing mechanism before the SR would exhaust its supply of Ca^{2+}. The fact that changes in $[Ca^{2+}]_{SR}$ occur in the same range in which $[Ca^{2+}]$ on the luminal side of RyR2 affects its open probability, supports the physiological relevance of modulation of RyR2 activity by luminal Ca^{2+}.

TERMINATION OF SR Ca^{2+} RELEASE AND RELEASE SITE REFRACTORINESS

During the SR Ca^{2+} release process, [Ca^{2+}] in the SR lumen decreases, whereas [Ca^{2+}] on the cytosolic side of the SR increases. Consequently, two types of mechanisms have been considered to explain Ca^{2+} release termination. According to one mechanism, binding of Ca^{2+} to the cytosolic inhibition sites on the RyR2 reduces channel activity through processes referred to as Ca^{2+}-dependent inactivation or adaptation.[200,219,220] According to the other mechanism, dissociation of Ca^{2+} from luminal regulatory sites decreases RyR2 open probability (a process termed luminal Ca^{2+} dependent deactivation).[202,209,221,222] To distinguish between these two possible mechanisms, we used low-affinity Ca^{2+} chelators entrapped into the SR in cardiac myocytes.[202] By clamping $[Ca^{2+}]_{SR}$ with these buffers we dramatically increased the size of electrically induced global Ca^{2+} transients and spontaneous Ca^{2+} sparks. Analysis of the rising phase and rate of change of these signals indicated that their augmented size was due to slowed termination of the underlying Ca^{2+} release fluxes to the cytosol. These results suggest that the duration of SR Ca^{2+} release depends on $[Ca^{2+}]_{SR}$ rather than on changes in cytosolic [Ca^{2+}]. More recently, we obtained similar results by overexpressing the native SR-resident Ca^{2+} buffering protein calsequestrin (CASQ2).[205] Namely, adenoviral mediated overexpression of wild type CASQ2 dramatically increased the magnitude and rise time of both cell averaged Ca^{2+} transients and Ca^{2+} sparks. Moreover, knocking down CASQ2 levels by CASQ2 antisense RNA expression led to Ca^{2+} signals that had a reduced amplitude and shortened rising phase. Together, these findings provide compelling evidence for the role of luminal Ca^{2+}-dependent deactivation of RyR2s in termination of SR Ca^{2+} release.

Following Ca^{2+} release a certain time must pass before another release event can be triggered again.[223] This refractoriness of the Ca^{2+} release mechanism is important for stability of CICR as it prevents the SR Ca^{2+} store from premature reactivation. Several pieces of experimental evidence suggest that similar to termination of SR Ca^{2+} release, this refractory behavior is also attributable to luminal Ca^{2+}-dependence of RyR2 activity. Endogenous (CASQ2) and exogenous (e.g., citrate) Ca^{2+} buffers introduced into the SR in addition to slowing release termination, delay the functional recovery of both global and focal Ca^{2+} release.[202,205] At the same time, reducing buffering (by inhibition of CASQ2 expression) accelerates restitution behavior of release sites.[205] Since the rate of recovery of $[Ca^{2+}]_{SR}$ is expected to be directly related to the concentration of Ca^{2+} binding sites inside the SR, these observations indicate that the functional recovery of the release mechanism after each release is controlled by $[Ca^{2+}]_{SR}$. In addition, Del Principe *et al.*[221] demonstrated that the SR Ca^{2+} release mechanism exhibit a much more prominent refractoriness following its activation on a global scale than following focal activation by photolysis of caged Ca^{2+}. Because the extent of depletion of the SR Ca^{2+} stores should be more complete following global than focal release, these findings might be also attributable to a functional depletion of the SR Ca^{2+} stores that leaves the stores unresponsive to activation until they are recharged with Ca^{2+}. Taken together these findings suggest that termination of Ca^{2+} release events and the subsequent restitution behavior of release sites in cardiac muscle is controlled by local intra-SR $[Ca^{2+}]$ regulating RyR2 openings.

DYNAMIC REGULATION OF SR Ca^{2+} DIASTOLIC LEAK BY LUMINAL Ca^{2+}

In addition to providing a robust mechanism for termination of CICR, the luminal Ca^{2+} sensor continuously regulates the functional size of the SR Ca^{2+} stores by linking the activity of Ca^{2+} release channels to the loading state of the SR. Evidence for such a dynamic control mechanism has come from measurements of spontaneous Ca^{2+} sparks at different SR Ca^{2+} loads in intact and permeabilized cardiac myocytes. Spontaneous Ca^{2+} sparks represent a substantial Ca^{2+} efflux (leak) that plays an important role in determining the SR Ca^{2+} content in cardiac myocytes.[224,225] The frequency of spontaneous Ca^{2+} sparks (and the amount of leak) increases at elevated SR Ca^{2+} loads and decreases at reduced Ca^{2+} loads.[223,224] Because of the dynamic changes in SR Ca^{2+} content associated with altered Ca^{2+} spark rates, any selective modulation of RyR2 channels by their inhibitors (tetracaine, Mg^{2+}) or agonists (caffeine) produce only transient effects (suppression or potentiation, respectively) on Ca^{2+} spark frequency.[224] The effects are transient because, for instance, inhibition of RyR2 by tetracaine decreases Ca^{2+} efflux though the RyR2 channels; this reduced Ca^{2+} efflux increases $[Ca^{2+}]_{SR}$, which in turn stimulates RyR2s at the luminal Ca^{2+} sensing sites, thereby countering the primary inhibitory effects of tetracaine on the RyR2 channels. The sequence of events is the opposite when the RyR2 agonist caffeine is applied. Therefore, regulation by luminal Ca^{2+} allows the store to self-adjust its functional size to stabilize CICR in the face of perturbations of RyR2s.[224]

Given such dynamic regulation of release, however, why do certain substances such as cyclic ADP ribose (cADPR), which is thought to interact specifically with RyR2s, have maintained potentiatory effects on SR Ca^{2+} release? It appears that cADPR does not act directly on RyR2, but, instead, influences the release channel indirectly via changes in intra-SR [Ca^{2+}].[226] Potentiation of Ca^{2+} release by cADPR is mediated by an increased SR Ca^{2+} load due to persistent enhancement of uptake, followed by luminal Ca^{2+}-dependent activation of RyR2s. This mechanism of indirect modulation of RyR2 activity via the luminal Ca^{2+} sensor could, therefore, serve as a paradigm for other effectors of Ca^{2+} release that show maintained effects.

MOLECULAR IDENTITY OF THE LUMINAL Ca^{2+} SENSOR

Although significant progress has been made in defining the molecular basis of regulation of ryanodine receptor by cytosolic Ca^{2+}, the molecular determinants of RyR2 channel responsiveness to luminal Ca^{2+} remain to be determined. Cardiac RyRs from the luminal side of the SR membrane are associated with a number of proteins, including the Ca^{2+} binding protein calsequestrin (CASQ2) and the putative "anchoring" proteins, triadin and junctin, forming together a multimolecular Ca^{2+} signaling complex in the junctional membrane.[227,228] To explore the potential role of these proteins in mediating RyR2 luminal Ca^{2+} sensitivity, we performed *in vitro* reconstitution experiments with purified RyR2s and using purified CASQ2, triadin 1 and junctin.[216] Purification of RyR2 by sucrose-gradient centrifugation led to a complete loss of RyR2 responsiveness to luminal Ca^{2+} (Fig. 7-1 B, upper and middle panels), suggesting that the effects of luminal Ca^{2+} are mediated by an auxiliary protein(s). Adding CASQ2 to the luminal side of the purified channels produced no significant changes in open probability (P_o), whereas luminal triadin and junctin increased RyR2 P_o. In RyR2s re-associated with triadin 1 and junctin, adding luminal CASQ2 decreased channel activity. Following re-association with all three proteins, RyR2s regained their ability to respond to rises of luminal Ca^{2+} by increasing their P_o (Fig. 7-1 B, lower panel). Based on these results, we hypothesized that a complex of CASQ2, triadin and/or junctin confers the luminal Ca^{2+}-sensitivity of the RyR2 (Fig. 7-1 C).[216] CASQ2 apparently serves as a luminal Ca^{2+} sensor while junctin and/or triadin, stimulatory by themselves, may be required to mediate the influences of CASQ2 upon the RyR2. Modulation of RyR2 by luminal Ca^{2+} appears to be through removal of an inhibitory influence that CASQ2 normally exerts on the RyR2 complex. This inhibition might be gradually relieved as the CASQ2 bindings sites become increasingly occupied with Ca^{2+} and the channel becomes maximally active when CASQ2 dissociates from the RyR2 complex at high luminal Ca^{2+}. Similar Ca^{2+}-dependent inhibition of RyR by CASQ has been demonstrated for the skeletal isoforms of these proteins.[229] Together, these results suggest the CASQ2 influences SR Ca^{2+} release not only in its capacity as a buffer but also more directly by serving as a luminal Ca^{2+} sensor for the RyR2.

ABNORMAL LUMINAL Ca^{2+} SIGNALING AND ARRHYTHMIA

Catecholaminergic polymorphic ventricular tachycardia (CPVT) is a familial arrhythmogenic disease characterized by syncope and sudden death inducible by exercise and catecholamine infusion (see Chapter 25).[230] To date four mutations in the cardiac calsequestrin gene have been linked to CPVT. One mutation converts a negatively charged aspartic acid into a histidine in a highly conserved region presumably involved in Ca^{2+} binding (D307H).[203] The three other mutations, a nonsense R33X, a splicing 532+1 G>1, and a 1 base-pare deletion, 62delA, are thought to induce premature stop codons, thus, potentially precluding CASQ2 from being synthesized.[204] The cellular mechanisms of adrenergic tachycardia were studied in myocytes in which CASQ2 levels were knock-down by adenoviral-mediated expression of CASQ2 antisense RNA.[205] In these myocytes, application of isoproterenol cause profound disturbances in rhythmic Ca^{2+} transients manifested by spontaneous "extrasystolic" Ca^{2+} transients. Since spontaneous SR Ca^{2+} release is arrhythmogenic (as a consequence of its ability to induce depolarizing currents and oscillations in the membrane potential, i.e. delayed after-depolarizations (DADs)),[231,232] the high incidents of spontaneous Ca^{2+} release could account for the pathogenesis of CPVT associated with reduced CASQ2 levels. The predisposition of CASQ2-underexpressing myocytes to spontaneous Ca^{2+} release was attributed to the premature recovery of the SR Ca^{2+} release channels from a luminal Ca^{2+}-dependent refractory state.[205] Due to a reduced concentration of Ca^{2+} binding sites, the restoration of $[Ca^{2+}]_{SR}$ by the Ca^{2+} ATPase occurs faster in CSQ2-underexpressing myocytes than in normal myocytes, thus accounting for the accelerated functional recovery of the release channels from luminal Ca^{2+}-dependent refractoriness in myocytes underexpressing CASQ2. $[Ca^{2+}]_{SR}$ recovery becomes even faster when the activity of SR Ca^{2+} pump is stimulated by PKA, potentially explaining the dependency of clinical episodes of CPVT on catecholamines.[205]

The cellular mechanisms of CPVT were further studied in myocytes overexpressing the arrythmogenic CASQ2 mutant D307H (Fig. 7-2).[206] Adeno viral-mediated expression of CASQ2.D307H reduced the Ca^{2+} storing capacity of the SR (Fig. 7- 2 A, top traces). In addition the amplitude, duration and rise-time of macroscopic I_{Ca}-induced Ca^{2+} transients and of spontaneous Ca^{2+} sparks were reduced in myocytes expressing CASQ2.D307H (Fig. 7-2 A, middle and lower panels).

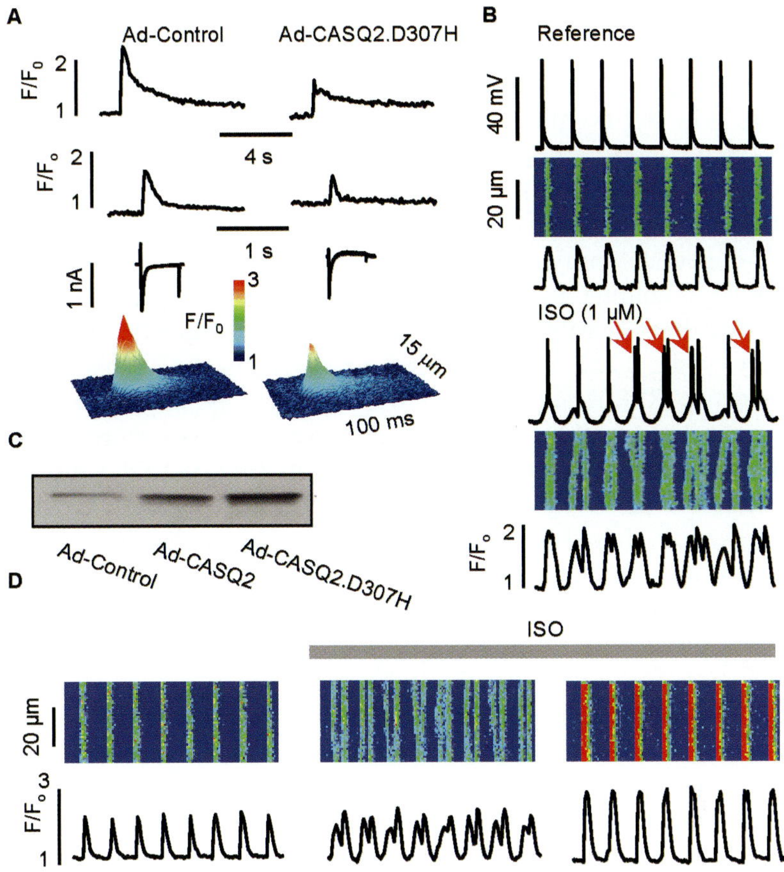

Figure 7-2. **Abnormal Ca^{2+} handling in myocytes overexpressing the arrhythmogenic CASQ2 mutant D307H. A**. Caffeine-induced Ca^{2+} transients (10 mM, top), depolarization-induced Ca^{2+} transients along with I_{Ca} (from -50 to 0 mV; middle), and images of averaged sparks (bottom) in control and D307H-expressing myocytes. **B**. Recordings of MP, along with line-scan images and time-dependent profiles of cytosolic [Ca^{2+}] in a myocyte expressing D307H before and after application of 1 μM isoproterenol (ISO). **C**. Representative immunoblots detecting wild-type and mutant CASQ2 in myocytes infected with the different adenoviral vectors. **D**. Restoration of normal rhythmic activity by intracellular dialysis with citrate in myocytes expressing CASQ2.D307H. Line-scan images and time-dependent profiles of cytosolic [Ca^{2+}] in a myocyte infected with Ad-CASQ2.D307H before and after exposure to 1 μM ISO. Pipette solution contained 5 mM of citrate. Recordings on the left and in the middle were made ~5 min after rupture of the membrane; recordings on the right were made 15 min later. Data are from Viatchenko-Karpinski *et al.*[206]

Myocytes expressing CASQ2.D307H also displayed drastic disturbances in rhythmic Ca^{2+} transients and membrane potential with signs of DADs when undergoing periodic pacing and exposed to isoproterenol (Fig. 7-2 B). Occasionally, DADs triggered irregular action potentials (arrows), resulting in "cellular arrhythmia". Since the effects of CSAQ.D307H occur on the background of a full complement of wild-type CASQ2 present in these myocytes (Fig. 7-2 C), these results suggest that the mutant protein disrupts normal CASQ2-dependent Ca^{2+} handling (i.e. dominant-negative effects).

There are two possible mechanisms for these effects of CASQ2.D307H.[206] One possibility is that the mutation impairs the process of Ca^{2+}-dependent polymerization of CASQ2 that is required for high capacity Ca^{2+} binding by CASQ2, making the SR less able to sequester Ca^{2+}.[233] The other possibility is that the mutation disrupts the interactions of CASQ2 with the RyR2 channel complex (via triadin and/or junctin), leading to hyperactive RyR2s and "leaky" SR Ca^{2+} stores with impaired ability to retain Ca^{2+}. Importantly, normal rhythmic activity was restored by loading the SR with the low-affinity Ca^{2+} buffer, citrate (Fig. 7-2 D), supporting the notion that the pathological mechanisms of CPVT involve reduced Ca^{2+} buffering and/or altered responsiveness of the release channel to changes in $[Ca^{2+}]_{SR}$. Studies with measurements of the effects of CASQ2.D307H on intra-SR $[Ca^{2+}]$ might help to distinguish between these possibilities.

CONCLUDING REMARKS

In summary, regulation of SR Ca^{2+} release by Ca^{2+} inside the SR has emerged as an important determinant of intracellular Ca^{2+} handling and excitation-contraction coupling in cardiac muscle. In general, this mechanism plays a restraining role by countering the intrinsic positive feedback of CICR, and is essential for stability of cardiac EC coupling. The control of Ca^{2+} release by luminal Ca^{2+} appears to involve coordinated interaction of at least several proteins within the junctional Ca^{2+} signaling complex, including calsequestrin, triadin and junctin. Genetic defects in these proteins lead to pathological states such as cardiac arrhythmia and sudden death. Future studies will have to define the exact molecular mechanisms whereby luminal Ca^{2+} controls SR Ca^{2+} release on a beat-to-beat basis and how defects in these mechanisms result in arrhythmia and other diseases associated with abnormal Ca^{2+} signaling in the heart.

Chapter 8

CYTOSOLIC CALCIUM REGULATION OF SINGLE RYANODINE RECEPTOR CHANNELS

Josefina Ramos-Franco and Michael Fill
Dept. of Physiology, Loyola University Chicago, 2160 South First Avenue, Maywood, IL

INTRODUCTION

The ryanodine receptor (RyR) is a Ca^{2+}-activated Ca^{2+} channel that resides on the surface of the sarcoplasmic reticulum (SR). The Ca^{2+} released from the SR by the RyR channel activates the contractile proteins. The RyR channel is activated by a cytosolic trigger Ca^{2+} signal. This trigger signal can arise from several different sources. It may arise from Ca^{2+} influx through surface membrane Ca^{2+} channels or Ca^{2+} released from nearby RyR channels. Additionally, the Ca^{2+} which passes through an open RyR channel, may even feedback and regulate the same channel.

Regardless of the source of the trigger Ca^{2+} signal, the effectiveness of that signal is critically dependent on both its speed and amplitude. In a now classical work in skinned cardiac myocytes, Fabiato (1985)[200] demonstrated that SR Ca^{2+} release was a bell-shaped function of trigger Ca^{2+} stimulus amplitude. He further showed that this function was scaled by the duration of the stimulus. These results were used to explain the Ca^{2+}-induced Ca^{2+} release (CICR) paradox. The paradox is that CICR, an inherently self-regenerating process, is precisely controlled in cells. This precise control implies that some negative feedback must exist to counter the inherent positive feedback of CICR. Fabiato suggested that this negative feedback was Ca^{2+} dependent inactivation.[200] Specifically, he proposed that SR Ca^{2+} release is governed by two cytosolic Ca^{2+} binding sites (i.e. activation & inactivation sites). The activation site has a fast on rate and a relatively low affinity. The inactivation site has a slower association constant and relatively high affinity. With this combination of sites, large fast Ca^{2+} signals transiently activate SR Ca^{2+} release because Ca^{2+} would activate before inactivation catches up. Slow small Ca^{2+} signals would not activate SR Ca^{2+} release because activation would "keep pace" with inactivation. Once the inactivation sites are occupied, the Ca^{2+} release process cannot respond to further Ca^{2+} stimulation. The recovery from this refractory state requires Ca^{2+} removal and time for the system to reprime. This general scheme SR Ca^{2+} release activation/inactivation is commonly applied to explain the Ca^{2+} regulation of many RyR-mediated Ca^{2+} signaling events. However, the existence of high affinity Ca^{2+} dependent inactivation of RyR-mediated Ca^{2+} release is still debated (see Chapter 7).

Patch-clamp studies on isolated cardiac myocytes have not definitively established that Ca^{2+} dependent inactivation occurs.[141,219,234] For example, the effectiveness of a 2nd trigger Ca^{2+} stimulus did not decrease when two stimuli were applied in rapid succession.[234] One interpretation is that the first did not inactivate release prior to the second. In another experiment, the SR release process did not become refractory during long duration stimuli.[219] Again, this is counter to what would be predicted if the release process inactivated. However, there is another possible explanation. It is possible that the 1st stimulus (or the prolonged stimulus) did not inactivate all the RyR channels present. Thus, the 2nd stimulus may have simply activated channels that had not been previously activated (or inactivated). These types of caveats have fueled the debate over the existence of Ca^{2+} dependent inactivation for years. The identification, isolation and functional characterization of single RyR channels in artificial planar lipid bilayers promised to resolve some of these questions.

The cytosolic Ca^{2+} regulation of the single RyR channel reconstituted in artificial planar bilayers is described here. The specific topics addressed are the steady state Ca^{2+} sensitivity, Ca^{2+} activation kinetics, feed-through Ca^{2+} activation, Ca^{2+} deactivation kinetics, Ca^{2+} inhibition as well as the modal gating (i.e. adaptation) of the RyR channel primarily the RyR channel found in the mammalian heart. Before going further, it is important to state that the bilayer method is a very simple model system with clear advantages and disadvantages. It allows important molecular RyR channel attributes (opening, closing, bursting, ligand regulation, blockade, etc.) to be directly measured in precisely controlled solutions. Thus, the bilayer studies have generated numerous insights into RyR-mediated Ca^{2+} signaling. The bilayer method, however, does not reproduce the cellular environment in which the RyR channel normally operates. Consequently, bilayer studies invariably fall short of definitively defining how the RyR channel functions in cells. The information presented here should be interpreted with this fact in mind.

STEADY STATE CYTOSOLIC Ca^{2+} SENSITIVITY OF SINGLE RYR2 CHANNELS

The steady state cytosolic Ca^{2+} dependency of single RyR1 and RyR2 channels has been defined in bilayer studies by several difference groups.[235-238] These studies show that there is little steady state RyR channel activity at low cytosolic free Ca^{2+} concentrations (<100 nM). This Ca^{2+} concentration corresponds to the resting Ca^{2+} level found in cells. Channel activity is defined in terms of the open probability (Po) of the channel. Low Po at resting cytosolic Ca^{2+} concentrations is entirely consistent with cellular observations. For example, the frequency of spontaneous RyR-mediated Ca^{2+} release events (Ca^{2+} sparks) in resting muscle cells is very low.[239,240]

Spontaneous RyR channel activity increases at higher steady state cytosolic Ca^{2+} concentrations. The EC_{50} of RyR channel Ca^{2+} activation is typically 0.5 to 5 μM. Maximal channel activity occurs when the cytosolic Ca^{2+} concentration reaches about 10 μM. These values are also consistent with cellular observations. In skinned cardiac muscle fibers,[200] the Ca^{2+} sensitivity of SR Ca^{2+} release activation was over this very same range. The cytosolic Ca^{2+} sensitivity of SR Ca^{2+} release activation also likely occurs over this range in intact cells as well.[63] The Ca^{2+} sensitivity of the RyR1 and RyR2 channels between 0.1 and 10 μM are quite similar. However, this is not the case at higher cytosolic Ca^{2+} concentrations.

The activity of the RyR1 channel falls to zero when the cytosolic Ca^{2+} concentration is raised to about the 1 mM mark.[235-237,241] The activity of the RyR2 (or RyR3) channels also falls but not completely when the cytosolic Ca^{2+} concentration is elevated above 1 mM.[235-237,241] This decrease in single RyR channel activity at high cytosolic Ca^{2+} levels is often interpreted as the molecular manifestation of Ca^{2+}-dependent inactivation. However, certain caveats must be considered. First, it is unlikely that the free Ca^{2+} levels in the cytosol of any mammalian cell ever exceeds 1 mM because the available Ca^{2+} sources (i.e. extracellular and intra-SR solutions) have only about 1 mM Ca^{2+}. Thus, this low affinity steady state Ca^{2+} inhibition of the RyR1 channel may be physiologically relevant. The low affinity Ca^{2+} inhibition of the RyR2 (and RyR3) channels may not be. Second, Fabiato proposed the existence of high affinity, not low affinity, Ca^{2+}-dependent inactivation.[200] Thus, it is difficult to reconcile observations in bilayers with the classical view of Ca^{2+}-dependent inactivation.

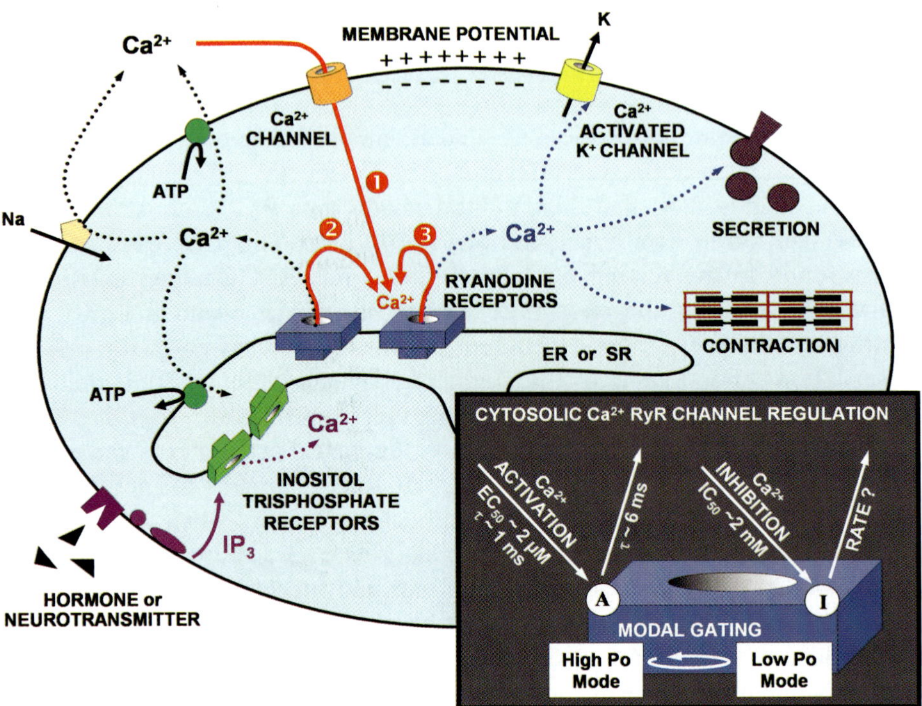

Figure 8-1. **Cytosolic Ca^{2+} regulation of the RyR channel.** The RyR channel is a Ca^{2+} activated Ca^{2+} channel that resides in the endoplasmic reticulum (ER) or sarcoplasmic reticulum (SR). When the RyR opens it generates local intracellular Ca^{2+} elevations (blue arrows) that act on many different cellular targets (e.g. Ca^{2+} activated K^+ channels, secretory apparatus, contractile proteins, etc.). The released Ca^{2+} is removed from the cytoplasm by different surface membrane and/or ER Ca^{2+} extrusion mechanisms (black arrows). The Ca^{2+} that activates the RyR channel (red arrows) can come from surface Ca^{2+} influx (1), neighboring RyR channels (2) and/or the open RyR channel itself (3). The inositol trisphosphate receptor (IP_3R) represents another class of intracellular Ca^{2+} release channels that mediate intracellular Ca^{2+} elevations (purple arrows). The crosstalk between RyR and IP_3R signaling is poorly understood. INSET: The cytosolic side of the RyR channel has activation (A) and inhibition (I) Ca^{2+} binding site (s). The steady state EC_{50} and IC_{50} of these sites are indicated. The time constants of Ca^{2+} activation and deactivation are also indicated. Upon Ca^{2+} activation, channel function is defined by a dynamic equilibrium between distinct gating modes.

CYTOSOLIC Ca^{2+} ACTIVATION KINETICS OF SINGLE RYR2 CHANNEL

The RyR channels operate in a dynamic (not stationary) cytosolic Ca^{2+} signaling environment (Fig. 8-1). Thus, the steady state cytosolic Ca^{2+} dependency of the RyR channel may not divulge important details concerning how Ca^{2+} regulates the RyR channel in cells. Several groups have applied fast cytosolic Ca^{2+} concentrations changes to single RyR channels reconstituted in bilayers.[242-248] Most of these studies have been focused on the RyR2 channel function.

Interpretation of these studies requires consideration of how the fast Ca^{2+} changes were generated because the nature of the applied Ca^{2+} stimuli varies dramatically between studies. Consequently, the response of the channel varies substantially between studies. When the nature of the Ca^{2+} stimulus is considered, the consistency of the data is remarkable. When laser flash photolysis of caged-Ca^{2+} is used to generate the Ca^{2+} stimulus,[242,247,248] the Ca^{2+} concentration change is very fast (<1 ms) and has a brief (~100 μs) Ca^{2+} spike at its leading edge. When the Ca^{2+} stimulus is generated by a physical solution change,[244-246] the Ca^{2+} concentration change is substantially slower (<20 ms) but does not have the Ca^{2+} overshoot. Interestingly, the fast Ca^{2+} overshoot generated by flash photolysis may reasonably reproduce the amplitude and kinetics of the free Ca^{2+} changes that initiate RyR2 channel activity in the cell (see below). Thus, the mechanical solution change studies reveal single RyR channel dynamics to monotonic Ca^{2+} stimuli while the flash photolysis studies may reveal how single RyR channel respond to more physiological Ca^{2+} stimuli. Details concerning this view can be found in a recent review.[211]

The RyR2 channel activates with a time constant of about 1 ms when the cytosolic Ca^{2+} change is applied by the flash photolysis method. The time constant of cytosolic Ca^{2+} activation is slightly slower (τ = 2 to 20 ms) when the Ca^{2+} change is applied mechanically. The difference likely reflects the differences in Ca^{2+} stimulus speed.[211] Generally, these values are consistent with cellular studies that conclude that large trigger Ca^{2+} stimuli induce very rapid activation of SR Ca^{2+} release (e.g. sparks) with very little delay perhaps <1 ms.[63] The cellular trigger Ca^{2+} stimuli are very localized and are generated when a surface membrane Ca^{2+} channels flickers open.[249] Theoretical estimates suggest that these triggers stimuli may reach very high levels (~100 μM) and may rise/fall very rapidly (10-100 μs).[250] The single channel studies described above suggest that the RyR channel has sufficiently fast Ca^{2+} activation kinetics to "see" and react to these trigger Ca^{2+} stimuli.

FEED-THROUGH Ca^{2+} ACTIVATION OF SINGLE RYR2 CHANNELS

It is also possible that some of the Ca^{2+} that interacts with the activation site is the Ca^{2+} that passes through the RyR channel itself. This is called feed-through Ca^{2+} activation. The idea here is that the RyR channel may operate in a local "common Ca^{2+} pool".[239,249,251-253] The single RyR channel studies described in the previous section were mostly done with a monovalent cation passing through the channel. Thus, feed-through Ca^{2+} activation can not complicate their interpretation. This is not the situation when single RyR channels studies are done with Ca^{2+} passing through the channel.[254-258] Consideration of feed-through Ca^{2+} activation is important because most single RyR channel studies in bilayers use huge Ca^{2+} driving forces (>50 times greater than those thought to exist in cells).

Is there evidence for feed-through Ca^{2+} activation at the single channel level? In simple solutions, the steady-state cytosolic Ca^{2+} sensitivity of the RyR1 and RyR2 channels are similar whether or not Ca^{2+} is the charge carrier.[237,258-260] One study has shown that the Po and open/closed dwell times of Ca^{2+} conducting RyR channels do not depend on the Ca^{2+} flux passing through the channel.[254] However, another study reports that the duration of single RyR channel open events are significantly longer if the channel carries even a small Ca^{2+} flux.[261] This latter study goes further to estimate that the activation site is about 75 nm distant from the RyR channel pore. This is about 3 times larger than the width of the channel itself.[56,57,106] To reconcile this fact, the authors argue that the activation site may be shielded in a protected pocket making the effective distance longer than the actual distance. Perhaps, the most compelling evidence of feed-through Ca^{2+} activation is the recent demonstration of intra-channel CICR between neighboring RyR channels in bilayers.[262] If Ca^{2+} passing through a RyR channel can activate neighboring RyR channels, then it clearly has the potential to activate itself. The important point here is that the existence of feed-through Ca^{2+} activation at the single channel level is a possibility. Whether or not, feed-through Ca^{2+} activation has physiologically relevant manifestations in the cell remains to be determined.

CYTOSOLIC Ca^{2+} DEACTIVATION KINETICS OF SINGLE RYR2 CHANNELS

Cytosolic Ca^{2+} binding to the RyR Ca^{2+} activation site clearly turn-on the channel.[242,245] Thus, cytosolic Ca^{2+} unbinding from the Ca^{2+} activation site will turn-off the channel. This latter process is called Ca^{2+} deactivation. This will take time because Ca^{2+} must fall off the activation site and the channel must transition into the close state. Both flash photolysis and mechanical solution changes have been applied to single RyR2 channels to define their Ca^{2+} deactivation kinetics.[245,246,248] One study reports that the time constant of Ca^{2+} deactivation is less than 10 ms.[246] Two other studies report time constants of Ca^{2+} deactivation of 5 to 6 ms. Thus, there is very good consensus concerning the speed of single RyR channel Ca^{2+} deactivation. This is not surprising considering that dissociation rates are Ca^{2+} independent and the Ca^{2+} stimuli applied were sufficiently fast in these particular studies. The significant point here is that the Ca^{2+} deactivation kinetics of single RyR channels will allow them to respond (turn off) rapidly to fast drops in local Ca^{2+} concentration. Considering the kind of Ca^{2+} stimuli that exist in cells, this may be a key feature of single RyR channel function.[249]

CYTOSOLIC Ca^{2+} INHIBITION OF SINGLE RYR2 CHANNELS

A long standing proposition is that there must be some sort of negative control mechanism to counter the inherent positive feedback of the RyR-mediated CICR process.[134,200,234,249,263-266] The role of cytosolic Ca^{2+} in this negative control has been extensively examined and the results are far from conclusive.

The most popular negative feedback mechanism, of course, is Ca^{2+} dependent inactivation as first defined in skinned ventricular myocytes.[200] A key feature of this work is that even a small elevation in resting cytosolic Ca^{2+} levels induced inactivation. However, a recent confocal imaging study in permeabilized ventricular myocytes showed that elevated Ca^{2+} levels increased, not decreased, the frequency of RyR-mediated Ca^{2+} sparks.[267] Thus, the existence of Ca^{2+} dependent inactivation remains controversial at the cellular level.

At the single RyR channel level, high cytosolic Ca^{2+} levels clearly inhibit channel activity. As described above, this inhibition requires steady state cytosolic Ca^{2+} levels (i.e. >1 mM) that are unlikely to be reached in cells, even in microdomains. Thus, the relationship between this phenomenon defined in vitro and the negative feedback that occurs in cells is unclear. Some fast solution change studies may clarify this relationship. Specifically, there are some mechanical solution change studies that have argued that Ca^{2+} dependent inactivation occurs following a fast Ca^{2+} stimulus.[244,254,265] In two of these studies,[244,254] the cytosolic Ca^{2+} level was quickly elevated to 100 μM (from 0.1 μM). Considering the steady state Ca^{2+} sensitivity of the channel, the jump to 100 μM Ca^{2+} should maximally activate the channel but should be well short of the Ca^{2+} levels that inhibit the channel. Nevertheless, one of these study reports partial voltage-independent Ca^{2+} inactivation.[244] The other study reports complete voltage-dependent Ca^{2+} inactivation.[254] Neither study determined if the inactivated channels became refractory. The third study applied a variety of different size Ca^{2+} stimuli.[265] This study also reports evidence of Ca^{2+} inactivation but attempts to demonstrate that the channels became refractory failed. The differences between these reports and the established steady state Ca^{2+} sensitivity of the channel suggest that there is more to this story than meets the eye. In other words, the cytosolic Ca^{2+} regulation of single RyR channel function may not simply reflect the interaction of activation and inhibition sites. It may involve complex interactions between multiple sites. Alternatively, it is possible that cytosolic Ca^{2+} dependent inactivation is a red herring or a vestigial concept of an earlier time.

Since the classic works of Fabiato, a lot has been learned about the geometry and local nature of the RyR-mediated Ca^{2+} release process.[200] The elemental unit of RyR-mediated Ca^{2+} release is the spark. As stated previously, the spark is generated by the concerted opening of several RyR channels. Although it can not be directly measured, it is reasonable to believe that the local Ca^{2+} level in the restricted space will quick reach very high levels. This may assure consistent uniform RyR channel activation within the RyR cluster while other factors (e.g. stochastic attrition, regulatory proteins, "fateful" inactivation, coupled gating, modal gating, and luminal Ca^{2+} regulation) may be responsible for turning off the channels.[211]

Ca^{2+} DEPENDENT MODAL GATING OF SINGLE RYR2 CHANNELS

Several research groups have reported modal gating of single RyR channel in planar bilayer studies.[268-271] Modal gating means that single channel activity occurs in bursts. A burst is a temporally clustered group of openings. The open events in a burst may be long or short. Bursts with long open events are classified as high Po. Bursts with short open events are classified as low Po. These bursts are clustered into modes. Trains of high Po bursts characterize a high Po mode. Trains of low Po bursts are characteristic of a low Po mode. Extended periods without channel openings represent a zero Po mode. Single RyR channel studies suggest that the channel can spontaneously shift between zero, low and high Po modes.[268-271] Interestingly, the likelihood of modal shifts is dependent on cytosolic Ca^{2+}

concentration. It appears that the RyR2 adaptation phenomenon is due to a transient shift in the Ca^{2+} dependent modal gating of the RyR2 channel.[269]

Why is Ca^{2+} dependent modal RyR2 channel gating important to consider? Its existence implies that the cytosolic Ca^{2+} regulation of the channels is much more complex than previously imagined. It also reconciles a large body of apparently contradictory single channel results (see discussion below).

Gating of single RyR channels can be classified into 3 distinct modes (zero, low and high Po). The zero Po mode (no activity mode) can occur at very low or very high Ca^{2+} levels. At low Ca^{2+} levels, the zero Po mode occurs because the channel is closed and its Ca^{2+} binding sites are largely unoccupied. At high Ca^{2+} levels, the zero Po mode occurs because the channel is inhibited (inactivated) and its Ca^{2+} binding sites are largely occupied. At all cytosolic Ca^{2+} levels, there is always a dynamic equilibrium between modes. In other words, changes in cytosolic Ca^{2+} level simply change the probability of being in particular modes. At very low steady state cytosolic Ca^{2+} levels, the equilibrium between modes favors the low Ca^{2+} zero Po mode. The equilibrium begins to favor the low and high Po modes as the steady state cytosolic Ca^{2+} level is elevated. At very high steady state cytosolic Ca^{2+} levels, the equilibrium between modes favors the high Ca^{2+} zero Po mode. Thus, the dynamic Ca^{2+} dependent equilibrium between modes explains the classical bell-shaped steady state Ca^{2+} sensitivity of the channel.[235,237,272]

When the cytosolic Ca^{2+} level is suddenly elevated, the dynamic equilibrium between modes is transiently upset until the system can spontaneous relax to a new equilibrium indicative of the higher Ca^{2+} level. Depending on the starting and ending Ca^{2+} levels, this can momentarily increase Po to levels well above those predicted by steady-state measurements. Interestingly, this can happen multiple times if the applied cytosolic Ca^{2+} elevations are small and fast enough. Indeed, transient activation to super steady state Po levels[242,244,247,273] and multiple transient activations by multiple Ca^{2+} elevations have also been experimentally observed.[242] If the applied Ca^{2+} elevation is slow, then the equilibration between modes will keep pace with the slowly changing cytosolic Ca^{2+} level. The result is the steady state cytosolic Ca^{2+} sensitivity of the channel described above. The point here is that Ca^{2+} dependent modal gating provides a robust interpretive context for understanding the cytosolic Ca^{2+} regulation of the RyR channel. It may be complex but we believe strongly that it will ultimately be an integral part of the final description of RyR channel cytosolic Ca^{2+} regulation.

CONCLUDING REMARKS

It should be noted that the cytosolic Ca^{2+} regulation of the RyR channel described here is from a single channel perspective. This current understanding is gained from studies using the planar lipid bilayer technique where the cellular environment is poorly represented. Thus, future studies will have to incorporate the missing endogenous factors (e.g. lumenal Ca^{2+}, Mg^{2+}, ATP, regulatory proteins) that may alter the cytosolic Ca^{2+} sensitivity of the channel. Although we have come a long way, we are far from the end of this journey. There are still many long-standing RyR channel mysteries to be solved.

Chapter 9

ELEMENTARY Ca^{2+} RELEASE EVENTS: RYANODINE RECEPTOR Ca^{2+} SPARKS

W. J. Lederer, Eric A. Sobie, Silvia Guatimosim, and Long-Sheng Song
Medical Biotechnology Center, University of Maryland Biotechnology Institute, Baltimore, MD

INTRODUCTION

The Ca^{2+} spark is the elementary Ca^{2+} signaling event in heart muscle that underlies excitation-contraction (EC) coupling.[240,274-276] Each Ca^{2+} spark reflects the release of Ca^{2+} from the sarcoplasmic reticulum (SR) that was either "triggered" by a brief local increase in $[Ca^{2+}]_i$ or that occurred spontaneously due to a variety of factors. Ca^{2+} sparks occur at distinctive sites within the heart cell, mainly at the junctions between the SR and the surface membrane or between the SR and the transverse tubule (TT) membrane.[277-280] At these junctions, specialized regions of the SR, the "junctional SR" or "jSR" contain RyR2 clusters that are organized in arrays. The L-type Ca^{2+} channels (dihydropyridine receptors, DHPRs) located in the sarcolemmal (SL) or TT membranes are thought to be located near the jSR so that Ca^{2+} flux through the DHPRs can influence the $[Ca^{2+}]_i$ at the jSR. The complex of the jSR, the associated array of RyR2s, the DHPRs, the TT or SL membrane and all of the proteins that are associated with these elements form a unit called "the couplon".[279] The primary input to the EC coupling machinery in heart muscle is the membrane voltage or "action potential" (AP) and the primary elementary output is the Ca^{2+} spark. The summation of Ca^{2+} sparks produces the cardiac Ca^{2+} transient.[281] There are, of course, many factors that are also important and we seek to discuss them in this review. However, the primary focus here is a discussion of RyR2s, Ca^{2+} sparks and our understanding of EC coupling.

THE Ca^{2+} SPARK AND THE $[Ca^{2+}]_i$ TRANSIENT

High-speed imaging of $[Ca^{2+}]_i$ within a quiescent heart cell reveals the occurrence of subcellular elevations of local Ca^{2+} that occur at a rate of about 100 per cell per second. These elevations, called Ca^{2+} sparks, are viewed using a confocal microscope and the Ca^{2+}-sensitive indicator fluo-3,[282] fluo-4 or rhod-2. Fig. 9-1 shows a line-scan image of Ca^{2+} sparks from a rat heart cell loaded with fluo-3. In an XY image, each Ca^{2+} spark appears to be nearly spherical with a diameter of about 2 micrometers (μm, microns).[240] The Ca^{2+} sparks arise from a quiescent $[Ca^{2+}]_i$ of about 100 nM and reveal local peak levels of 200 to 300 nM. The slight eccentricity that may be seen in the XY image of Ca^{2+} sparks[277] may reflect the asymmetric distribution of diverse proteins in the transverse plane (along the z-lines and parallel to the TTs) versus the longitudinal plane (along the long axis of the cell and parallel to the contractile filaments). Fig. 9-1 A depicts signal averaged line scan images of Ca^{2+} sparks. The Ca^{2+} sparks rise to a peak in about 10 ms and fall with a half-time of decay of about 20 ms.[240,276,277,281] Because Ca^{2+} sparks arise as a cluster of RyR2s are activated at a couplon, they are predominantly located along the Z-lines of the sarcomere and at the TTs which reside on the Z-line.[277,278] Fig. 9-1 B shows a signal-averaged view of the TTs obtained at the same time as the Ca^{2+} sparks and reveals the location of the Ca^{2+} sparks along the TTs. The longitudinal TTs (TT extensions that are parallel to the long axis of the cell and that connect Z-line TTs) are relatively sparse compared to the transverse TTs and the abundance of couplons and Ca^{2+} sparks along these longitudinal TTs remains unstudied. Fig. 9-1 C shows a surface plot of Ca^{2+} sparks from Fig. 9-1 A with respect to the TTs (Fig. 9-1 B).

At "rest" or under non-stimulated conditions Ca^{2+} sparks arise in heart cells due to the spontaneous opening of RyR2s in the cluster at the couplon. With roughly a million RyR2s within a single rat heart cell, a Ca^{2+} spark rate of 100 per cell per second is equivalent to a spontaneous opening rate of an isolated RyR2 (e.g. in a planar lipid bilayer) of about 10^{-4} per second. For a single RyR2, this would mean an opening once every 10,000 seconds. Thus, the spontaneous Ca^{2+} spark rate is consistent with the hypothesis that these Ca^{2+} sparks are due to the spontaneous openings of RyR2s within the cluster and that these openings of RyR2s are sufficient to activate the entire couplon to produce a Ca^{2+} spark.

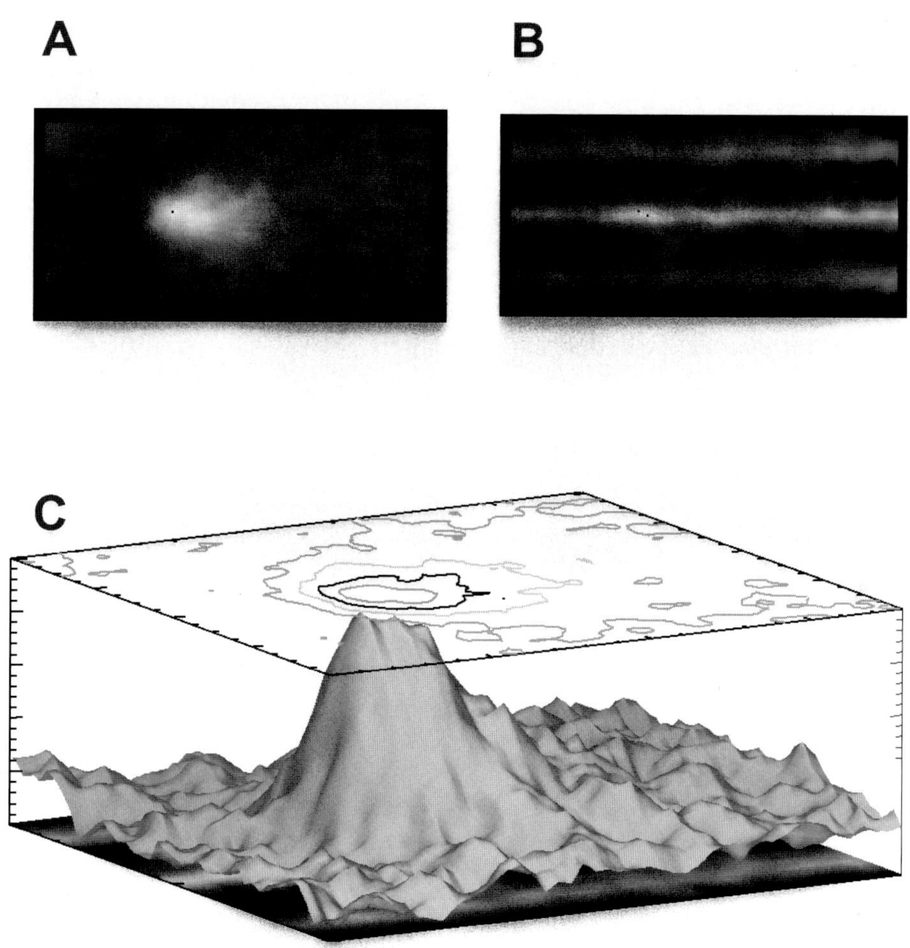

Figure 9-1. **Ca^{2+} sparks in heart**. **A**. Signal averaged line scan images of Ca^{2+} sparks collected from rat heart cells loaded with fluo-3. **B**. Signal averaged line-scan images of cardiac TTs filled with sulforhodamine B. **C**. Shaded surface plot of signal-averaged Ca^{2+} sparks (**A**) plotted in relation to the TTs (**B**). Taken from Cheng *et al.*[277]

Triggered Ca^{2+} sparks are also readily studied.[275,276,281,283] Triggering Ca^{2+} sparks, even at a low rate, vastly increases the Ca^{2+} spark rate over that which is observed at rest. The rate is sufficiently high so that Ca^{2+} sparks are triggered in and out of the confocal imaging plane. Those that appear in the confocal imaging plane look like Ca^{2+} sparks observed at rest.[274] However, those that are activated outside of the plane of focus are not normally seen as Ca^{2+} sparks but instead contribute to the background $[Ca^{2+}]_i$ elevation.[281] This background $[Ca^{2+}]_i$ elevation has the kinetics of the cell-wide (or "global") $[Ca^{2+}]_i$ transient, with a time to peak of 20 - 30 ms and a half-time of decay of 100 - 200 ms. The kinetics of individual Ca^{2+} sparks are much faster and reflect the time-course of Ca^{2+} release (a decreasing function with time with a duration of about 20 ms - see model below) and also the normal and facilitated diffusion of Ca^{2+} away from the couplon that gave rise to the Ca^{2+} spark.[222,284] Thus the half-time of decay of the Ca^{2+} spark is about 20 ms. As the number of triggered Ca^{2+} sparks increased, individual Ca^{2+} sparks are no longer easily viewed and one sees only the global $[Ca^{2+}]_i$ transient. In this manner the Ca^{2+} sparks sum to produce the voltage-gated $[Ca^{2+}]_i$ transient that underlies the contraction.

ISSUES IN EXCITATION-CONTRACTION (EC) COUPLING

There are many important molecular features that contribute to EC coupling, the $[Ca^{2+}]_i$ transient and contraction itself. These have been nicely reviewed by D. M. Bers[1,63,285] and others.[286-293] There are a number of exciting, yet controversial issues in EC coupling that merit a brief discussion in this review. Each, in some manner, focuses on subcellular signaling.

Issue 1: Does phosphorylation of RyR2 by protein kinase A (PKA) affect EC coupling *per se*? On-going experiments examine the matter and yet excellent work by different groups appears to lead to very different results. This is an area where paradox resolution may prove exciting for all. Some features are discussed in the next section of this review.

Issue 2: What happens to EC coupling in heart failure? Important but apparently contradictory results have been published in the literature. The controversy involves issue 1 (above) but also involves the role of the sarcoplasmic reticulum - endoplasmic reticulum Ca^{2+} ATPase (SERCA or Ca^{2+} pump), phospholamban and "pump-leak" balance for two related systems: (i) the heart cell and (ii) the SR. A question related to this issue is: "What does it mean for the RyR2 to be leaky?"

Issue 3: How does the release of Ca^{2+} from the SR through the Ca^{2+} spark terminate? While we know that Ca^{2+} sparks have very limited durations (e.g. about 40 ms), the mechanism of Ca^{2+} spark termination remains uncertain. This question involves RyR2 gating, SR Ca^{2+} content, cross-signaling among RyR2s in a cluster and interactions among lumenal, cytosolic and transmembrane proteins.

Does phosphorylation of RyR2 by protein kinase A (PKA) affect EC coupling *per se*?

The effects of PKA phosphorylation on the RyR2 have been involved in many controversies over the past two decades. Valdivia *et al.* (1995)[247] provided a relevant perspective. Fig. 9-2 shows how RyR2 responds to rapid changes in $[Ca^{2+}]_i$ and how PKA phosphorylation affects the open probability (P_o) of RyR2. This result, modified from Valdivia *et al.* (1995)[247], shows how step increases in $[Ca^{2+}]_i$ in the region surrounding the cytoplasmic face of RyR2 can change the gating of this channel. Fig. 9-2 A shows the set-up. A planar lipid bilayer containing RyR2 was bathed by a cytoplasmic solution ("cis") that contained ATP, Mg^{2+} and caged Ca^{2+} (NP-EGTA). Cs^+ (in the lumenal or "trans" side of the bilayer) was used as the charge carried through the RyR2. As shown in the diagram, a fiber optic element delivered the pulsed UV light to the bilayer to produce photolysis and thereby rapidly increase $[Ca^{2+}]_i$ on the cytoplasmic side of the bilayer near the RyR2. By this means $[Ca^{2+}]_i$ increased from 100 nM to 10 μM in less than a millisecond. The photolysis of the caged Ca^{2+} occurred only between the end of the fiber optic and the planar lipid bilayer. This rapid increase in $[Ca^{2+}]_i$ activated the RyR2 to increase the P_o of the channel as revealed in Fig. 9-2 B. There was a clear and rapid increase in P_o that appeared to decline with time. Following PKA phosphorylation, the same procedure led to an even greater increase in P_o of RyR2 instantaneously with the increase in $[Ca^{2+}]_i$. With a sustained increase in $[Ca^{2+}]_i$ there was an even greater decline than there had been under control (i.e. without PKA phosphorylation). A comparison of the signal averaged effects under control and PKA-phosphorylated conditions is shown in Fig. 9-2 C.

Three important features should be pointed out. First, the openings of the DHPRs are brief and would normally occur during the time when the large increase in P_o occurs following the photolysis. This increase in P_o is clearly enhanced following PKA phosphorylation. Second, there is little, if any, change in P_o at resting $[Ca^{2+}]_i$ (around 100 nM) following PKA phosphorylation. Third, the sustained step increase in $[Ca^{2+}]_i$ produces a lower increase in P_o following PKA phosphorylation of RyR2 than is observed in control. Such a steady-state increase in $[Ca^{2+}]_i$ does not occur physiologically.

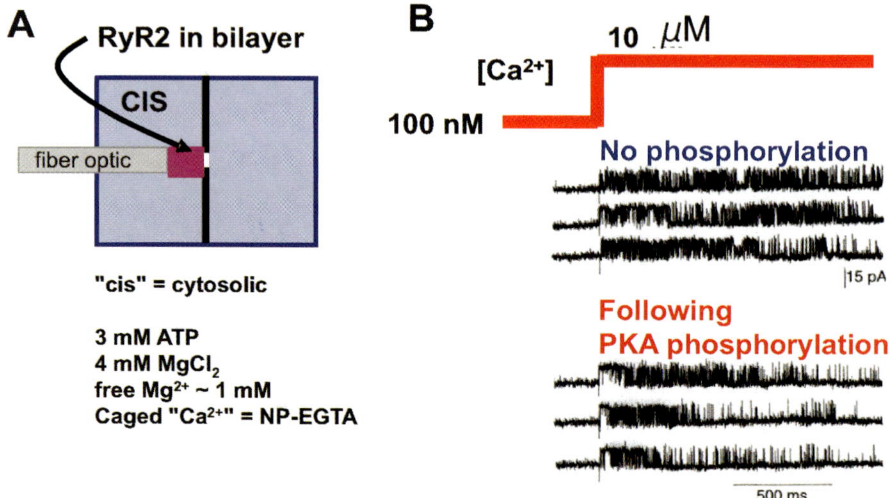

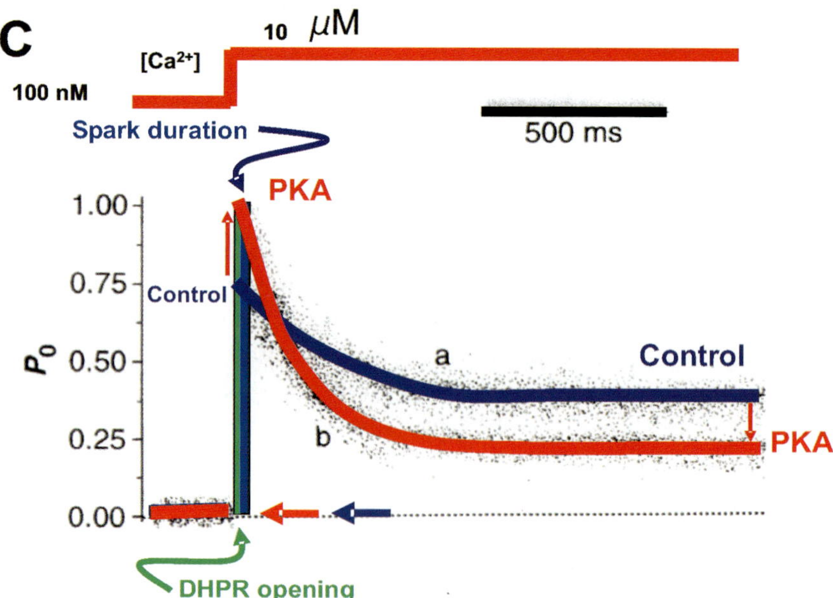

Figure 9-2. **Activation of RyR2 by Ca^{2+}. A**. Experimental set-up. A planar lipid bilayer was established with the cis (cytoplasmic) site episodically illuminated by a pulsed frequency-tripled Nd:YAG laser producing a 5 nS 355 nm flash. The UV pulse is used to uncage Ca^{2+}. **B**. Sample records of single channel membrane current before and after $[Ca^{2+}]_i$ increased from 100 nM to 10 μM. **C.** Signal averaged records from B using 17 (control) and 21 (PKA) sweeps. Taken from Valdivia *et al.*[247]

The results of Wehrens *et al.* (2003)[294] showed changes in P_o in RyR2 due to PKA phosphorylation that were similar to those shown by Valdivia *et al.* (1995),[247] when comparison was possible. Fig. 9-3 shows a re-plot of the findings of RyR2 from normal animals. PKA phosphorylation of these RyR2s produced a small but clear increase at low $[Ca^{2+}]_i$ but the investigation only examined the P_o under steady-state conditions.[294] The experiments by Valdivia *et al.* (1995)[247] did not examine intermediate $[Ca^{2+}]_i$ levels. At high steady-state levels, the data of Valdivia *et al.* (1995)[247] and Wehrens *et al.* (2003)[294] largely agree.

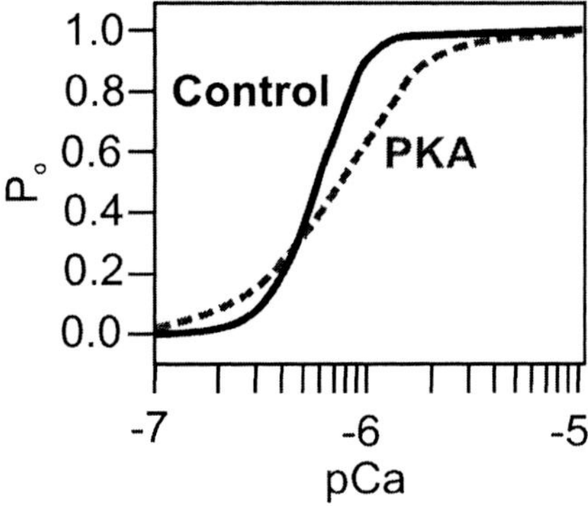

Figure 9-3. **RyR2 P_o as a function of steady-state $[Ca^{2+}]_i$.** Normal mouse RyR2 was studied in the absence of PKA phosphorylation and after it was complete. Data replotted from Wehrens *et al.*[294]

Examination of Ca^{2+} sparks under similar conditions is quite difficult, but work continues to provide a robust and clear answer. PKA increases SR Ca^{2+} content, which has an important and positive effect on SR Ca^{2+} release and increases the Ca^{2+} current through L-type Ca^{2+} channels, which enhances the Ca^{2+} trigger. Cross-talk between other systems that may enhance Ca^{2+} release (e.g. CaMK) and changes in kinetics of triggering and release, as well as changes in RyR2 properties, may contribute to or complicate the investigation in intact cells.[295-299] Consequently the actions of PKA and CamKII on Ca^{2+} sparks remains a topic of active investigation. From the planar lipid bilayer work noted above, however, there is reason to believe that the RyR2 clusters will be significantly influenced by PKA phosphorylation.

What happens to EC coupling in heart failure?

The triggering of SR Ca^{2+} release depends on multiple factors, each one of which appears to be "non-linear". By this it is meant that the release is not simply scaled by the total amount of "trigger Ca^{2+}" that is delivered to the RyR2. Such non-linearities in the Ca^{2+} signaling system may make it hard to determine, in a simple or consistent manner, how Ca^{2+} releases (i.e. Ca^{2+} sparks) are regulated under pathological conditions. There are changes in Ca^{2+} sources such as the Na^+/Ca^{2+} exchanger; the total amount of Na^+/Ca^{2+} exchanger expressed frequently increases during heart failure.[300-303] The widely observed decrease in SERCA in heart failure leads to a decrease in the amount of Ca^{2+} in the SR Ca^{2+} stores and a reduced sensitivity of the system.[286,304-307] In addition, there are possible changes in the spatial organization between TTs and the remaining components on the cell.[308,309] Moreover, the resting or diastolic $[Ca^{2+}]_i$ may change.[285,310,311] The PKA and CaMK-dependent chages in RyR2 gating may increase the mean open time of the RyR2 Ca^{2+} channels and make them, in effect, leaky. Together these changes and others make the Ca^{2+} signaling complicated in heart failure.

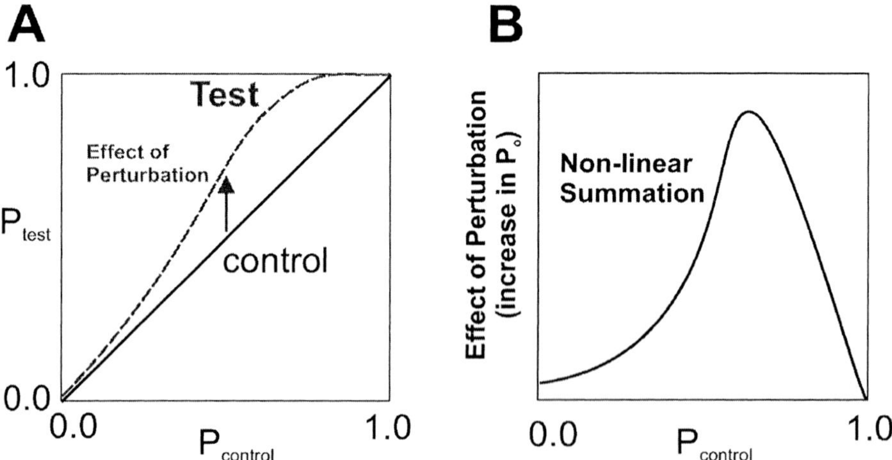

Figure 9-4. **Non-linear summation of Ca^{2+} signaling.** This diagram illustrates how non-linear summation of several Ca^{2+} signals may work in principle. **A.** The effect of "triggering" the signal that activates RyR2 compared to a "line of unity". The abscissa shows the probability that RyR2 is activated before the perturbation ($P_{control}$). The ordinate shows how a perturbation (test) may influence the probability that the RyR2 will open (P_{test}). The effect of a perturbation depends on many factors, including where on the $P_{control}$ axis it occurs. **B.** This panel shows the relative effect of the perturbation as a function of $P_{control}$. This curve therefore reflects the non-linear summation of the perturbation.

Fig. 9-4 shows diagrammatically how non-linear summation of trigger signals may occur and how they may affect the triggering of RyR2s. There are two curves. The top curve shows a plot of the relationship between the RyR2 P_o (P_{test}) under conditions of a "triggering" perturbation as a function of the P_o under control conditions ($P_{control}$). A "unity" ($P_{test}=P_{control}$) reference line is drawn. The plot shows how there is increasing efficacy as a function of control P_o followed by a region of decreasing efficacy. This is the kind of curve that one may observed if the "condition" were a Ca^{2+} influx as one may observed through a DHPR Ca^{2+} channel activated by depolarization. At low control P_o, the efficacy may increase as control P_o increases and this would reflect the increasing ability of the trigger to activate RyR2s. At the high end of P_o, there may be a decline in efficacy as the additional "test" intervention may be excessive in amount. The curve in the right panel is drawn to suggest the general shape of the effect of such simple "non-linear" summation effects as one might expect to observe. An example of non-linear summation may be activation of Ca^{2+} release by Na^+/Ca^{2+} exchanger and DHPRs.[312] Through non-linear summation and other mechanisms, physiological and pathophysiological changes can produce significant complexities in RyR2 gating.

How does the Ca^{2+} spark terminate?

SR Ca^{2+} release is a positive feedback system. As Ca^{2+} is released from the SR via RyR2 Ca^{2+} release channels, it can activate not only the channel that is involved in the release but its neighboring RyR2s. Thus a couplon will tend to remain a source of Ca^{2+} until some termination mechanism is activated. Although there is evidence that RyR2s may "inactivate" under some conditions, these conditions appear to be largely non-physiological. The conditions of RyR2 inactivation include very high $[Ca^{2+}]_i$ and very long periods of exposure. Fig. 9-2 provides a context for the requirements. The green and blue bars on Fig. 9-2 C reflect the duration of the Ca^{2+} spark. Virtually no change in RyR2 P_o occurs over that time-scale. The very slow reduction of P_o with the sustained elevation of $[Ca^{2+}]_i$ shown in Fig. 9-2 is called "adaptation"[242,247,269] and may reflect a different process than that which is responsible for terminating the Ca^{2+} spark. While there has been some controversy about the flash photolysis methods used in the investigations,[269,313] Fig. 1 of Valdivia *et al.* (1995)[247] provides an internal control for many of the concerns.

An alternative approach to account for Ca^{2+} spark termination has been suggested by Sobie *et al.* (2002).[222] This work includes the idea that RyR2 P_o depends on the amount of Ca^{2+} within the SR ("lumenal Ca^{2+}" or "SR Ca^{2+} load")[201,212,314] and depends on cooperativity among the RyR2 channels.[315,316]

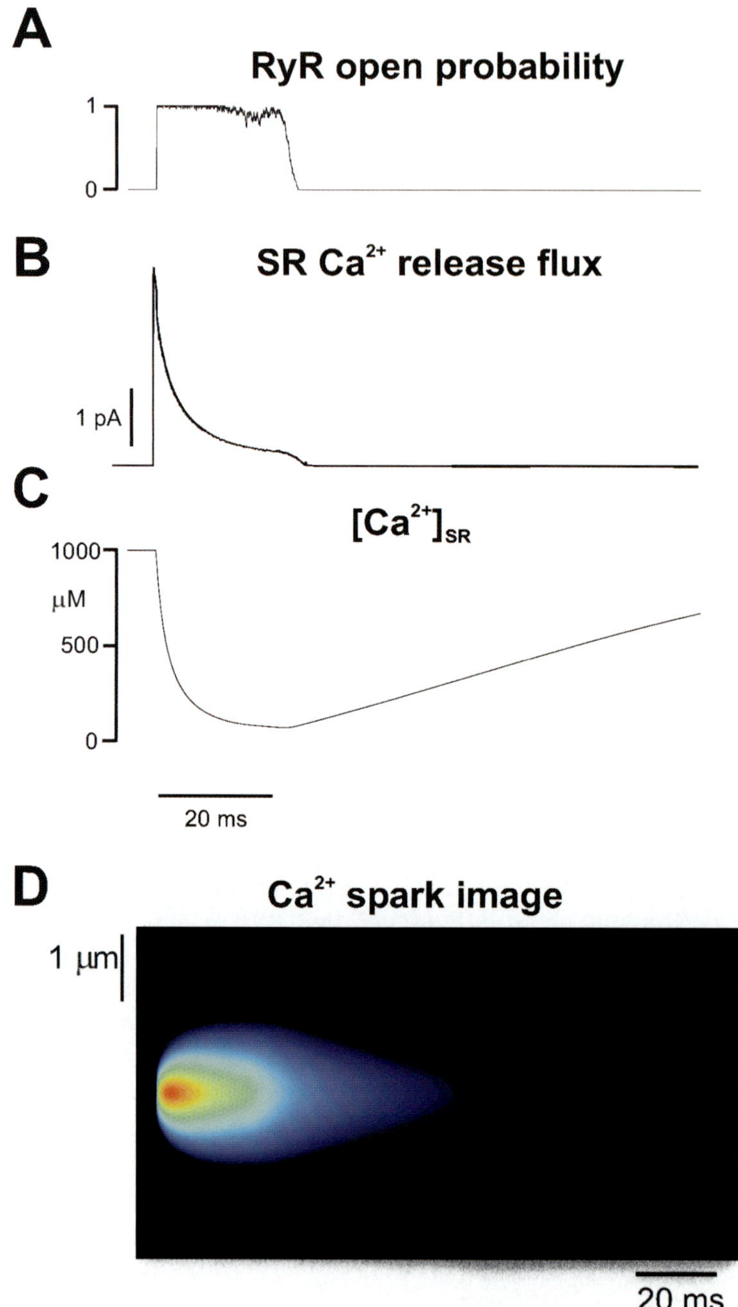

Figure 9-5. **Model Ca^{2+} spark.** **A**. Composite P_o of 50 RyR2s in a cluster. **B**. SR Ca^{2+} release flux, **C**. Depletion from the SR Ca^{2+} stores during the Ca^{2+} spark. **D**. Line-scan image of the "mock" spark. Taken from Sobie *et al.*[222]

Fig. 9-5 shows how a model using these principles performs.[222] This simulation of a couplon reveals that even with 50 RyR2s in the couplon, RyR2 P_o can be managed. As the SR Ca^{2+} content falls due to lumenal depletion, the efflux is a decreasing function with time. When the SR Ca^{2+} content is sufficiently decreased, the RyR2 clusters close. The cooperativity is discussed in terms of the reported "coupled gating", a feature also found in skeletal muscle.

There are two important experimental approaches that must be carried out to adequately address Ca^{2+} spark termination. The first is that a careful restitution experiment must be completed. Arguably the best to date was one of the first[223] although it, too, is incomplete. If the restitution can be shown to depend on refilling, then a central role for lumenal Ca^{2+} will be better established. More work is clearly needed. Other important investigations of this question have been carried out inconclusively.[220,221] The second area of investigation that must still be done is an investigation of the SR Ca^{2+} content in the terminal cisternae (i.e. junctional SR). If depletion is an important factor, it should occur and be measurable. An excellent beginning was made by the Bers group using the low affinity Ca^{2+} indicator, fluo-5N.[218]

The Sobie model[222] provides for robust spark termination and does not depend significantly on the numbers of RyR2s or the initial Ca^{2+} loads. It can accommodate prolonged Ca^{2+} spark duration under special conditions and can reproduce many other features of SR Ca^{2+} release. Nevertheless, the above two tests have the possibility of supporting or denying this model and may enable refinements for this or other models.

CONCLUDING REMARKS

Ca^{2+} sparks are the elementary units of SR Ca^{2+} release. They can occur at a low spontaneous rate or be triggered by elevations of local $[Ca^{2+}]_i$ and are sensitive to cellular geometry and organization, RyR2 phosphorylation and SR Ca^{2+} content. Improved understanding of Ca^{2+} signaling in health and disease will depend on the current investigations of the structure of the couplons, of RyR2 biophysics and biochemistry, of Ca^{2+} spark termination mechanisms and of the proteins that organize and support the TTs.

Chapter 10

Ca^{2+} RELEASE FROM THE SARCOPLASMIC RETICULUM IN INTACT CARDIOMYOCYTES

Donald M. Bers, and Kenneth S. Ginsburg
Dept. of Physiology, Loyola University Chicago, Stritch School of Medicine, Maywood, IL

INTRODUCTION

The cardiac ryanodine receptor (RyR) is the SR Ca^{2+} release channel and is the centerpiece of a macromolecular complex of regulatory proteins. This chapter focuses on how certain RyR modulators affect Ca^{2+} release and excitation-contraction coupling in intact ventricular myocytes, where the RyR complex in the sarcoplasmic reticulum associates closely with sarcolemmal Ca^{2+} channels. We consider the effects of protein kinase A, calmodulin/Ca^{2+}-calmodulin dependent protein kinase, and protein phosphatases on RyR function in intact ventricular myocytes. There are multiple inherent feedback systems and parallel pathways which can complicate the effects of these and other RyR modulators, integrating into a cellular response. To determine experimentally how any given RyR modulator affects the RyR function specifically in the intact cell setting, it is necessary to control factors which can independently influence RyR function, especially the SR Ca^{2+} content and cytosolic $[Ca^{2+}]$ or triggering Ca^{2+} current.

NEGATIVE FEEDBACK STABILIZES EXCITATION-CONTRACTION COUPLING

During cardiac excitation-contraction (E-C) coupling, Ca^{2+} influx via sarcolemmal L-type Ca^{2+} channels (or dihydropyridine receptors, DHPRs) triggers the release of Ca^{2+} from the sarcoplasmic reticulum (SR) via ryanodine receptors (RyRs).[1] Ca^{2+} release via RyR entails several- or more fold amplification, but E-C coupling is normally stable, due to local control[249] whereby the highly amplified Ca^{2+} release is confined spatially to single junctions. Local control is mediated structurally, since the SR and sarcolemmal membrane come into very close apposition only at periodic regions along the surface membrane, including the transverse (T) tubules of ventricular myocytes. Each of the ~10,000 couplons in a ventricular myocyte is normally activated independently by Ca^{2+} influx from its own DHPRs. Pacemakers and atrial cells lack T-tubule structures, so Ca^{2+} release is not governed as strictly by the local Ca^{2+} influx, but local control still operates and affords stabilization.

These local SR Ca^{2+} release events at each couplon are synchronized in time due to action potential-dependent near-simultaneous activation of Ca^{2+} current (I_{Ca}) at each junction and thus sum to produce rapid relatively homogeneous increases in $[Ca^{2+}]_i$. As described extensively by Diaz *et al.* (Chapter 11), this global Ca^{2+} release is stabilized by negative feedbacks. Any increase in Ca^{2+} influx leads to increasing SR Ca^{2+} release (a direct consequence of greater activation of RyRs). However, the increased SR Ca^{2+} release inhibits further Ca^{2+} influx (via Ca^{2+}-dependent I_{Ca} inactivation and decreasing Ca^{2+} influx via Na^+/Ca^{2+} exchange, NCX) and enhances Ca^{2+} extrusion from the cell via NCX, thereby limiting the increase in SR Ca^{2+} content which would otherwise result from the initially enhanced Ca^{2+} influx. Feedback appears also to help terminate Ca^{2+} release through local depletion of Ca^{2+} stores, whereby regulatory action of lower intra-SR $[Ca^{2+}]$ reduces the RyR open probability.[202,212,218,317]

The negative feedbacks that moderate and stabilize E-C coupling can be described as autoregulatory,[318] but this regulation cannot be absolute, as evidenced by the normal adaptive responses of E-C coupling to demand. In ventricular cells these would include graded contraction, inotropy, frequency dependent staircases and acceleration of relaxation, rest decay of Ca^{2+} load, and others. In pacemaker cells regulation may also directly affect firing frequency. The consequence of negative feedback for E-C coupling is that its properties can be modulated in predictable fashion.

RYR MACROMOLECULAR COMPLEXES AND Ca^{2+} RELEASE IN INTACT CELLS

As part of a large macromolecular complex,[319,320] RyRs are influenced by regulators including calmodulin, Ca^{2+}-dependent calmodulin kinase (CaMKII), FK-506 binding proteins, sorcin, protein kinase A (PKA), and protein phosphatases 1 (PP1) and 2A (PP2A), which can evoke a large repertoire of dynamic responses, including changes in open probability and/or duration, appearance of subconductance states, and greater or lesser coordination among subunits within an RyR tetramer and/or among tetramers.[315] RyRs also respond to cofactors which have a structural or stabilizing, rather than a dynamic role, including calsequestrin and other SR Ca^{2+} binding proteins, junctin, triadin, Mg, and ATP.

To reveal key properties of these varied modulations has required experiments on bilayer and vesicle preparations where RyRs are removed from the intact cell environment. In such experiments RyRs are bereft not only of the negative feedbacks described above, but also of the dyadic or couplon structure which could control the access of regulators to their sites of action. The subcellular preparations of course both require and allow artificial control of the concentrations of relevant regulators.

To understand the implications of RyR modulation, we need to know how it works in intact cells, but this is difficult because modulators (such as PKA and CaMKII) can by themselves activate other pathways which can independently influence function of the RyR. Dominant among these feedback influences are the SR Ca^{2+} load and the Ca^{2+} influx via I_{Ca}, which directly and strongly modulate RyR properties and E-C coupling independently of all other factors.[208,295,317,321] Indeed, both PKA and CaMKII simulate I_{Ca} and SR Ca^{2+} uptake directly, enhancing both the SR Ca^{2+} content and the trigger for release. To study RyR responses in intact cells, we need to defeat the inherent autoregulation and parallel regulation experimentally. In this way we can assess how RyR itself participates in complex regulatory responses due to PKA and CaMKII.

In our laboratory we have employed several approaches to functional dissection. In normal intact cells we have controlled SR Ca^{2+} loading by stimulating to steady state with pulses of varying frequency or (under voltage clamp), amplitude and/or duration. We have largely prevented the intrinsic regulation of SR Ca^{2+} uptake and load caused by phospholamban (PLB) phosphorylation by using transgenic mice where PLB cannot be phosphorylated,[322] as well as knockout mice entirely lacking PLB.[323] Fine control of resting cytosolic $[Ca^{2+}]$ can also be attained by permeabilizing cells (e.g. with saponin) and using heavily Ca^{2+} buffered solutions. We have also similarly controlled Ca^{2+} influx and I_{Ca}, by abrupt changes in external

$[Ca^{2+}]$, choice of test potentials or by reducing I_{Ca} availability by agents (e.g. nifedipine) or by partially pre-inactivating I_{Ca}.[295] These manipulations can separately affect I_{Ca} /DHPR open probability, unitary current and/or Ca^{2+} influx.

Protein kinase A

Marx *et al.*[5,6] showed that protein kinase A (PKA) is anchored to the cardiac RyR via mAKAP, an A kinase anchoring protein, from where it may phosphorylate its target RyR2 site (Ser-2809). Two phosphatases (PP1 and PP2A) also associate specifically with RyR2 via their own respective targeting proteins (spinophilin and PR130). Thus, the requisite molecular machinery for dynamic control of RyR phosphorylation and dephosphorylation is anchored directly to the protein (see Chapter 15). Conceivably, the associated PP1 and PP2A can dephosphorylate distinct sites or oppose phosphorylation due to different kinases. DHPR, though nearby (≤10 nm away), appear to have their own distinct PKA-dependent regulatory responses (as well as their own characteristic CaM/CaMKII dependent phosphorylation responses). PKA-dependent regulation of I_{Ca}[324] can dramatically increase I_{Ca} amplitude and shift its activation E_m dependence negative. Although the pathway of PKA-dependent RyR phosphorylation is not yet known in detail, separate PKA signaling of DHPR and RyR is possible.

PKA-dependent RyR phosphorylation alters RyR gating in bilayers. Valdivia *et al.*[247] found that PKA slightly decreased basal open probability (P_o) at 100 nM $[Ca^{2+}]$, but greatly increased peak P_o (to nearly 1.0) during a rapid photolytic increase of $[Ca^{2+}]$. PKA also accelerated the subsequent decline in P_o (attributed to adaptation). In contrast, Marx *et al.*[5], measuring only steady state behavior, found that PKA-dependent RyR phosphorylation enhanced open probability of single RyRs in bilayers, but also caused the appearance of prominent subconductance states. They attributed this dual effect to displacement of FKBP12.6 from the RyR, although other groups have found that FKBP12.6 still binds to RyRs after PKA-dependent phosphorylation.[325,326] It is less clear how total Ca^{2+} flux changes when PKA phosphorylates RyRs. If open probability is enhanced, but mean conductance is reduced (due to substates), the net effect on total steady state Ca^{2+} flux may be at least partially mitigated.

In intact cells at rest, steady state Ca^{2+} spark frequency and characteristics reflect leak from the SR via stochastic opening of RyR clusters. In resting adult ventricular myocytes (either permeabilized, Fig. 10-1 A,B or intact, Fig 10-1 C) Ca^{2+} spark frequency and characteristics were unaffected by PKA-dependent RyR phosphorylation, as long as SR Ca^{2+}

load was closely controlled. The needed control was achieved by regulating SR Ca^{2+} uptake (using mice with either nonphosphorylatable PLB or PLB knockout) and the SR Ca^{2+} content was measured.[297] Despite this, adrenergic inotropy in heart tissue is one of its best established responses,[327] and needs to be explained at the intact cell level. Apparently, in normal myocytes direct PKA-mediated changes in resting RyR Ca^{2+} leak are small, especially compared to the effects of PKA on the SR Ca^{2+}-ATPase function which are mediated by PLB phosphorylation (and indirectly enhance Ca^{2+} spark frequency due to elevated intra-SR [Ca^{2+}]).

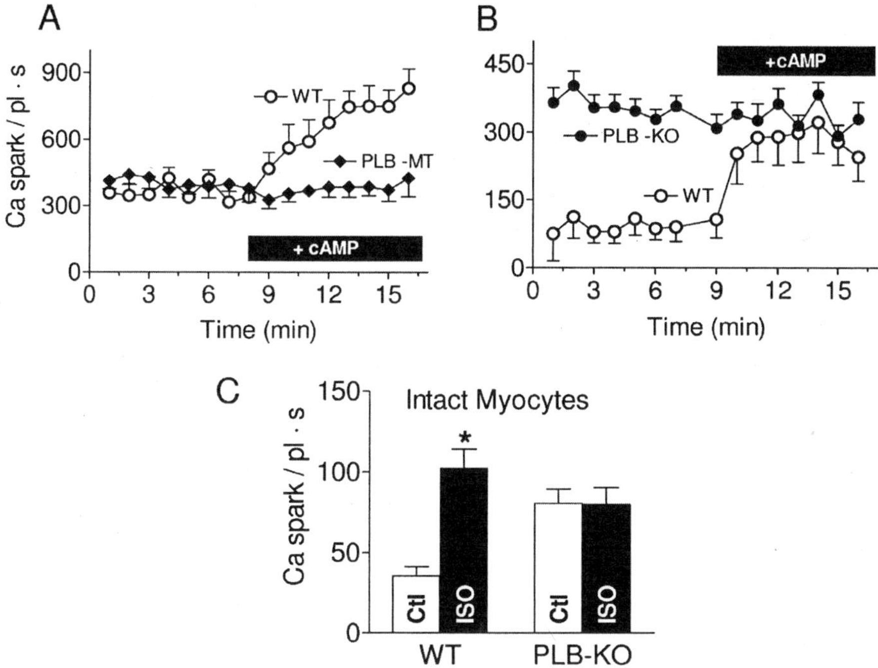

Figure 10-1. **PKA effects on Ca^{2+} sparks** (modified from Li *et al.*[297]). **A,B**. Steady state spark frequency increased on adding cAMP in permeabilized cells of WT mice where SR Ca^{2+} load also increased, but not in permeabilized cells of nonphosphorylatable phospholamban mutant mice (**A**) or phospholamban knockout mice (**B**), where SR Ca^{2+} load did not change on adding cAMP. **C**. Steady state spark frequency increased with isoproterenol addition in intact cells of WT mice, but not in intact cells of phospholamban knockouts, where SR Ca^{2+} load was rigorously controlled (not shown).

On PKA activation in beating cells, both I_{Ca} and SR Ca^{2+} uptake (and hence SR Ca^{2+} loading) normally increase (Fig. 10-2 A), such that PKA could enhance Ca^{2+} transients even if there were no independent RyR effect.

The E-C coupling gain (dimensionless ratio of SR Ca^{2+} released to integrated I_{Ca}) can be considered a fundamental measure of E-C coupling and we have used it to provide a metric for RyR modulation. Recent studies of voltage-clamped ventricular myocytes showed either enhanced or depressed gain with PKA activation,[328,329] but in these studies SR Ca^{2+} load was not measured under the same conditions and I_{Ca} amplitude was not controlled. It is most revealing to compare E-C coupling gains ±β-adrenergic receptor activation at the same I_{Ca} trigger and same SR Ca^{2+} load, as well as the same membrane voltage, since the E-C gain depends profoundly on all of these, independently of adrenergic state. We recently characterized the effect of PKA activation over a broad range of SR Ca^{2+} loads and I_{Ca} trigger amplitudes.[295] At a given SR Ca^{2+} load and I_{Ca} amplitude, PKA activation did not affect Ca^{2+} release (Fig. 10-2 B) and had no effect on gain as measured by the amount of SR Ca^{2+} released divided by I_{Ca} integral (Fig. 10-2 C). The profound loss of gain with increasing I_{Ca} trigger and increase of gain with increasing SR Ca^{2+} load were preserved (Fig. 10-2 C). Thus, the amount of RyR-mediated SR Ca^{2+} released for a given I_{Ca} and SR Ca^{2+} content was remarkably unaltered by PKA. On the other hand, PKA activation consistently increased the initial rate of SR Ca^{2+} release (Fig. 10-2 D) and rate of shut-off of release (not shown) at all triggers and loads.

Thus, PKA-dependent modulation of RyR may be more important in speeding the rate of SR Ca^{2+} release rather than increasing the total amount released. The normal robust PKA-dependent enhancement of I_{Ca} and SR Ca^{2+} content (when not experimentally controlled) are likely to be mainly responsible for the large increase in amount of SR Ca^{2+} release. The increased I_{Ca} and SR Ca^{2+} content caused by PKA may also contribute to speeding up the rate of SR Ca^{2+} release. During sympathetic stimulation, relaxation and $[Ca^{2+}]_i$ decline are also accelerated, and this is mediated by phosphorylation of both PLB (speeding SR Ca^{2+} uptake) and troponin I (hastening Ca^{2+} dissociation from troponin C). Thus, PKA-dependent effects on RyR may work synergistically with I_{Ca}, PLB and troponin I to cause even larger and faster Ca^{2+} transients and contractions during the urgent fight or flight responses activated by the sympathetic nervous system.

Ca^{2+}-dependent calmodulin kinase II

Calmodulin (CaM) binds to RyR with an affinity that increases as more of its four Ca^{2+} binding sites become occupied.[330] At physiological $[Ca^{2+}]_i$, especially in the beating heart, CaM binding sites on RyR may remain almost fully occupied, and this reduces P_o at all $[Ca^{2+}]$ and also shifts the Ca-dependence of activation to higher $[Ca^{2+}]$.[331,332] CaM may exert its own effects on RyR gating, but here we are most interested in its activation of

Ca^{2+}-dependent calmodulin kinase (CaMKII).[333-335] CaMKII is expressed in the cytosol of cardiac cells as the δ_c isoform[336,337] and co-immunoprecipitates with RyR2,[338] but the molecular site of interaction is not known. CaMKII and CaM together can mediate target phosphorylation with unique complex dynamics. CaM-free CaMKII can rest in an autoinhibited state, but when Ca^{2+}-CaM binds to the regulatory region of CaMKII it displaces the autoinhibitory domain so that the catalytic site can phosphorylate targets. CaMKII also becomes auto-phosphorylated, resulting in autonomous Ca^{2+}-independent activity (and trapping of CaM), maintained even after $[Ca^{2+}]_i$ declines.[339] Even after CaM dissociation, autophosphorylated CaMKII remains partially active (20-80%).[340-343]

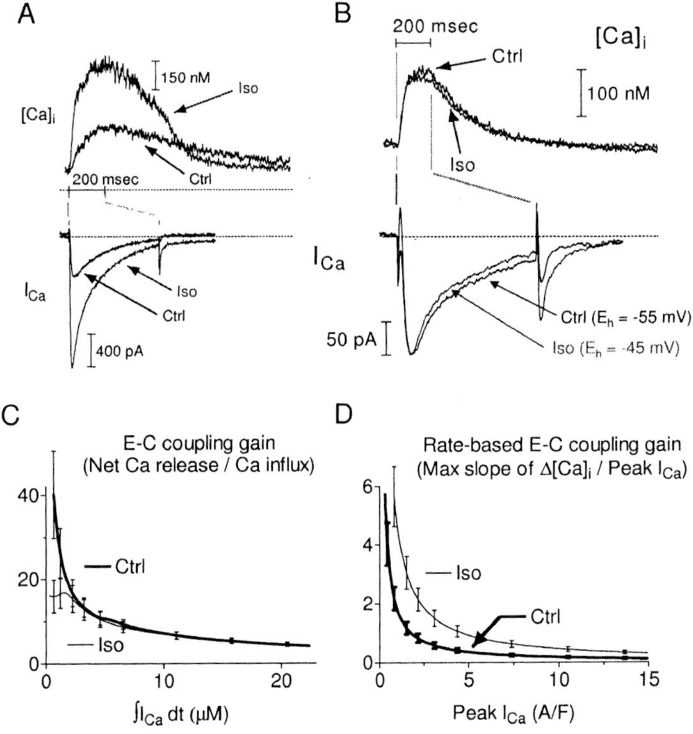

Figure 10-2. **PKA effects on E-C coupling** (modified from Ginsburg *et al.*[295]). **A**. Classic inotropic and lusitropic response to isoproterenol (iso), rabbit cell. Both I_{Ca} trigger and SR Ca^{2+} load (not shown) increased, causing larger $[Ca^{2+}]_i$ transient. **B**. With I_{Ca} and SR load (not shown) controlled to match ±iso, $[Ca^{2+}]_i$ transient did not change; mouse cell with nonphosphorylatable phospholamban. **C**. Dimensionless E-C coupling gain, measured as total Ca^{2+} release vs Ca^{2+} influx, was unaffected by iso. **D**. E-C coupling gain, measured as peak $d[Ca^{2+}]_i/dt$ vs peak Ca^{2+} influx, increased with iso.

CaMKII may phosphorylate RyR2 at up to six consensus sites,[344-349] including Ser-2809, the site of PKA-dependent phosphorylation. Multisite phosphorylation would support complex potent effects on RyR gating. Recently, Wehrens *et al.*[298] reported that CaMKII phosphorylates RyR2 at Ser-2815 and not at the PKA-dependent phosphorylation site Ser-2809. The maximum CaMKII:RyR2 stoichiometry was reported to be 1.5:1,[298] but evidence from another study also supports a higher (4:1) value.[349] In any case, CaMKII-mediated phosphorylation may well occur at multiple RyR sites.

Although decreased RyR P_o with CaMKII phosphorylation has been reported in bilayer and vesicle preparations,[350] several studies have reported increases[298,345,346] as well as increased Ca^{2+} sensitivity;[298] prolonged openings occur and unlike the case with PKA-dependent phosphorylation there do not seem to be subconductance states.[298,345]

A preponderance of data in intact myocytes indicates that CaMKII increases both resting Ca^{2+} leak from stores and SR Ca^{2+} release during E-C coupling, reflecting the increased RyR fluxes seen in bilayers. In intact voltage clamped ventricular myocytes endogenous CaMKII (assessed using the CaMKII inhibitor KN-93) increased Ca^{2+} release, measured with both I_{Ca} and SR Ca^{2+} load held constant ±KN-93, as shown in Fig. 10-3 A,B and C.[351] Notably, when the conditioning pulses gave weak Ca^{2+} transients (perhaps not activating CaMKII), KN-93 was without effect. In particular these cellular results suggested that dynamic regulation of RyR function may be expected to be associated with changes in heart rate and Ca^{2+} transient amplitude.

Transgenic overexpression of CaMKIIδ_C in mice[296] increased diastolic Ca^{2+} spark frequency and spark signal mass (Fig. 10-3 D,F and E), indicating substantial increase in diastolic Ca^{2+} leak. This increase of Ca^{2+} spark frequency occurred despite the fact that both diastolic $[Ca^{2+}]_i$ and SR Ca^{2+} content were reduced (both of which would independently reduce Ca^{2+} spark frequency). Moreover, the higher SR Ca^{2+} leak probably contributed to the reduced SR Ca^{2+} content. The acute CaMKII dependency of these changes in transgenic mice was verified by the observation that acute application of KN-93 reduced Ca^{2+} spark frequency such that there was no difference between wild type and transgenic myocytes.

Fractional SR Ca^{2+} release during E-C coupling also increased in these CaMKIIδ_C transgenic mice,[296] as seen in normal ferrets upon activation of endogenous CaMKII.[351] We have further tested these CaMKII effects by short term adenoviral transfection of rabbit ventricular myocytes with CaMKIIδ_C[352] and by acute application of pre-activated CaMKII to permeabilized mouse ventricular myocytes lacking PLB.[353] In both cases Ca^{2+} spark frequency was enhanced by CaMKII when normalized for SR Ca^{2+} content.

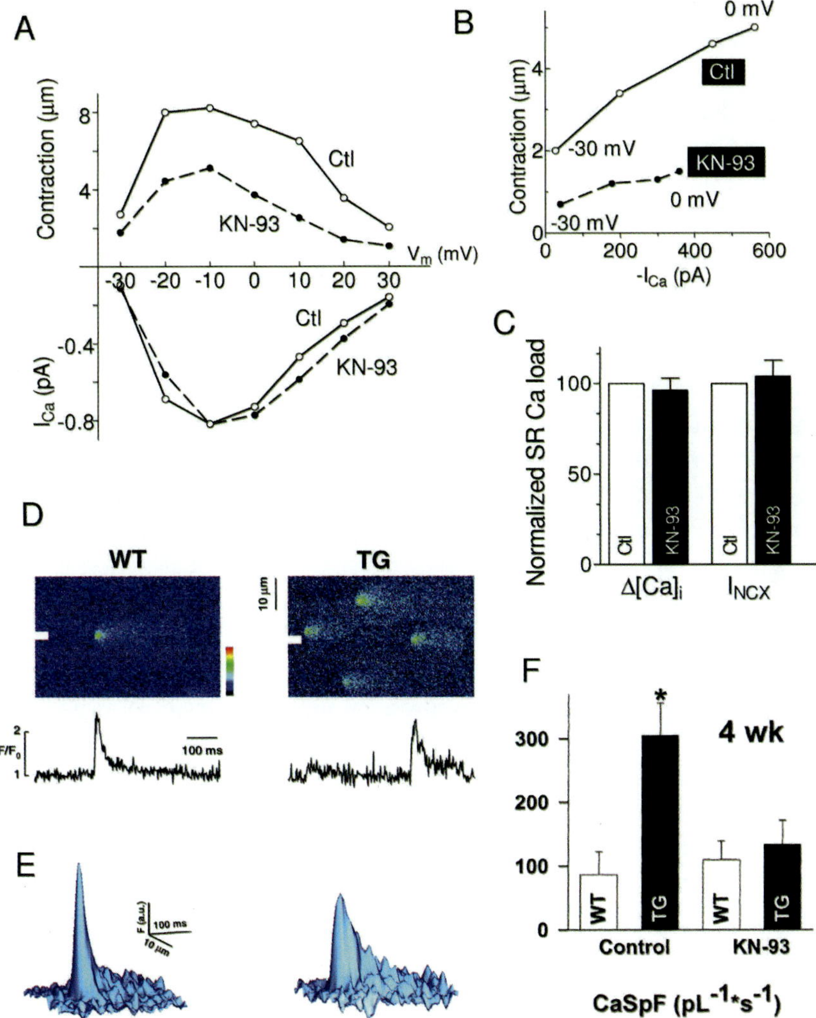

Figure 10-3. **CaMKII-induced RyR phosphorylation**. **A**. for a given I_{Ca} trigger with SR Ca^{2+} load were held constant, contraction was larger with CaMKII (ferret cells; modified from Li *et al.*[351]). **B**. Ascending limb of (**A**) replotted as contraction vs I_{Ca} influx to show E-C coupling gain increase. **C**. SR Ca^{2+} loading, as measured by caffeine-induced $[Ca^{2+}]_i$ transient amplitude and integral of I_{NCX}, did not change in the experiments of A. **D,E**. With CaMKII overexpression, resting spark frequency, width and duration increased, consistent with larger Ca^{2+} leak flux. **F**. Acute application of the CaMKII inhibitor KN-93 to CaMKII overexpressing myocytes renormalized spark frequency, indicating a specific CaMKII-related effect (modified from Maier *et al.*[296]).

Intact cell responses to CaMKII activation differ substantially from those of PKA-dependent phosphorylation, despite both pathways tending to increase SR Ca^{2+} release. CaMKII activation in intact myocytes causes dramatic changes in RyR function with more modest changes in I_{Ca} and SR Ca^{2+} loading, while the reverse is true for PKA effects. It is important to recognize that activation of RyR by CaMKII alone would ultimately feed back to reduce SR Ca^{2+} content (as reported in Maier *et al.*[296]) and thereby renormalize or even reduce overall release.

As for PKA, not all cellular results with CaMKII agree. For example, reduced SR Ca^{2+} release and E-C coupling gain has also been reported with adenoviral expression of constitutively active CaMKII[354] or (in native cells) with specific inhibition by AC3-I.[354] Thus, considerable diversity remains in observations on CaMKII actions in intact cells. CaMKII effects on RyR function lead to complex intact-cell CaMKII effects, such as the frequency dependence of contractility and relaxation[355,356] because of the inherent Ca^{2+} dependence and memory of the Ca^{2+}-CaM-CaMKII system, as well as (in analogy with PKA) simultaneous phosphorylation of multiple targets, including DHPR and PLB.

Dual role of phosphatases

E-C coupling is controlled by a dynamic balance between phosphorylated and dephosphorylated states of key proteins including RyR, PLB and DHPR. In intact cells, the basal state of phosphorylation seems to be partial, as evidenced by depression of Ca^{2+} release with phosphatases PP1 or 2A[357] or enhancement with corresponding phosphatase inhibitors.[358] This seems parallel and consistent with the effects of PKA and CaMKII activation to be generally stimulatory with respect to to E-C coupling (as above). Surprisingly, application of exogenous phosphatase has been reported to increase P_o in bilayers and Ca^{2+} spark frequency in permeabilized cells.[359] It is not clear how these interesting results can be reconciled with the activation by kinases. One might speculate that strong phosphatase activity might destabilize RyR by dephosphorylating a site that is otherwise always phosphorylated (e.g. perhaps a structural site which allows the RyR to function normally). Of course normal phosphatase function in intact cells, like PKA- and CaMKII-mediated phosphorylation, is subject to the same feedbacks and autoregulation, and parallel effects on Ca^{2+} influx and SR Ca^{2+} loading in the steady state.[318,359]

CONCLUDING REMARKS

As part of a massive macromolecular complex, the cardiac RyR channel is physically located to mediate and regulate a key step in E-C coupling, amplified Ca^{2+} release. Although the potent direct effects of dynamic regulators such as PKA and CaM/CaMKII on isolated RyRs may be partially limited by negative feedbacks inherent in intact cells, they are still evident and appear to participate in the orchestration of a control strategy which achieves finely graded regulation of global E-C coupling during physiological activity.

ACKNOWLEDGEMENTS

Supported by NIH grants HL-30077, HL-64098 and HL-64724.

Chapter 11

STABILITY AND INSTABILITY OF Ca^{2+} RELEASE FROM THE SR

Mary E. Díaz, Stephen C. O'Neill, Andrew W. Trafford, and David A. Eisner
Unit of Cardiac Physiology, University of Manchester, 1.524 Stopford Building, Oxford Rd, Manchester M13 9PT, UK

INTRODUCTION

As discussed in many other chapters in this book, release of calcium during systole occurs through the ryanodine receptor (RyR) via the process of calcium-induced calcium release (CICR). On this mechanism (Fig. 11-1 A), the entry of a small amount of Ca^{2+} into the cell via the L-type Ca^{2+} current results in the release of a considerably larger amount from the sarcoplasmic reticulum (SR) (see Bers[1] for review). The amount of calcium released depends on at least three factors: (1) The size of the L-type Ca^{2+} current; (2) the properties of the RyR and, in particular, their sensitivity to activation by Ca; (3) the calcium content of the SR. It is changes in these factors that will be important in disease. In this article we focus on these control points and how they affect systolic Ca^{2+}. In particular, we emphasize the factors that determine the stability of control. First, however, it is important to discuss how SR Ca^{2+} content is controlled.

THE CONTROL OF SR CA^{2+} CONTENT

At its simplest, the SR Ca^{2+} content depends on the balance between the amount released (via the RyR) and the amount taken up from the cytoplasm (by the SR Ca^{2+}-ATPase, SERCA). Therefore anything which increases the opening of the RyR would be expected to decrease SR Ca^{2+} content.

Conversely, agents that increase the rate of SERCA (by phosphorylation of the regulatory protein phospholamban)[360] increase SR content. However it is also clear that, while modulation of SERCA and the RyR will affect the actual level of SR Ca^{2+} reached, other factors are responsible for the fact that SR Ca^{2+} can be controlled and, as we will see later, whether or not this control is stable.

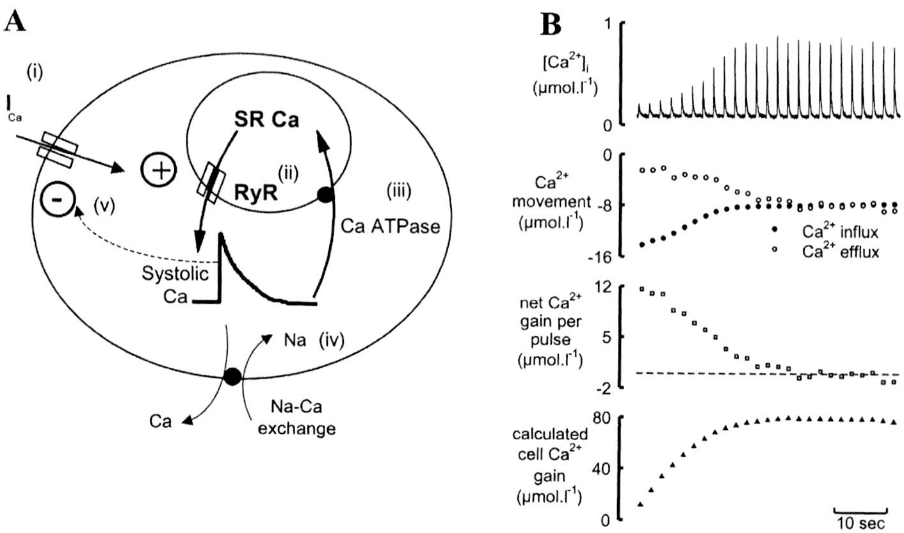

Figure 11-1. **Steps involved in calcium induced calcium release and regulation of SR content. A**. The diagram shows: (i) entry of Ca^{2+} via the L-type current (I_{Ca}); (ii) release of Ca^{2+} from the SR through the ryanodine receptor (RyR); (iii) uptake of Ca^{2+} into the SR by the Ca^{2+}-ATPase; (iv) efflux of Ca^{2+} from the cell via Na^+-Ca^{2+} exchange. As the amplitude of the Ca^{2+} transient increases more Ca^{2+} is pumped out of the cell (iv) and there is greater Ca^{2+}-dependent inactivation of the Ca^{2+}-current decreasing Ca^{2+} entry (v). The three control points described in the text (I_{Ca}, SR Ca^{2+} content and RyR) are shown in bold. **B**. Measurement of sarcolemmal Ca^{2+} fluxes during recovery of SR Ca^{2+}. Caffeine had previously been added to deplete SR Ca^{2+} and then removed. Stimulation was begun at the start of the record shown. Panels show (from top to bottom): $[Ca^{2+}]_i$; sarcolemmal Ca^{2+} fluxes (influx on L-type Ca^{2+} current, efflux on NCX); net gain per pulse calculated as influx – efflux; cumulative Ca^{2+} gain calculated by summing net gains per pulse. Modified from Trafford *et al.*[361]

It is important to realize that SR Ca^{2+} content can only be kept at a constant level if the entry of Ca^{2+} into the cell from the extracellular fluid (largely via the L-type Ca^{2+} current) has exactly the same magnitude as the efflux (largely via Na^+-Ca^{2+} exchange, NCX). If the entry is larger than the efflux then the cell and therefore the SR will gain Ca^{2+}. The interaction between the control of SR and cytoplasmic Ca^{2+} is shown in Fig. 11-1 B. In this experiment the SR had previously been emptied of calcium by exposure to caffeine. Caffeine was removed and then, at the start of the record shown, stimulation recommenced. The Ca^{2+} transient was initially small, presumably because the SR Ca^{2+} content was low. However, over the time-course of a few beats, the Ca^{2+} transient increased in amplitude to a steady level (top panel). These changes of the amplitude of the calcium transient are accompanied by changes of membrane current. As shown in the second panel of Fig. 11-1 B, as the amplitude of the Ca^{2+} transient increases, the Ca^{2+} entry via the L-type Ca^{2+} current decreases and the efflux on NCX efflux increases.[361] In the steady state, efflux and influx are exactly balanced. The lower panels of Fig. 11-1 B show that, at first there is a net influx of Ca^{2+} on each pulse and, in the steady state there is no net flux. These changes of net flux result in a calculated SR gain of Ca^{2+} (bottom panel). This result shows that measured changes of Ca^{2+} influx and efflux account for significant changes of SR Ca^{2+} content. The decrease of entry of Ca^{2+} is due to increased Ca^{2+}-dependent inactivation of the L-type Ca^{2+} current due to the increased Ca^{2+} transient.[362-364] The increase of efflux is a result of the larger Ca^{2+} transients, thereby increasing the activation of the NCX. The fact that an increase of amplitude of the systolic Ca^{2+} transient increases Ca^{2+} efflux and decreases influx provides an important mechanism for controlling SR Ca^{2+} as follows. An increase in SR Ca^{2+} content will increase the amplitude of the Ca^{2+} transient and this, in turn, will increase Ca^{2+} efflux and decrease Ca^{2+} influx (steps iv and v respectively of the scheme of Fig. 11-1 A). These changes of membrane flux will therefore tend to lower SR Ca^{2+} back towards the initial level. While the exact level of SR Ca^{2+} reached will depend on the properties of the RyR and SERCA, the ability to maintain a steady SR content depends on this simple homeostatic mechanism whereby changes of SR Ca^{2+} content affect the amplitude of the systolic transient and hence the sarcolemmal fluxes.

CONTROL POINTS FOR REGULATING THE AMPLITUDE OF THE CA^{2+} TRANSIENT

In the introduction we pointed out the three factors that affect the amplitude of the Ca^{2+} transient. We will briefly consider these in turn.

The SR Ca^{2+} content

As shown in Fig. 11-1 B (an increase of SR Ca^{2+} content results in an increase of the amplitude of the systolic Ca^{2+} transient. Several studies have shown that the relationship can be steep)[208,317,361,365] and we have found that the amplitude of the Ca^{2+} transient is proportional to the cube of SR content.[366] This steep dependence may be due, in part, to the fact that the open probability of the RyR is increased by an increase of the Ca^{2+} content of the SR.[213,367] The SR Ca^{2+} content, in turn will depend on the balance between Ca^{2+} entry into the cell and efflux from the cell. Therefore maneuvres that decrease Ca^{2+} efflux result in Ca^{2+} overload of the SR, spontaneous release and arrhythmias.[368]

The properties of the RyR

Agents that increase the open probability (P_o) of the RyR (such as caffeine or BDM) produce a *transient* potentiation of the amplitude of the systolic Ca^{2+} transient.[366,369,370] In the steady state the amplitude of the Ca^{2+} transient in the presence of these agents is the same as in the control. The transient nature of these effects arises because the potentiation of release decreases SR Ca^{2+} content. Conversely, depressing RyR opening with either tetracaine or acidification results in only a transient decrease of the Ca^{2+} transient.[371,372]

The amplitude of the L-type Ca^{2+} current

The L-type current has two roles in calcium induced calcium release. First, it triggers Ca^{2+} release from the SR and second it contributes to loading the cell and therefore the SR with Ca^{2+}.[373] We have found that changes of external Ca^{2+} concentration that have large effects on the amplitude of the L-type Ca^{2+} current and the Ca^{2+} transient have very little effect on the SR Ca^{2+} content. Indeed lowering external Ca^{2+} from 2.0 to 0.2 mM resulted in a small *increase* of SR Ca^{2+} content.[321] The relative lack of effect of external Ca^{2+} on SR content reflects the fact that the increased trigger function (which will tend to decrease SR content- like caffeine) is balanced by the increased loading (which will increase content).

INSTABILITY AND ALTERNANS

In the previous sections of this article, we have emphasised how simple homeostatic mechanisms regulate SR Ca^{2+}. However, it is a general property of such feedback mechanisms that they do not always behave in a stable manner. Indeed if there are delays in the system and the gain is too high then instabilities can result. In the case of the system shown in Fig. 11-1 A, the gain is equivalent to the change of net sarcolemmal flux divided by the initiating change of SR Ca^{2+} content. This, in turn, depends on a combination of (a) the dependence of Ca^{2+} release from the SR on the Ca^{2+} content and (b) the fraction of this released Ca^{2+} that is pumped out of the cell rather than returned into the SR. Previous modelling has shown that if relationship (a) is made steeper then instabilities result.[374,375] One can argue that the advantage of a steep dependence of Ca^{2+} release on SR content is that it provides a sensitive means whereby small changes of SR content can have large effects on the amplitude of the Ca^{2+} transient. The disadvantage of a very steep relationship is that instabilities may result.

One form of instability is that of mechanical alternans in which identical stimuli alternately produce large and small contractions (see Euler[376] for review), associated with alternans of the amplitude of the underlying Ca^{2+} transients.[377] Alternans is seen clinically in heart failure[378-380] and experimentally in ischaemia and acidosis.[381,382] One obvious question is whether the above model of alternans (couched in terms of increased feedback gain) can account for the fact that acidosis and related conditions produces alternans. Indeed it is not immediately obvious how this model can explain the fact that acidosis[381] or metabolic inhibition[383] produce alternans since both manoeuvres would be expected to decrease RyR P_o.[272] The question then is what effect does decreasing RyR P_o *per se* have on the probability of alternans occurring?

The effects of reducing RyR P_o on alternans

In order to investigate this question, we have investigated the effects of specifically decreasing RyR P_o with the local anaesthetic tetracaine. As shown by the confocal linescans of Fig. 11-2 A, this results in a subcellular alternans. Thus the region with the greatest Ca^{2+} release in c has little release in d and, conversely, those regions that release in d did not do so in c. The traces labelled as i and ii below emphasise the discordant nature of this subcellular alternans. Fig. 11-2 B shows another line-scan in tetracaine. This shows that there are two phases of Ca^{2+} release. The first is more or less uniform throughout the cell whereas the second spreads as a wave through part of the cell. The superimposed specimen traces below demonstrate that the second phase of release reaches region i before ii and never enters region iii. Similar results were found when intracellular acidification was used to decrease RyR P_o.[384] These results therefore show that the large local responses in this alternans require wave propagation. This is important because wave propagation is known to occur only above a threshold SR Ca^{2+} content.[385] This result therefore raises the possibility that the threshold nature of wave propagation produces a steepening of the relationship between SR content and Ca^{2+} release. Wave propagation (in this case radially into the cell) has also been observed in alternans in atrial cells.[383]

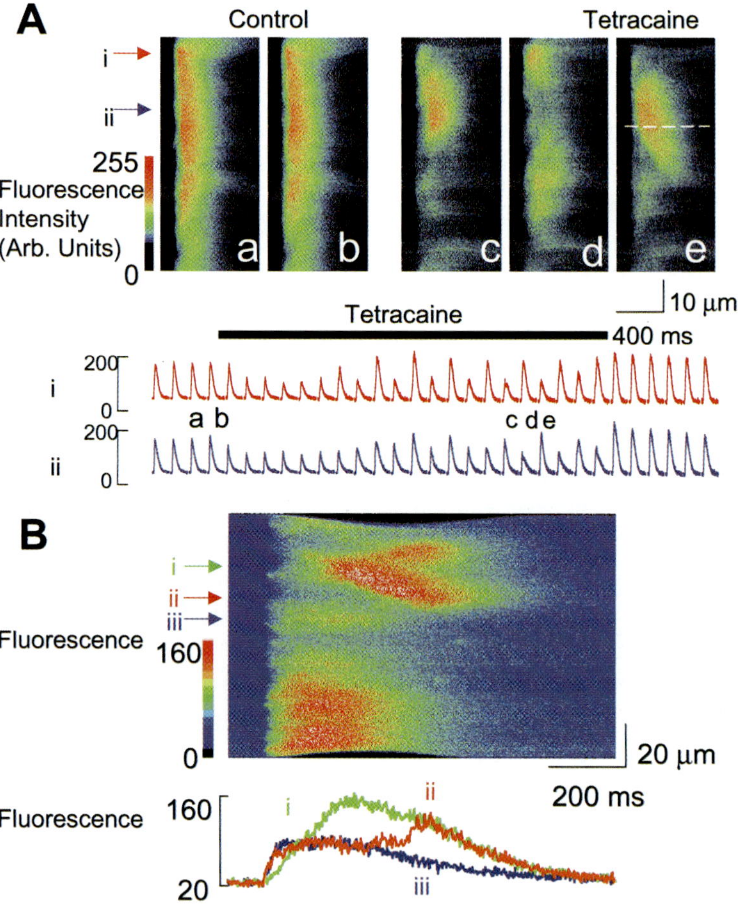

Figure 11-2. **Local alternans produced by tetracaine. A**. Linescans a and b were obtained in control and the others in 50 μM tetracaine. In each panel a 100 ms duration depolarizing pulse was applied from –40 to 0 mV. Traces i & ii (below) represent the fluorescence measured at the points indicated. **B**. Linescan in the presence of tetracaine with (below) three specimen fluorescence records from the points indicated. Modified from Diaz *et al.*[384]

Does SR Ca^{2+} content alternate?

As described above, the hypothesis for alternans depends on a beat-to-beat alternation of SR Ca^{2+} content. However it has also been suggested that alternans may be due to beat-to-beat alternation of the release process of calcium from the SR rather than the content.[383]

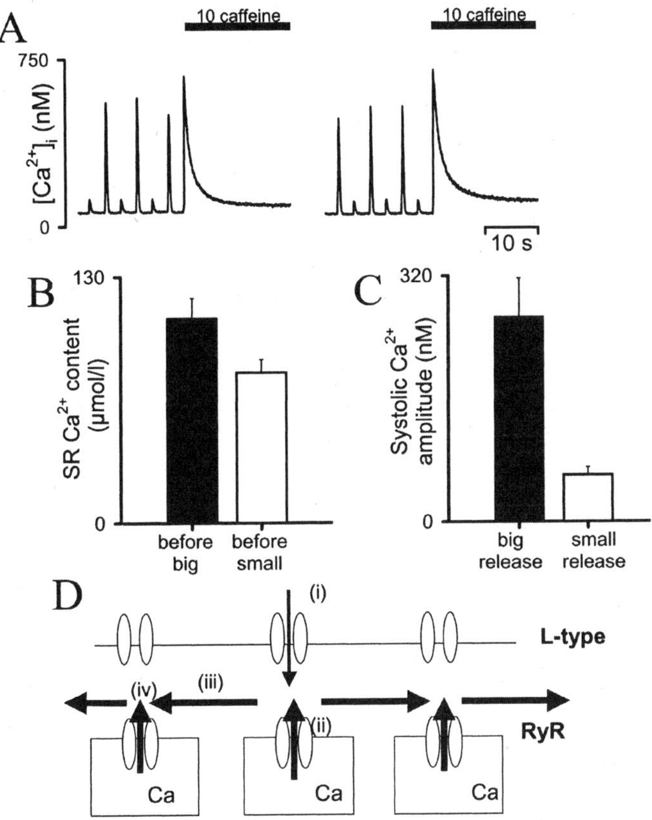

Figure 11-3. **Alternation of SR Ca^{2+} content. A**. Original data. The cell was stimulated with a 10 mV depolarizing pulse (see text) resulting in alternans. Stimulation was stopped after either a large (left) or small Ca^{2+} transient (right pulse) in order to measure SR content. Note that the caffeine response is larger following the small transient. **B.** SR Ca^{2+} content is greater before a big than a small transient but the fractional change is less than that of systolic Ca^{2+}. **C**. Data taken from.[386] **D**. Model. Ca^{2+} enters via the L-type current (i) inducing Ca^{2+} release from a "coupled" RyR (ii). On the first pulse SR Ca^{2+} content is above a threshold value and this Ca^{2+} spreads as a wave (iii) and activates release from other RyRs (iv). As a result of consequent loss of Ca^{2+} from the cell, on the next pulse the SR Ca^{2+} content will be below threshold and the initial release of Ca^{2+} (ii) will not be able to produce a wave. The smaller response will therefore lead to an increase of SR content and thence alternans.

Measurement of SR Ca^{2+} content during alternans induced by tetracaine or acidification is complicated by the subcellular heterogeneity of the alternans. We have therefore recently developed an alternative model of alternans. To do this we use small amplitude (10 mV) depolarizing pulses from a resting potential of –40 mV (in the presence of elevated external Ca^{2+} concentration, 5 mM). As shown in Fig. 11-3, this stimulation protocol results in alternans.[386] This figure also shows that the SR Ca^{2+} content is greater at the time of the large than the small Ca^{2+} transient and, therefore, that the alternans of Ca^{2+} transient amplitude is, indeed, accompanied by alternans of SR content. Figs. 11-3 B+C show that the rather small fractional alternation of SR Ca^{2+} content is accompanied by a much larger change of Ca^{2+} transient amplitude. As discussed in the original paper,[386] this is a steeper dependence of Ca^{2+} transient amplitude on SR content than is seen under control conditions. Again, this steep dependence seems to be due to the fact that the larger Ca^{2+} transients require wave propagation and a small change of SR Ca^{2+} content about the threshold level therefore determines whether or not propagation occurs. A diagram of what may be happening in alternans is shown in Fig. 11-3 D. With small depolarizing pulses, only a small fraction of L-type Ca^{2+} channels open (i) and therefore only a small fraction of RyRs are activated (ii). If the SR Ca^{2+} content is above the threshold level then Ca^{2+} release will spread as a wave from the open RyR (iii) and activate other RyRs (iv) leading to wave propagation. The Ca^{2+} wave will decrease SR Ca^{2+} as some Ca^{2+} is pumped out of the cell thereby decreasing SR content to below the threshold level. As a consequence wave propagation will not occur on the next stimulus. Little Ca^{2+} will be lost and the SR will therefore refill with Ca^{2+} to a level at which wave propagation can occur on the next beat. Repetition of these events will thereby produce alternans. In this model of alternans, the fact that only a small fraction of the L-type channels are opened results in the opening of only a small fraction of RyRs. This model can also account for the fact that agents such as acid pH and tetracaine also produce alternans associated with wave propagation. In this case many L-type Ca^{2+} channels will open, however the intrinsic depressed P_o of the RyR means that only a small number of RyRs will be activated. In contrast, when small depolarizing pulses are used, the RyR has a normal sensitivity but the reduced opening of the L-type channel results in reduced RyR opening. The common factor in the two circumstances is therefore the decreased opening of the RyR.

CONCLUDING REMARKS

As reviewed above, the SR Ca^{2+} content is a major factor determining the amplitude of the systolic Ca^{2+} transient and hence the heart beat. Since the Ca^{2+} transient affects sarcolemmal fluxes, this provides an important mechanism to control SR Ca^{2+} content. However, we suggest that excessive feedback gain may result in alternans. One circumstance that produces increased feedback gain is a decrease in the open probability of the RyR. Here, the increased feedback gain is due to the fact that, when the RyR P_o is decreased, only a small fraction of RyRs are initially activated and activation of the majority of RyRs depends on propagation of waves of CICR. Future work needs to address the question of whether this experimental model of alternans is relevant to clinically observed *pulsus alternans*. Furthermore it is as yet unclear how alternans is synchronized between cells in the heart.

ACKNOWLEDGMENTS

Work from the author's laboratory was funded by The British Heart Foundation.

Chapter 12

RYANODINE RECEPTORS IN SMOOTH MUSCLE

Steven O. Marx
Division of Cardiology and Center for Molecular Cardiology; Depts. of Medicine and Pharmacology, Columbia University College of Physicians and Surgeons, New York, NY

INTRODUCTION

Ca^{2+} signaling in smooth muscle is complex and is important for the regulation of diverse cellular processes including differentiation, proliferation, gene expression, contraction and apoptosis. The high incidence of stroke and hypertension in the United States remains a leading indication for visits to physicians, and the use of prescription drugs and morbidity/mortality. Chronic blood pressure elevation leads to end-organ damage, including the eye, cardiac, and central nervous system. Blood pressure for instance is dependent upon smooth muscle tone within resistance vessels. Smooth muscle cell contractile tone is critically dependent upon intracellular Ca^{2+} ($[Ca^{2+}]_i$).

Ca^{2+} enters the smooth muscle cytoplasmic compartment through plasma membrane ion channels[387] and Ca^{2+} release channels (ryanodine receptor (RyR) and inositol 1,4,5 trisphosphate receptor (IP_3R)) on the sarcoplasmic reticulum (SR). External Ca^{2+} can enter the cell through voltage dependent Ca^{2+} channels (VDCC) on the membrane or Ca^{2+} permeable cation channels. In smooth muscle, the spatiotemporal pattern of Ca^{2+} release is believed to enable the specificity of Ca^{2+} signaling. The architecture of the smooth muscle is thought to play an important role in this process through the localization of ion channels and pumps, contractile elements, mitochondria and SR[388]. Three distinct Ca^{2+} signaling modalites have been identified in smooth muscle: global cytosolic Ca^{2+}, propagating Ca^{2+} waves and Ca^{2+} sparks.[389]

Global intracellular Ca^{2+} levels lead to smooth muscle cell contraction. However, compared to striated muscle, contraction is slower and myofilaments do not demonstrate the organized patterns seen in striated muscle. Ca^{2+} binds to calmodulin, which then activates myosin light chain kinase (MLCK), which phosphorylates serine19 of myosin light chain, thereby releasing inhibition of myosin ATPase.[390-392] ATP hydrolysis ensues, leading to the sliding of myosin on actin filaments to generate force. In vascular smooth muscle, the dynamic range of $[Ca^{2+}]_i$ is narrow, ranging from approximately 100 nM when the artery is maximally dilated to 350 nM when arteries are maximally constricted.[393] In arterial myocytes, the opening of the L-type Ca^{2+} channel, modulated by the membrane potential plays a critical role in the establishment of global Ca^{2+} concentration. Neurotransmitters, hormones and other agonists cause the release of Ca^{2+} from internal stores after the activation of phospholipase C, which generates both diacylglycerol (DAG) and IP_3, which activates IP_3R.[390] Thus IP_3R play an important role in pharmaco-mechanical coupling. While the role of IP_3R in agonist induced contraction has been well-established in the literature, the role of the RyR in smooth muscle has only recently been elucidated.[394] In general, the role for the internal stores of Ca^{2+} is limited in smooth muscle, responsible for the initial phase of contraction.

Propagating Ca^{2+} waves are the result of intracellular Ca^{2+} release through the RyR and/or IP_3R. They can be induced by caffeine, pH changes and vasoconstrictors such as norepinephrine and UTP.[395-399] Most reports suggest that the waves occur asynchronously within the vessel wall although synchronization with neighboring smooth muscle cells to modulate vasomotion has been reported.[398,400] In addition, Ca^{2+} waves have been reported to lead to both depolarization (potentially through activation of chloride channels) or hyperpolarization/relaxation (through activation of large conductance Ca^{2+} activated K^+ channels; BKCa, Maxi-K; see below). Therefore, the physiologic significance of Ca^{2+} waves has not been definitively determined.

Ca^{2+} sparks are transient local increases in intracellular Ca^{2+} that occur through the coordinated opening of a group of RyR located on the SR.[394] The global Ca^{2+} concentration does not materially change from a Ca^{2+} spark, but modulate the neighboring plasma membrane BKCa channels, thereby causing hyperpolarization of the membrane (Fig. 12-1). In cerebral artery myocytes, Ca^{2+} sparks lead to activation of the BKCa channel, thus providing an important feedback role in the regulation of pressure-induced constriction.[394] Vasodilators may act in part through increasing the frequency of Ca^{2+} sparks. Moreover, recent studies have suggested that Ca^{2+} sparks may influence gene expression (see below).[401,402]

The SR Ca^{2+} stores in smooth muscle are classified based on the arrangement of IP_3R and RyR. Conflicting evidence exists regarding their number and types. For instance, a single Ca^{2+} store has been proposed, based upon the findings that caffeine prevented IP-mediated Ca^{2+} release.[398,403-405] Two separate stores have also been proposed, based upon the findings that depletion of RyR-sensitive stores failed to abolish agonist dependent IP_3 mediated Ca^{2+} release.[406] Other arrangements are possible for instance, with two stores, one expressing both intracellular Ca^{2+} release channels and the other store only expressing one. Diversity can exist in the source of Ca^{2+} uptake, for instance in colonic myocytes, the existence of two Ca^{2+} stores has been proposed, with one containing only RyR and refilled from cytoplasmic Ca^{2+}, whereas the other store expressing both RyR and IP_3R and is dependent upon external Ca^{2+} for refilling.[403]

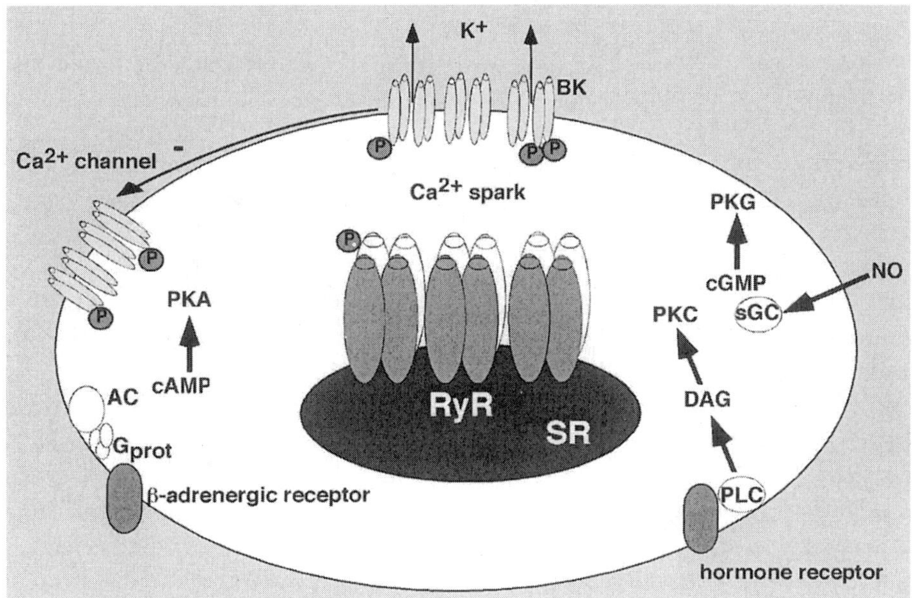

Figure 12-1. **Schematic of smooth muscle cell demonstrating relationship between RyR and BK channel.** Ca^{2+} sparks lead to activation of BK channel, causing inhibition of the L-type Ca^{2+} channel. All three ion channels are regulated by phosphorylation by PKA, PKC and PKG.

RYR ISOFORMS IN SMOOTH MUSCLE

Initially, the identification and characterization of RyR in smooth muscle was performed with pharmacological tools, such as caffeine and ryanodine. The presence of RyR in smooth muscle was first suggested utilizing caffeine, which caused transient contractures of the muscle in the absence of extracellular Ca^{2+}.[407] Micromolar administration of ryanodine in combination with caffeine produced almost a complete depletion of caffeine-sensitive stores in skinned guinea pig smooth muscle of pulmonary artery, portal vein and taenia caeci.[408] The effect of ryanodine on smooth muscle RyR have been studied in the planar lipid bilayer with different findings; in toad smooth muscle, RyR display the typical subconductance state in response to micromolar ryanodine;[409] in contrast, ryanodine was not reported to induce the subconductance state in RyR isolated from aorta or coronary artery smooth muscle, but millimolar concentrations did fully inhibit the channel activity (up to 10 μM activated channel activity without subconductance state).[410,411] It is not clear why differences in ryanodine sensitivity and effects were demonstrated.

All three RyR isoforms have been reported in smooth muscle[10,12,412] although the relative proportion of each isoform varies between tissues. The determination of the isoform expression has mostly been shown using northern or non-quantitative RT-PCR techniques from tissues with multiple cell-types.

The expression of RyR2 and RyR3 has been demonstrated using immunoblot analysis.[409] The identification of particular RyR isoforms needs to be interpreted with caution since contamination by other cells is possible.[413] Channels from aortic and visceral smooth muscle have been recorded, consistent with the biophysical and pharmacologic properties of the RyR.[409,410,414]

Immunofluorescence and immunoelectron microscopy have confirmed the expression of RyR in smooth muscle.[415-417] In the aorta and vas deferens, a mesh-like immunostaining was observed and in vascular smooth muscle myocytes, peripheral expression of RyR2 was noted, which overlapped with the location of the L-type Ca^{2+} channel.[414,418] In the vas deferens, a more punctate RyR expression was noted, which contrasted with the more diffuse staining of the L-type Ca^{2+} channel.[417] In non-pregnant myometrial cells, only RyR3 was noted, diffusely expressed throughout the cytoplasm.[419] The diffuse expression pattern in smooth muscle is in marked contrast to the organized arrangement of RyR in skeletal and cardiac muscle.[279]

The physiologic role of each of the isoforms of the RyR is lacking. Arterial smooth muscle derived from a RyR3 null mouse demonstrated a normal contractile response to caffeine and norepinephrine.[51] However, in another study, Ca^{2+} spark frequency was markedly higher in cerebral artery smooth muscle derived from the RyR3 null mice, suggesting that RyR3 can inhibit spark frequency.[420,421] Further study of RyR3 function is clearly warranted. The respective roles of RyR2 and RyR1 in smooth muscle have been incompletely elucidated,[23,422] in part because RyR2 null mice are lethal.[423]

In rat portal vein myocytes, antisense oligonucleotides targeting each of the RyR isoforms demonstrated that both RyR1 and RyR2 are required for myocytes to respond to membrane depolarization with Ca^{2+} sparks and global increase in intracellular Ca^{2+}.[424]. However, in contrast to the RyR3 null animal data, antisense of RyR3 did not alter Ca^{2+} spark frequency, which may be due to the fact that RyR3 may only respond to caffeine in conditions of increased SR Ca^{2+} loading.[413,419,424,425]

IDENTIFICATION OF RYR-MEDIATED Ca^{2+} RELEASE

Initial functional studies identified caffeine-induced ryanodine-sensitive Ca^{2+} release in vascular and non-vascular smooth muscle preparations.[426-428] Prior to the identification of Ca^{2+} sparks, electrophysiology studies suggested the presence of an interaction between Ca^{2+} released from the SR and large conductance K^+ channels on the plasma membrane.[389] Spontaneous transient outward currents (STOC) were first described in smooth muscle by Bolton and coworkers[429,430] and have been shown in a diverse group of vascular and non-vascular smooth muscle.[394,416,431-436] Activation of the BKCa channel underlie the transient outward current induced hyperpolarization of the plasma membrane. Each transient outward current represents the activation of 10-100 BKCa channels.[437] BKCa channel current was abolished by ryanodine[410] and depletion of SR Ca^{2+} stores by thapsigargin.[438] The finding that BKCa channel activity can be dissociated from global Ca^{2+} concentrations suggested that the localized Ca^{2+} release from the RyR may occur in smooth muscle in the absence of a detectable change in global Ca^{2+}.[439]

Nelson and colleagues obtained the first evidence of Ca^{2+} sparks in smooth muscle, which were found to occur at a frequency of 1 Hz near the cell membrane.[394] Similar findings have been shown in numerous smooth muscle cells derived from arteries, portal vein, urinary bladder, gastro-intestinal tract, airway and gallbladder.[440-446] The sparks had a spatial spread of a few square microns, were transient, with a rise time of 20 ms and half time of decay of 50 ms. Therefore, each spark was calculated to cause < 2 nM rise in global Ca^{2+}.[394] The sparks were abolished by ryanodine, and agents that depleted SR Ca^{2+} stores also reduced Ca^{2+} spark frequency.

Although the sparks can occur for a period of time in the absence of extracellular Ca^{2+} or blockade of L-type Ca^{2+} channel, Ca^{2+} spark activity is not independent of the level of Ca^{2+} influx into the cytosol or the global Ca^{2+} levels.[394,447] RyR activity increases in response to cytosolic and luminal SR Ca^{2+} levels. For instance, when SR Ca^{2+} levels reach >80% capacity, a very steep relationship exists between SR Ca^{2+} and spark frequency, and thus indirectly BKCa channel activity.[447] Consistent with the influence of SR Ca^{2+} load, arterial smooth muscle derived from phospholamban null mouse demonstrated an increased Ca^{2+} spark frequency.[448] Depolarization of the membrane (thereby increasing Ca^{2+} stores) increased both Ca^{2+} spark frequency and amplitude; in urinary bladder smooth muscle, the increase of Ca^{2+} spark frequency is likely due to both an increase in SR Ca^{2+} load as well as increase in RyR activity due to elevated cytoplasmic Ca^{2+} (loose coupling; see below).[389,442,449]

PHYSIOLOGIC ROLE OF RYR IN SMOOTH MUSCLE

The role of RyR's in smooth muscle is not clearly elucidated. RyR has been demonstrated to be involved in the amplification of the Ca^{2+} transient originating from activation of L-type Ca^{2+} channel or IP_3R, and/or participate in relaxation through BKCa channel activation. In this section, we will review the physiologic relevance of RyR activation.

Excitation-contraction coupling

As stated above, membrane depolarization increases $[Ca^{2+}]_i$ through VDCC opening. However, this Ca^{2+} is insufficient to induce contraction, potentially due to Ca^{2+} buffering.[450,451] Therefore, the existence of an additional source of Ca^{2+} is required, most likely through the SR. Several possible mechanisms for the amplification have been investigated: (1) Ca^{2+} from the VDCC and membrane depolarization leads to increased IP_3 production, thereby activating IP_3R[452-454]. However, heparin, an IP_3R antagonist did not reduce the Ca^{2+} transient in response to membrane depolarization.[449,455] (2) Activation of RyR by CICR, which has been shown in cardiac muscle.[200] The first direct evidence of CICR in smooth muscle was derived in experiments in skinned smooth muscle bundles (taenia caeci), in which a Mg^{2+} and pH dependent Ca^{2+} release was observed that was steeply dependent upon Ca^{2+} and augmented by caffeine.[456] However, it was suggested that CICR might not be a primary release mechanism because of the high Ca^{2+} concentration (~ 1 μM) required for activation of CICR and to induce contraction.[414,456] The CICR in smooth muscle has been termed "loose coupling" to indicate the non-obligate characteristics, in contrast to the "tight coupling" seen in cardiac and skeletal muscle. The loose coupling provides an effective way to integrate the degree of neural, humoral or local activation of the VDCC.[414] CICR is not universally present in all smooth muscle cells.[413] The characteristics of loose coupling are:

(1) release is focal, arising from individual areas of the cell.[457]

(2) CICR is delayed in smooth muscle, as the amplication is only evident 50-100 ms after VDCC activation, as compared to a time constant ~7 ms in cardiac cells.[449,458,459]

(3) The coupling is non-obligate; CICR is dependent upon net Ca^{2+} flux rather than VDCC open probability.[414]

There are several concerns with the loose coupling hypothesis: the RyR Ca^{2+} sensitivity may be insufficient to activate the channels and that an unstable condition may develop due to the lack of adequate RyR control.[413] Furthermore, the interactions between the IP_3R and RyR remain controversial, perhaps dependent upon the cell-type and conditions utilized.

Smooth muscle cell relaxation

Arterial blood pressure is determined by several factors, including vascular tone, which represents the contractile activity of smooth muscle within the walls of resistance vessels (small arteries and arterioles). The modulation of the contractile state of smooth muscle is organized through the interplay of vasoconstrictor and vasodilatory neurohormones and by blood pressure itself (the Bayliss effect; constriction of the vessel after an increase in transmural pressure).[460-462] The autoregulatory Bayliss effect is based upon graded membrane depolarization in response to pressure, which activates VDCC, causing vasoconstriction.

It has been proposed that increased global $[Ca^{2+}]_i$ not only triggers contraction, but a compensatory increase in Ca^{2+} spark frequency, thereby activating the BKCa channels, leading to relaxation (Fig. 12-1).[394] Thus, the RyR (Ca^{2+} spark)-BKCa channel can be viewed as a mechanism to limit smooth muscle contraction. Ca^{2+} spark frequency is increased when intravascular pressure is elevated from 10 to 60 mm Hg in rat cerebral arteries.[463] Inhibition of RyR or BKCa channels has been demonstrated to lead to pressure-induced cerebral artery constriction.[418,464] Consistent with the functional effects, co-localization studies have confirmed zones within smooth muscle in which RyR and BKCa channels are very close situated spatially.[465] However, BKCa channels can also be activated by Ca^{2+} influx through VDCC; Ca^{2+} sparks can also activate Ca^{2+} dependent chloride channels, which can induce membrane depolarization and smooth muscle contraction.[466] The source of Ca^{2+} for activation of the BKCa channel has been the subject of significant investigation. Several studies have suggested a functional linkage between the BKCa channel and VDCC and/or RyR.[394,467] In vascular smooth muscle, the activation of L-type Ca^{2+} channel can increase $[Ca^{2+}]_i$ in the environment of a neighboring BKCa channel leading to its activation.[465] Activation of BKCa channels was independent of RyR activity and could be inhibited by nifedipine. In urinary bladder smooth muscle, steady state BKCa channel activity was found to be highly dependent upon Ca^{2+} entry through VDCC, whereas transient activity required local communication with RyR through Ca^{2+} sparks.[467] Consistent with these findings, recently we have identified a macromolecular complex between L-type Ca^{2+} channel and BKCa channels, mediated by the β2-adrenergic receptor (β2AR) in brain and smooth muscle (Fig. 12-2).[468] Targeting of β2AR to the BKCa channel can therefore serve two purposes: (1) anchoring of phosphorylation modulatory proteins to the channel and (2) recruitment of VDCC to the complex to contribute a source of Ca^{2+} for BKCa channel activation (Fig. 12-2).

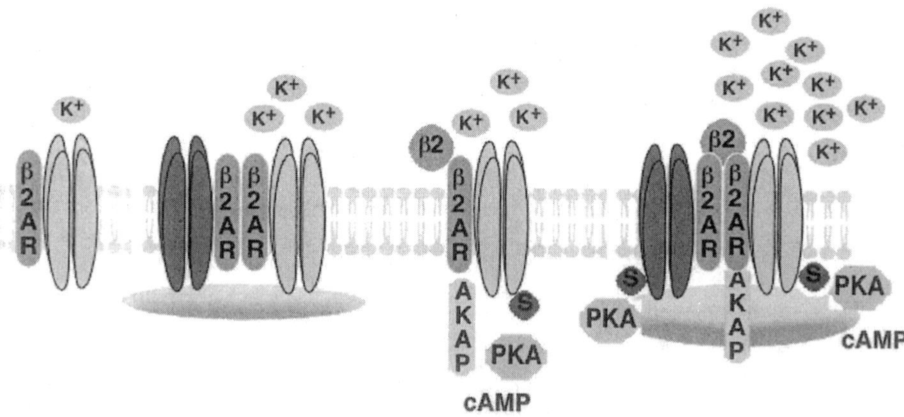

Figure 12-2. **Schematic representing interaction between β2-adrenergic receptor (β2AR), BKCa (light grey) and L-type Ca^{2+} (dark grey) channels within the plasma membrane.** β2AR associates with the BKCa channel, thereby recruiting an AKAP into the macromolecular complex. A β2 agonist can activate adenylyl cyclase (not shown) thereby increasing cAMP in the environment around the channel. PKA is activated, phosphorylating both the L-type Ca^{2+} and BKCa channels, leading to increased efflux of K^+, and hyperpolarization of the plasma membrane. Concomitantly, RyR and phospholamban (not shown) may be phosphorylated, leading to further increases in Ca^{2+} spark frequency and activation of BKCa channels. The association of L-type Ca^{2+} channel with the BKCa channel complex can lead to phosphorylation-dependent and –independent modulation of the channel.[468]

Quantitative evidence of a functional coupling between RyR and BKCa channels demonstrated that at –40 mV, greater than 96% of Ca^{2+} sparks were associated with the initiation of a transient BKCa current.[469] In general, Ca^{2+} spark and BKCa channel amplitudes were found to correlate in cerebral artery myocytes, although ~50% of BKCa currents were not associated with a detectable spark,[469] although given the techniques utilized, a small spark may have been missed. In non-vascular smooth muscle, the correlation between sparks and BKCa channel activity was significantly less than in vascular tissue.[389] Thus, Ca^{2+} sparks can deliver micromolar Ca^{2+} to localized areas of the membrane containing BKCa channels.

Recent studies utilizing the BKCa channel β1 subunit null mice have significantly increased our understanding of the interdependence of RyR and BKCa channels. Co-expression of the β1 subunit with the BKCa channel α subunit leads to ~10 folder higher Ca^{2+} sensitivity as compared to α subunit alone. BKCa channel from vascular smooth muscle cells derived from the β1 subunit knockout animals demonstrated ~100 fold lower probability of opening and Ca^{2+} spark induced BKCa channel current was significantly reduced and >1/3 of sparks failed to elicit a BKCa channel activation.[470] Moreover, both thoracic aorta and cerebral arteries from the β1 subunit null animals demonstrated more constriction compared to wild type control animals. Mean arterial pressure was elevated in the β1 subunit null animals, leading to left ventricular hypertrophy.[470] Thus, the ability of the BKCa channel to sense the Ca^{2+} sparks was impaired by the loss of the β1 subunit.

Activation of the PKA and PKG signal transduction pathways leads to 2-3 fold increases in both Ca^{2+} spark and BKCa channel activity.[436,448] Ryanodine reduced dilation to forskolin by 80%, consistent with the importance of Ca^{2+} sparks. In arterial smooth muscle derived from phospholamban null mice, forskolin had little effect compared to the ~2 fold increase in Ca^{2+} spark frequency in wild type animals.[448] Vasoconstrictors may also act in part through inhibition of Ca^{2+} sparks and BKCa channels (Fig. 12-1).[471]

Ca^{2+} sparks and gene expression in smooth muscle

Ca^{2+} entry through the VDCC leads to increased expression of immediate early response genes such as c-fos in neuronal tissues.[472,473] Likewise in myocytes, membrane depolarization leads to an increase in activated nuclear cAMP responsive element binding (CREB) and increased c-fos expression. Ca^{2+} spark inhibition by ryanodine in mouse cerebral arteries caused an increase in the percentage of nuclei staining positive for the active form of CREB and enhanced c-fos expression.[401] These effects were inhibited by a

L-type Ca^{2+} channel blocker. Increased Ca^{2+} spark activity decreases nuclear NFAT levels, but does not appear to be mediated through changes in membrane potential (as opposed to CREB/c-fos). In contrast, increased IP_3R mediated Ca^{2+} release promotes nuclear accumulation of NFAT.[402] The apparent paradox has not been completely elucidated, but suggests a complex role for SR Ca^{2+} regulation of smooth muscle gene expression.

CONCLUDING REMARKS

The role for the RyR in smooth muscle has been recently elucidated. Through a series of elegant reports, RyR have been shown to be critical for the excitation-contraction coupling, relaxation and gene expression in smooth muscle. Whereas RyR mediated Ca^{2+} release in striated muscle causes contraction, in smooth muscle it leads to relaxation in several cell-types, through the activation of the BKCa channel.

ACKNOWLEDGMENTS

This work was supported in part by grants from the N.I.H. and American Heart Association.

Chapter 13

FUNCTIONS OF RYR3 HOMOLOGUES

Yasuo Ogawa, Takashi Murayama, and Nagomi Kurebayashi
Dept. of Pharmacology, Juntendo University School of Medicine, Tokyo 113-8421, Japan

INTRODUCTION

Ryanodine receptor (RyR) is the Ca^{2+}-induced Ca^{2+} release (CICR) channel protein, which is named because of its high affinity for ryanodine in the open state. Three genetically distinct isoforms are known in mammals: RyR1, the primary isoform in skeletal muscle; RyR2, the main isoform in cardiac muscle; and RyR3, ubiquitously expressed in a minuscule amount.[110,134,228,474] In many non-mammalian vertebrate skeletal muscles, on the other hand, RyR1 and RyR3 homologues which are referred to as α-RyR and β-RyR, respectively, have been detected almost in equal amounts.[134,135,474,475] Rapidly contracting muscles such as the swimbladder muscle of fish, however, express α-RyR alone.[134] RyR3 is detected in neonate mammalian skeletal muscles, and increases in amount up to 2 weeks after birth, followed by decrease to nil in adult skeletal muscles except for diaphragm and soleus.[474]

Animals which lack RyR1 or α-RyR cannot survive after birth because of asphyxia.[23,134] RyR3 knockout mice, however, look normal except for their high speed of locomotion. They can grow up to fertile adults and have litters as usual.[51,474] During the course of growth, muscle contraction of RyR3-deficient mice was reported to be smaller than the wild type at 2 weeks after birth, but there was no difference at the adult stage.[476] Involvement of RyR3 was also suggested in the mechanism of behavior associated with hippocampal activity, because hippocampus is its preferential expression site in the brain.[474] Although important contributions such as those by Balschum *et al.*[477] and Futatsugi *et al.*[478] have been made concerning LTP, more rigid correlation between the cellular basis in hippocampal LTP and the behavioral changes is required to understand the role of RyR3. The function of RyR3 in smooth muscles is discussed in Chapter 12. In this chapter, we will be concentrate on the role of RyR3 (or β-RyR) in its coexistence with RyR1 (or α-RyR) in skeletal muscle, comparing the characteristics of these two RyR isoforms.

OCCURRENCE OF RYR3 AND β-RYR ISOFORMS

Homotetramers of RyR molecules form the Ca^{2+} release channel, the cytoplasmic part of which is referred to as the foot.[228] RyR3 cannot form a heterotetramer with RyR1, but it could do so with RyR2, at least in HEK293 cells when they were co-expressed.[479] It is notable that RyR3 purified from the brain as well as from skeletal muscle was a homotetramer.[480]

Dysgenic and dyspedic skeletal muscles which lack dihydropyridine receptor (DHPR), the voltage sensor in the T-tubule, and the RyR1 isoform, respectively, cannot contract with electrical stimulation but do show caffeine contracture. This means that RyR1 and α-RyR can release Ca^{2+} (depolarization-induced Ca^{2+} release, DICR) through voltage dependent interaction with DHPR (orthograde signaling) as well as through CICR activated by caffeine. Consistently restoration of RyR1 increases Ca^{2+} influx through DHPR and induces tetrad formation, a cluster of 4 DHPR molecules (retrograde signaling). RyR3 does not show either orthograde or retrograde signalling.[131,134,228]

Knowledge of the arrangement of RyR isoforms in the junctional SR in reference to that of DHPR in the T-tubule is critical for understanding the mechanism of excitation-contraction (EC) coupling. Feet were characteristically aligned longitudinally in two rows on the junctional face of SR in the triad.[228] The tetrads were in precise synchrony with each alternate foot (i.e., α-RyR or RyR1) in the SR. RyR3 and β-RyR were reported to be co-localized within the same triad.[481] Recently additional feet-like structures, termed parajunctional feet, were identified in one or two rows on either side of the junctional feet.[138] Interestingly, the packing arrangements were different between the two arrays. It was assumed that the parajunctional feet were made of RyR3 or β-RyR, because their occurrence was well correlated with their contents in vertebrate skeletal muscles including mammals (see Chapter 4). RyR3 heterologously expressed in 1B5 cells also formed an ordered array in a cluster.[131]

PROPERTIES OF CICR ACTIVITY OF PURIFIED RYR3

Because RyR3 heterologously expressed in 1B5 cells did not interact with DHPR, RyR3 should serve as the CICR channel.[482] Ca^{2+} dependent [^{3}H]-ryanodine binding and cation channel activity on lipid bilayer membrane were the common methods to evaluate CICR activity of RyR. As shown in Fig. 13-1, however, characteristics of Ca^{2+} dependent activity of RyR3 depend on the methods by which determinations were performed.[195] Ca^{2+} dependent [^{3}H]-ryanodine binding showed biphasic Ca^{2+} dependence: stimulatory at a range of less than 100 μM, whereas inhibitory at higher concentrations. RyR1, in comparison with RyR3, showed a higher sensitivity to activating Ca^{2+}, whereas similar sensitivity to inactivating Ca^{2+}. Takeshima *et al.*[422] reported similar results of CICR with skinned neonatal mouse skeletal muscles. β-RyR from bullfrog skeletal muscle was very similar in its Ca^{2+} dependence not only to bullfrog α-RyR but also to mammalian RyR3.[475]

In lipid bilayer membranes, in contrast, RyR3 showed entirely different channel activity.[195] The channel activity increased steeply with increase in Ca^{2+} concentration from 0.1 to 1 μM (pCa 6) where Po became ~1. In the range of pCa 6-3, Po was near 1. We can say that the Ca^{2+} dependence should be almost monophasic, and that inactivation by Ca^{2+} is very weak and can conclude that RyR3 would be more sensitive to Ca^{2+} than RyR1 on the basis of channel activity. Similar results were also reported by other investigators with purified RyR3,[483] recombinant RyR3 expressed in HEK293 cells and β-RyR from chicken and fishes (see also Murayama et al[195]). These results indicate that no stimulation by ATP or caffeine at pCa 6-5 could be observed at variance with the reported results.[422] Hereafter discussion on Ca^{2+} dependence of CICR will be primarily based on the results from Ca^{2+}-dependent [^{3}H]-ryanodine binding, because its characteristics were very similar to those for CICR in skinned fibers from neonate dyspedic mice.[422]

In Table 13-1, characteristics of RyR3 are summarized in comparison with RyR1. There was no marked difference between RyR1 and RyR3 in responses to stimulatory and inhibitory modulators. ATP and other adenine nucleotides stimulate RyR, resulting in increased activity without change in Ca^{2+} dependence. When calibrated with the peak activity, the Ca^{2+} dependence curves for various concentrations of the nucleotide were homologous. This means that Ca^{2+} is necessary for the activation, but not a sufficient condition. The adenine nucleotides also stimulate Ca^{2+} release activity in the virtual absence of Ca^{2+}.[475] Caffeine, on the other hand, has dual stimulatory actions: Ca^{2+}-sensitizing and increase in the peak activity (ATP-like effect). The Ca^{2+} sensitization is saturated at 10 mM caffeine, whereas the ATP-like action is not saturated.[475] The magnitude of stimulation, therefore, depends on the Ca^{2+} concentration where the determination was made. 4-chloro-*m*-cresol (CMC) was reported to stimulate RyR1, being ineffective on RyR3 up to 500 μM.[482] Inhibition by procaine was independent of Ca^{2+} concentration upon determination. Mg^{2+} is a competitive antagonist to activating Ca^{2+} and also an agonist to inactivating Ca^{2+}.[110,475] Therefore, the magnitude of inhibition depended on the Ca^{2+} concentration on determination. The oxidation-reduction state in the cytoplasm is also an important modulator (see Chapter 20).[484]

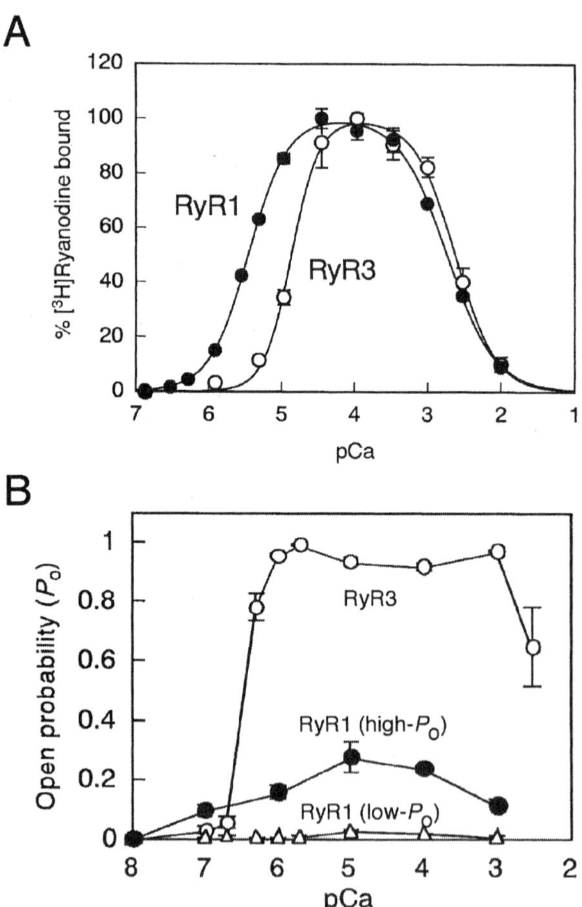

Figure 13-1. **Ca^{2+} dependent activity of purified RyR1 and RyR3.** [^{3}H]-ryanodine binding (**A**) and channel activity on lipid bilayer membrane (**B**) may show different results. In panel **A**, 100% of [^{3}H]-ryanodine binding corresponds to B/B_{max} (an averaged fractional activity of a single molecule) of 0.25 and 0.29 for RyR1 and RyR3, respectively (see also Table 13-1). Reproduced with permission from *J Biol Chem.*[195]

Table 13-1. **Comparison of properties of purified RyR1 and RyR3.**[135,195]

	RyR1	RyR3
B/B_{max} [a)]	0.25	0.29
Ca^{2+} dependence		
EC_{50} (μM)	3.5	14
IC_{50} (mM)	1.9	2.9
Mg^{2+} dependence with 0.1 mM Ca^{2+}		
IC_{50} (mM)	2.5	2.1
Other modulators		
stimulatory	ATP, caffeine, 4-CMC, oxidizing -SH reagents	ATP, caffeine, oxidizing -SH reagents
inhibitory	procaine, reducing -SH reagents, ruthenium red	procaine, reducing -SH reagents, ruthenium red
Ryanodine (≤ 10 μM) [b)]	sustained opening at subconductance state	

[a)] B/B_{max} ([^{3}H]-ryanodine binding calibrated with the maximum binding sites) stands for the averaged fractional activity of a single channel in the medium containing 0.17 M KCl and 1mM AMPPCP at pH6.8. These values for RyR1 and RyR3 correspond to 100% in Fig. 13-1 A. [b)] Effect of a higher concentration of ryanodine was controversial: some investigators claimed it closed the channel while others claimed it sustained the opening with the empty Ca^{2+} store.

PROPERTIES OF CICR ACTIVITY OF RYR1 AND RYR3 HOMOLOGUES IN THE SR MEMBRANE

CHAPS and phospholipids which were reagents necessary for solubilization and purification of RyR were found to affect [^{3}H]-ryanodine binding of RyR. The activity of each isoform *in the SR membrane*, therefore, was determined.[485] The results obtained were a complete surprise: the [^{3}H]-ryanodine binding (B) of α-RyR was markedly low at only 4% that of β-RyR in an isotonic medium containing 1 mM AMPPCP, a non-hydrolyzable ATP analog (Fig. 13-2 A) in spite of similar numbers (45 : 55) of their maximum binding sites (B_{max}) (Fig. 13-2 B). The Ca^{2+} dependence of α-RyR and β-RyR were similar as shown in the inset (Fig. 13-2 A). The relative extent of effects of CICR modulators, adenine nucleotides and caffeine were also indistinguishable. These results are in marked contrast to those of purified isoforms which showed very similar [^{3}H]-ryanodine binding (Table 13-1). The parameter B/B_{max} then stands for the averaged fractional activity of a single CICR channel molecule. The B/B_{max} value for α-RyR is much lower than that for β-RyR, although they are very similar in Ca^{2+} dependences and responses to AMPPCP and caffeine: α-RyR has an amplification gain lowered for CICR. Here, this state is referred to as a stabilized state.

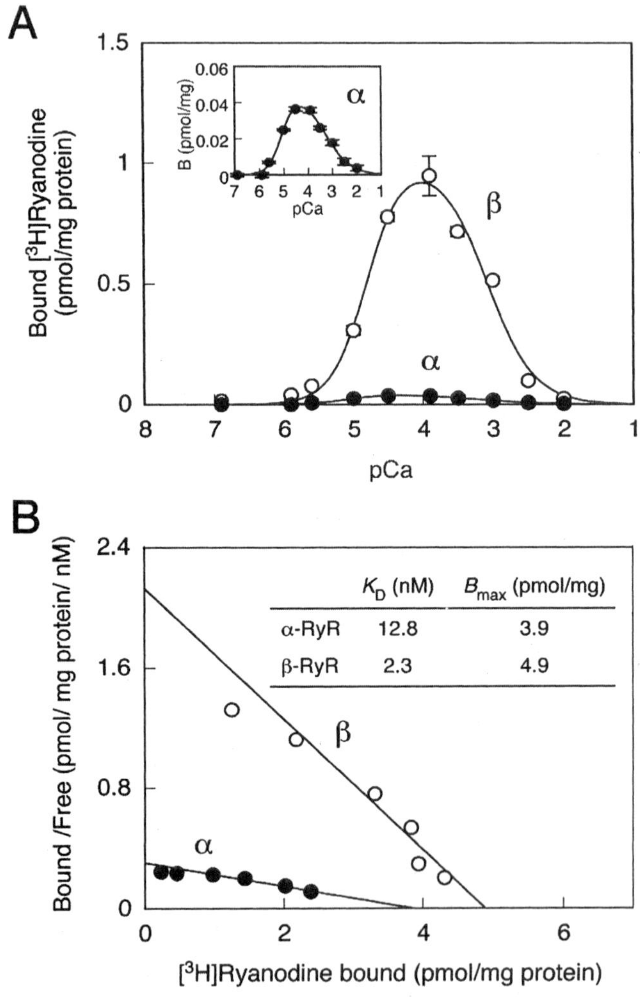

Figure 13-2. **[³H]-ryanodine binding of α-RyR and β-RyR in the SR vesicles from frog skeletal muscle.** Note that the peak activity of α-RyR (B/B_{max} = 0.009) is very low in comparison with that of β-RyR (0.19) although there is no difference in their Ca^{2+} dependences (**A**, and inset). Scatchard plot analysis (**B**) shows that the ratio of their B_{max} values was 45:55, which corresponded to the ratio of contents of the two isoforms as estimated from band densities on SDS-PAGE. Responses of α-RyR to AMPPCP and caffeine as well as to Ca^{2+} were very similar to those of β-RyR. In the SR membrane, α-RyR has a lowered gain for CICR, i.e., it is "stabilized" (see also Table 13-2). Reproduced with permission from J Biol Chem.[485]

Similar conclusions were obtained with RyR1 and RyR3 in the SR from bovine diaphragm.[486] Whereas RyR3, 4% of total RyR, is not stabilized, RyR1, the major isoform, is stabilized. Although B/B_{max} values for β-RyR and RyR3 are similar (0.20-0.25), these values for RyR1 and α-RyR were 0.03 and 0.009, respectively, α-RyR being more strongly stabilized than RyR1(Table 13-2).

Table 13-2. **Properties of RyR1 and RyR3 homologues in SR vesicles from adult skeletal muscle.**[135,475,485]

	Bovine diaphragm SR		Frog SR	
	RyR1	RyR3	α-RyR	β-RyR
Content (%) [a)]	96	4	45	55
B/B_{max}	0.03-0.04	0.20-0.30	0.009	0.20-0.25
Ca^{2+}				
EC_{50} (μM)	6	13	11	16
IC_{50} (mM)	0.3	0.8	0.8	0.8
Mg^{2+} [b)]				
IC_{50} (mM)	0.15	0.14	similar to those of RyR1/RyR3	
ATP				
EC_{50} (mM)	0.3	0.3	0.3	0.3
Caffeine				
Ca^{2+} sensitizing effect	Δ(pCa)≈1 at 10 mM		Δ(pCa)≈1 at 10 mM	
ATP-like effect	2-3 fold at 10 mM		4-7 fold at 10 mM	
Destabilizing treatment [c)]				
control	0.025	0.22	0.009	0.20
FK506	0.04	0.19	0.009	0.20
CHAPS	0.12	0.19	0.3	0.47 [d)]
combined	0.18	0.21	-	-

[a)] Contents of RyR3 in adult mammalian diaphragm depended on species: rabbit, 0.6%; bovine, 4-5%. Except for diaphragm and soleus, adult mammalian skeletal muscles showed no or very minor amount of RyR3. [b)] IC_{50} value for Mg^{2+} depends on the Ca^{2+} concentration where determinations of Mg^{2+}-effect are made. Determinations were made in the presence of 30μM Ca^{2+}, which was near optimum. The condition is comparable to that in Table 13-1. [c)] Effects of destabilizing treatments were expressed in terms of B/B_{max}. [d)] The reason the ryanodine binding to β-RyR from frog skeletal muscle was increased by CHAPS remains to be elucidated.

The B/B_{max} value for RyR1 was increased 1.6-fold by FK506 treatment, indicating partial contribution of FKBP12 to the stabilization. CHAPS and phospholipids increased B/B_{max} for RyR1 about 5-fold, indicating that protein-protein interaction and/or protein-lipid interaction may be important for stabilization. The combined effects of these two treatments nearly restored the destabilized state. The two kinds of reagents work additively, indicating that the mechanisms of the two are distinct. It should be noted that these destabilizing agents were also effective in similar magnitudes in a 1M NaCl medium where [^{3}H]-ryanodine binding was augmented. RyR3, on the other hand, was not significantly affected either by treatment with FK506, with CHAPS and phospholipids, or their combination. FKBP12 was not co-immunoprecipitated with RyR3, although the isoform showed the capability of binding FKBP12. Considering the case with frog α-RyR, CHAPS and phospholipids should be more important in destabilization, because the treatment stimulated α-RyR, whereas FK506 treatment had no effect (Table 13-2). FKBP12-like protein was detected with α-RyR in the SR, but its N-terminal partial sequence indicated that it is rather similar to mammalian FKBP12.6. Frog FKBP12-like protein has a minor effect on α-RyR. The reason β-RyR was stimulated by the treatment with CHAPS and phospholipids (Table 13-2) remains to be elucidated.

None of the coexisting RyR3, calmodulin or DHPR is the cause of the stabilization. Recently Lee *et al.* reported that DHPR exerted a negative regulatory effect on RyR1 expressed in 1B5 cells, reducing its sensitivity to caffeine.[487] The reduction in caffeine sensitivity, however, was eliminated by external addition of La^{3+} and Cd^{2+} which should not affect skeletal muscle-type EC coupling. Caffeine sensitivities of RyR1/RyR2 chimeras did not correspond to the results of restoration of skeletal muscle-type EC coupling. Further investigation is required.

When Ca^{2+} dependences of purified RyR1 (Table 13-1) and RyR1 in SR (Table 13-2) are compared, the Ca^{2+} sensitivity to the inactivating Ca^{2+} is increased about 6-fold with RyR1 in SR, in contrast to similar sensitivity to the activating Ca^{2+}. Correspondingly, the IC_{50} value for Mg^{2+} was decreased about 17-fold. These changes may be related to the underlying mechanism for stabilization.

DP4, a peptide fragment of RyR1 (2442-2477), selectively stimulated RyR1, whereas DP4-mut with a replacement of R2458C did not.[180] The authors claimed that DP4 should disturb the interdomain interaction within RyR1, causing activation of RyR1 and that this perturbation may be the underlying mechanism for malignant hyperthermia (see Chapter 6). We hypothesize that a similar interdomain interaction causes stabilization of RyR1. In this context, it is interesting that no disease caused by mutation in RyR3 has been reported, whereas diseases related to mutations of RyR1 and RyR2 are of record.

PHYSIOLOGICAL RELEVANCE OF COEXISTENCE OF A STABILIZED RYR1 AND UNSTABILIZED RYR3 HOMOLOGUE IN THE SR

Stabilization of RyR1 homologues implies that CICR should primarily be performed by RyR3 homologue in skeletal muscles, although RyR1 homologue can release Ca^{2+} through DICR. The hypothesis that RyR1 homologues uncoupled to tetrads may serve as amplifiers of Ca^{2+} release through the CICR mechanism can be excluded. The rate of CICR with skinned frog skeletal muscle would not exceed 100 min^{-1} even in the absence of Mg^{2+} in a medium simulating the physiological ionic strength, pH and ATP concentration. The rate is much smaller than the expected rate of DICR (1000-2000 min^{-1}), indicating that CICR is too slow to explain DICR.[475]

Functional contribution of RyR3 to CICR or drug-induced Ca^{2+} release should be greater than the expected magnitude on the basis of its content. Some examples are discussed in the following. Ca^{2+} sparks (transient, restricted and localized Ca^{2+} release) can more easily be observed with frog skeletal muscle, whereas it is very rare with mammalian skeletal muscle.[488] This is consistent with the findings that many adult mammalian skeletal muscles except diaphragm or soleus contained little or no RyR3.

Caffeine stimulates CICR by sensitizing RyR to the activating Ca^{2+} and also by ATP-like effect. Caffeine easily causes contracture with frog skeletal muscle, but it often is abortive with mammalian skeletal muscle.[489] β-RyR in frog skeletal muscle is about half of the total RyR, whereas RyR3 is at most 5% in the mammalian skeletal muscle. The response of the coexisting α-RyRand RyR1 would be minor. Therefore, overall Ca^{2+} release action in excess of Ca^{2+} pump activity should be much weaker on mammalian than on frog skeletal muscle.

CICR activity of skinned fiber from neonate mouse dyspedic skeletal muscle appeared to be much greater than that expected from the residual RyR3 (about 5%) when compared with CICR in the wild-type animal.[51] This is reasonable if RyR1, but not RyR3, in neonate skinned fiber is stabilized. Furthermore, the distribution of RyR3 is expected to be heterogenous, because loss of RyR3 during growth was reported to be due to the disappearance of fibers containing RyR3.[481]

Caffeine contracture of neonate skeletal muscle was reported to be parallel to the amount of RyR3.[490] Ca^{2+} sparks in mouse embryonic myotube (E18) appeared to be dependent on the content of RyR3, and RyR3 was claimed to be more sensitive to caffeine than RyR1.[491] RyR3 heterologously expressed in 1B5[482,492] and HEK293[493] cells is reported to be more sensitive to caffeine than RyR1, although Takeshima *et al.*[51] indicated no difference in caffeine sensitivity with skinned fibers between RyR1 (wild type) and RyR3

(RyR1-deficient). An explanation for this discrepancy could be as follows. Transfected RyR3 was more abundantly expressed in 1B5 cells than transfected RyR1.[482] This tendency was observed also with HEK293 cells.[493] The cytoplasmic Ca^{2+} change was determined by fluorescent transient of a Ca^{2+} indicator dye, e.g. fluo-3, which was so sensitive that the response was easily saturated at a low Ca^{2+}. Transfected RyR1 in 1B5 and HEK293 cells can also be assumed to be in the stabilized state. Taken together, the apparent higher sensitivity to caffeine of RyR3 is consistent with our conclusion that RyR1 is stabilized in the SR membrane. Our discussion so far has been made assuming a constant Ca^{2+}-pump activity. However, in some cases, secondary changes in the Ca^{2+}-pump activity might be involved.

It was reported that electrical stimulation induced Ca^{2+} propagation from the cell periphery to the center in RyR3-deficient mouse myotubes at a rate comparable to the rate of CICR by RyR2 in cardiac myocytes, concluding that the propagation was due to CICR by RyR1[494] These findings suggest that RyR1 in myotubes might not be stabilized unlike the case with adult skeletal muscle. Considerable amounts of T-tubule, however, were shown to be running transversely in mouse myotubes at the corresponding developmental stage.[495] The Ca^{2+} propagation, then, could be due to the electrical propagation along the T-tubule. Further studies are required.

Comparisons of functions between cells with and without RyR3 expression often lead to the conclusion that RyR3 may modulate the function of the other isoforms. Further investigations are required to confirm that the underlying mechanism is attributable to formation of heterotetramers.

CONCLUDING REMARKS

RyR3 is ubiquitously distributed, albeit in a minuscule amount. Especially in the brain, the localization is fascinating. Whereas RyR1 is stabilized in CICR activity in the SR, RyR3 is *not* stabilized. Therefore RyR3 can contribute to CICR in skeletal muscle to a greater extent than its content. Although CICR plays a minor role in physiological contraction of skeletal muscles, it takes the crucial part in drug–induced contracture. In this sense, the functional roles of RyR3 in the brain and smooth muscles, which are targets of many drugs are intriguing issues to be clarified. On this occasion, secondary modulations by Ca^{2+}-activated K^{+} channel, Ca^{2+}-activated Cl^{-} channel, Ca^{2+}-calmodulin dependent protein kinase, and calcineurin dependent phosphatase should be taken into consideration in addition to direct impacts by increased Ca^{2+} concentrations.

Chapter 14

KNOCKOUT MICE LACKING RYR AND JUNCTOPHILIN SUBTYPES

Hiroshi Takeshima
Dept. of Medical Chemistry, Tohoku University Graduate School of Medicine, Sendai, Miyagi 980-8575, Japan

INTRODUCTION

Cytoplasmic Ca^{2+} regulates important cellular functions including muscle contraction, neurotransmitter release, cell growth and cell death. In excitable cells, the depolarization signal activates voltage-dependent Ca^{2+} channels (VDCCs) on the plasma membrane, and the resulting Ca^{2+} influx basically produces intracellular Ca^{2+} signals. Ca^{2+}-induced Ca^{2+} release (CICR) is shared by excitable cell types and is considered to be an amplification mechanism of cellular Ca^{2+} signaling, by which Ca^{2+} influx triggers Ca^{2+} release from the intracellular Ca^{2+} store, the endoplasmic or sarcoplasmic reticulum (ER/SR). Ryanodine receptors (RyRs), expressed throughout excitable cells, basically mediate CICR from intracellular stores, and are thus involved in a variety of physiological functions. During the CICR process, Ca^{2+} derived from the extracellular space binds to RyR and facilitates its channel opening. Therefore, the activation of RyRs by Ca^{2+} influx likely requires a close association between VDCCs and RyRs which are located on different membrane systems, to overcome strong Ca^{2+} buffering effects in the cytoplasm which may inhibit the communication between both Ca^{2+} channel types. Indeed, it has been observed in striated muscles that VDCCs and RyRs are co-localized in junctional membrane complexes composed of the plasma membrane and the SR, referred to as 'triads' in skeletal muscle and 'diads' in cardiac muscle, respectively. Our recent studies have provided evidence that junctophilins (JPs) contribute to the formation of junctional membrane complexes in excitable cells by interacting with the plasma membrane and spanning the ER/SR membrane. Furthermore, results from knockout mice also indicate that JPs are essential for functional communication between VDCCs and RyRs. Fig. 14-1 schematically shows the proposed subcellular localization of VDCC, RyR and JP in the junctional membrane structure.

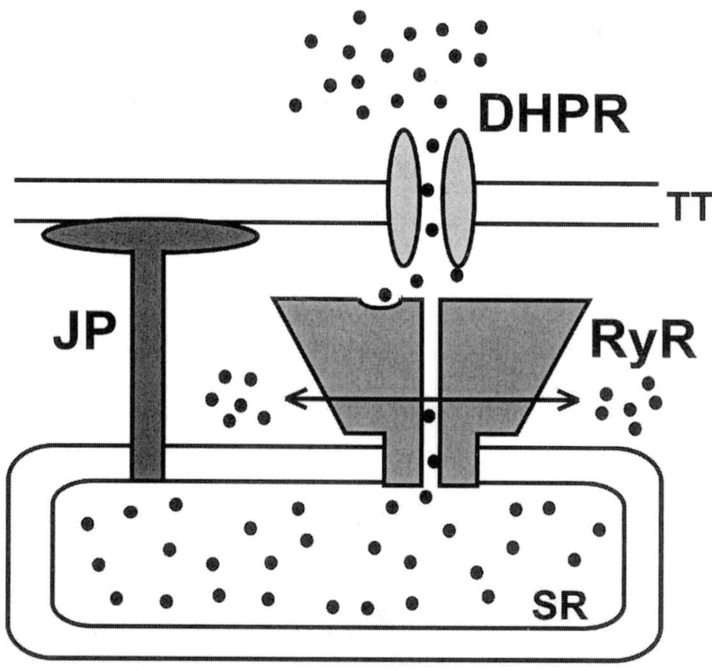

Figure 14-1. **Schematic presentation of major molecules contributing to cardiac E-C coupling.** DHPR, dihydropyridine receptor; RyR, ryanodine receptor; JP, junctophilin; TT, transverse tubule; SR, sarcoplasmic reticulum. During E-C coupling, DHPRs activated by depolarization produce Ca^{2+} influx, and RyRs activated by the CICR mechanism generate Ca^{2+} release. This Ca^{2+} signal amplification probably requires functional coupling between DHPR and RyR within the junctional membrane complex composed of JPs, namely, "diad" and "peripheral coupling".

In recent years, the analysis of knockout mice lacking RyR subtypes has demonstrated their essential contribution to physiological functions in skeletal muscle, cardiac muscle and neurons. In this chapter, the biological roles of RyR subtypes are reviewed on the basis of abnormal phenotypes observed in knockout mice. On the other hand, four JP subtypes are differentially distributed in excitable cell types, and this chapter also focuses on knockout mice lacking JP subtypes.

KNOCKOUT MICE LACKING RYR SUBTYPES

DNA cloning studies have demonstrated that the vertebrate genome contains three RyR genes, namely RyR1, RyR2 and RyR3.[496] Some general features of RyR subtypes are listed in Table 14-1. Knockout mice lacking the respective RyR isoforms have been described, and revealed the essential contribution of RyRs to muscle and brain function as described below. As described in Chapters 22-25, mutations in RyR genes have been associated with several human genetic diseases, including malignant hyperthermia, central core disease, and familial ventricular tachycardia. On the other hand, there are no RyR genes found in yeast, and invertebrates only express a single RyR gene (see Chapter 1).[17] Mutant nematodes and fruit flies lacking a normal RyR gene display abnormal motor function and defects in muscle excitation-contraction (EC) coupling.[497]

Table 14-1. **Features of mammalian RyR subtypes**

Subtype	Locus	Tissue distribution	Knockout mice	Human genetic disease
RyR1	Mouse 7A2-B3	Skeletal muscle, brain	Muscle dysfunction (neonatal lethality)	Malignant hyperthermia, central core disease
RyR2	Mouse 13A1-2	Cardiac and smooth muscle, brain	Heart failure (embryonic lethality)	Ventricular tachycardia, ventricular dysplasia
RyR3	Mouse 2E5-F3 Human 15q14-15	Skeletal and smooth muscle	Impaired memory, hyperlocomotion	-

RyR1-knockout mice

RyR1 is expressed predominantly in skeletal muscle and weakly in the brain.[3] During skeletal muscle contraction, depolarization is converted into intracellular Ca^{2+} signaling without the requirement of extracellular Ca^{2+}. During skeletal muscle EC coupling, the dihydropyridine receptor (DHPR) functions as a voltage sensor rather than a voltage-dependent Ca^{2+} channel, and it has been proposed that direct coupling between DHPRs and RyRs converts depolarization into Ca^{2+} release through RyRs. This idea is based on the fact that DHPR and RyR are co-localized in the triad junction, and that a null mutation in either skDHPR or RyR1 results in dysfunction of skeletal muscle E-C coupling in mice. On the other hand, the role of RyR1 in the brain is still uncertain.

Mutant mice lacking RyR1 survive during fetal developmental stages but die immediately after birth.[23] The death is probably due to respiratory failure because the knockout neonates fail to breathe and do not move. In RyR1-

deficient skeletal muscle, myofibril content was significantly reduced and electron-microscopic analysis frequently found abnormal triad junctions lacking 'foot' structures.[23,127] Skeletal muscle EC coupling under physiological conditions is totally abolished in RyR1-knockout neonates, but their muscles showed weak contraction in an artificial extracellular solution containing a VDCC agonist and high extracellular Ca^{2+} concentration. These results show that Ca^{2+} release after DHPR activation is impaired in RyR1-knockout muscle, demonstrating that RyR1 functions as a physiological Ca^{2+} release channel during muscle EC coupling. On the other hand, RyR1-knockout muscle still retained caffeine-evoked Ca^{2+} transients. Biochemical experiments showed the predominant expression of RyR1 and the weak expression of RyR3 in skeletal muscle, suggesting that RyR3 is responsible for the caffeine-induced transients in RyR1-knockout muscle.[422] The absence of depolarization-evoked Ca^{2+} transients in RyR1-knockout muscle strongly indicates that RyR1 contributes to skeletal muscle EC coupling but that RyR3 cannot couple with skDHPR under physiological conditions.

In RyR1-knockout muscle cells, voltage-gated Ca^{2+} current density via skeletal muscle DHPR (skDHPR or Cav1.1) was remarkably diminished.[133,498] Moreover, strong and long-lasting depolarization, which normally produced excessive tail currents upon repolarization in normal muscle cells, failed to do so in RyR1-knockout muscle cells. These abnormalities are not due to reduced channel protein levels, because Northern blot analysis revealed apparently normal levels of skDHPR mRNA and that muscle membranes from RyR1-deficient neonates did not show a significant reduction of dihydropyridine (DHP) binding. Therefore, the impaired skDHPR channel activity in RyR1-deficient muscle is likely caused by the absence of its direct coupling with RyR1, suggesting the presence of retrograde signaling from RyR1 to skDHPR. This retrograde signaling is probably unique to skeletal muscle, since VDCC currents were not obviously impaired in mutant cardiac myocytes from RyR2-knockout neonates (see below).

Cultured muscle cells from RyR1-knockout mice or double-knockout mice lacking both RyR1 and RyR3 provide us with an important assay system for examining physiological functions of RyR subtypes when cDNAs for mutant RyRs are functionally expressed. Using the cultured cell system, several functional domains of RyRs, for example regions essential for muscle EC coupling and retrograde signaling to skDHPR, have been mapped within their primary structures.[192,194,499,500]

RyR2-knockout mice

RyR2 is expressed predominantly in cardiac muscle, and moderately in smooth muscle and the brain. Although all of the three RyR subtypes are expressed in the brain, RyR2 is the most abundant subtype. During EC coupling in mature cardiac muscle, RyR2 functions as a physiological partner of the cardiac DHPR, also known as the L-type Ca^{2+} channel (cardDHPR or Cav1.2). Ca^{2+} influx through cardDHPR triggers the activation of Ca^{2+} release via RyR2 by the CICR mechanism, and the amplified Ca^{2+} signaling causes cardiac muscle contraction. The amplification factor of cardDHPR/ RyR2 is defined as the amount of Ca^{2+} released from the SR relative to Ca^{2+} influx through cardDHPR, and an average amplification factor of ~20 in rat ventricular myocytes has been reported.[501] Therefore, RyR2-mediated Ca^{2+} release is essential for composing cardiac EC coupling. On the other hand, the physiological role of RyR2 in smooth muscle cells and neurons remains unclear, although it is proposed that RyR2-mediated Ca^{2+} release takes part in both Ca^{2+} signaling by the CICR mechanism and the regulation of Ca^{2+}-dependent ionic transport systems including Ca^{2+}-dependent K^+ channels on the cell surface membrane.

In contrast to mature heart muscle, embryonic cardiac myocytes exhibit immature SR functions and RyR2-mediated Ca^{2+} release does not contribute well to cardiac EC coupling during fetal developmental stages. Knockout mice lacking RyR2 showed cardiac arrest and lethality at about embryonic day E10.5.[423] Ultrastructural analysis showed that the ER/SR elements were partly swollen in E8.5 RyR2-deficient cardiac myocytes and were further vacuolated at E9.5 and E10.5, suggesting that the vacuolated ER/SR was Ca^{2+}-overloaded in RyR2-knockout myocytes.[502] Moreover, mitochondria exhibited tubular cristae and were swollen in knock-out cardiac myocytes. Degenerated mitochondria produce cell-death signals by releasing cytochrome c, which may underlie the cardiac arrest in RyR2-knockout embryos. In embryonic cardiac myocytes, spontaneous contractions and Ca^{2+} oscillations were still retained under store-depleted conditions in the presence of both caffeine and ryanodine, although a slightly reduced amplitude of Ca^{2+} oscillations was observed. Therefore, the loss of CICR mediated by RyR2 does not abolish E-C coupling in the heart at early embryonic stages. In the RyR2-knockout cardiac myocytes, cytoplasmic Ca^{2+} derived from the extracellular fluid during EC coupling may gradually accumulate in developing SR. Cytoplasmic Ca^{2+} that cannot be sequestered by the overloaded SR may then flow into mitochondria, causing defective organelles and/or abnormal Ca^{2+} homeostasis that leads to cellular dysfunctions. Therefore, it is likely that RyRs can function as a safety valve of the intracellular Ca^{2+} store to prevent abnormal overloading.

The above conclusion is supported by the result that the vacuolated SR is shared by mutant skeletal muscle from double-knockout mice lacking both RyR1 and RyR3.[503] Skeletal muscle contains RyR1 and RyR3 as the major and minor components, respectively, but mutant muscle cells lacking either RyR1 or RyR3 do not exhibit such severe ultrastructural defects of the SR. Because Ca^{2+}-overloading alone cannot produce obvious osmotic changes between the SR lumen and the cytoplasm, the molecular mechanism for the vacuolated SR is unclear. One possibility is that luminal Ca^{2+}-sensitive K^+ or Cl^- channels may be involved in this mechanism.

RyR3-knockout mice

It has been reported that RyR3 is weakly expressed in skeletal muscle, smooth muscle, neurons, and certain non-excitable cells including epithelial cells and lymphocytes. The features of RyR3 channels were first characterized using RyR1-knockout skeletal muscle,[422] and we now know that RyR3 shares pharmacological properties with other RyR subtypes; for example, RyR3 is sensitive to both caffeine and ryanodine. Based on its expression pattern and channel properties, RyR3 likely participates in the CICR-mediated amplification of Ca^{2+} signaling in a variety of cell types. However, RyR3 functions are as yet poorly understood at the whole-animal level, although RyR3-knockout mice have been established.

RyR3-knockout mice show normal growth and reproduction.[51] Skeletal muscle from RyR3-knockout mice retained the skeletal-muscle type of EC coupling, but the Ca^{2+} signaling and force generation may be slightly weakened in comparison with those in wild-type muscle.[477,491,504] Increased locomotor activity,[51] impaired learning and memory,[505] and abnormal electrophysiological and biochemical properties of hippocampal neurons were observed in RyR3-knockout mice.[506] The observations indicate that RyR3-mediated Ca^{2+} release contributes to physiological modulation in several neuronal circuits. On the other hand, abnormalities caused by the loss of RyR3 in the brain might be compensated by residual RyR1 and RyR2. In the liver from double-knockout neonates lacking both RyR1 and RyR3, glycogen accumulates in excess amounts, whereas there is no irregular glycogen accumulation in either RyR1- or RyR3 single knockout mice.[507] The collaborative contribution of RyR1 and RyR3 may be suggested in a certain neural network responsible for glucose metabolism. The physiological roles of RyR subtypes in the brain are still unclear, and tissue-specific gene knockout strategy to overcome the lethality in RyR1- and RyR2-knockout mice is absolutely required for future studies.

KNOCKOUT MICE LACKING JUNCTOPHILIN SUBTYPES

As described above, junctional membrane structures between the plasma membrane and the ER/SR are likely an important structural ground for RyR-mediated Ca^{2+}-signal amplification. Since RyRs are observed as "foot" proteins in the junctional gap between the T-tubule and the SR of the triad junction, it may be proposed that RyRs can produce the junctional membrane structure. However, mutant muscle expressing no RyR proteins still retained triad junctions,[503] and cultured cells stably transfected with RyR cDNAs did not show the junctional membrane structure between the cell membrane and the ER.[125] Thus, we found no contributions of RyRs to the formation of junctional membrane structures.

Table 14-2. **Features of mammalian JP subtypes**

Subtype	Locus	Tissue distribution	Knockout mice	Human genetic disease
JP-1	Mouse 1A2-5 Human 8q21	Skeletal muscle	Impaired muscle contraction (neonatal lethality)	-
JP-2	Mouse 2H1-3 Human 20q12	Skeletal, cardiac and smooth muscle	Heart failure (embryonic lethality)	-
JP-3	Mouse 8E Human 16q23-24	Brain	Motor discoordination	Huntington's disease (HDL-2)
JP-4	Mouse 14C1-2 Human 14q11.1	Brain	-	-

In our recent survey for protein components in the triad junction,[121,508] junctophilin (JP) subtypes have been identified as the best candidate for the protein participating actively in junctional membrane formation. JP subtypes are composed of 628-744 amino acid residues, carry conserved MORN-motif sequences of 14 residues repeated eight times in the amino-terminal regions, and possess a transmembrane segment spanning the ER/SR membrane.[121,509] cDNA expression studies demonstrated that the MORN-motif region interacts specifically with the plasma membrane, and that JP can generate the junctional membrane complex between the plasma membrane and the ER in amphibian embryonic cells. The vertebrate genome contains four JP subtype genes activated in distinct tissues, namely JP-1, JP-2, JP-3 and JP-4.[121,509,510] Some general features of JP subtypes are listed in Table 14-2. The knockout mice lacking the subtypes were previously generated, revealing that JP subtypes are essential for the physiological functioning of RyR subtypes as described below. On the other hand, there are no JP genes in yeast, and there is a single JP gene in invertebrates. Nematode with a defective JP gene showed motor defects, and JP seems to be important for muscle EC coupling in invertebrates.[511]

JP-1-knockout mice

JP-1 is abundantly expressed in skeletal muscle cells and specifically localized in the triad junction. Immature muscle at fetal stages and mature adult muscle contain JP-2, while JP-1 expression starts and its level remarkably increases after birth correlating well with the formation of triad junctions.[512] The JP-1-knockout neonatal mice have a weak voice and weak movements after birth, exhibited a suckling defect, and die within one day after birth.[513] Skeletal muscle from neonatal mice contains both triads and diads as junctional membrane complexes, however, mutant muscle from the JP-1-knockout neonates showed the deficiency of triad junctions. In the measurements of muscle contraction, JP-1-knockout muscle generated normal maximum force at tetanus stimuli, but developed less force at low-frequency stimuli. Therefore, the force-frequency curve of JP-1-knockout muscle shifted downward, demonstrating that the loss of JP-1 reduces the efficiency of muscle EC coupling. The insufficient EC coupling is likely due to the deficiency of triad junctions where functional coupling occurs between skDHPR and RyR1. Moreover, irregular responses to extracellular Ca^{2+} changes were observed in JP-1-knockout muscle, suggesting that the deficiency of triad junctions interferes with the functions of the T-tubular and SR systems.

Triads are usually detected in skeletal muscle expressing both JP-1 and JP-2, while diads are formed in cardiac muscle predominantly expressing JP-2. This observation, together with results obtained from JP-1-knockout muscle, may indicate that JP-1 is essential for the formation of triad junctions, and that JP-1 and JP-2 have different roles in the formation of junctional membrane complexes in skeletal muscle. Assuming that the expression of JP-1 is the major determinant for the structural maturation of the junctional membrane complex from diads to triads in skeletal muscle, diads may be converted into triads by JP-1 cDNA expression in cardiac myocytes containing endogenous JP-2. However, this idea is not supported by our current study demonstrating that no typical triads ware detected in transgenic mice expressing JP-1 specifically in cardiac myocytes.[514] It is possible that triad formation requires highly complex cellular mechanisms specific for skeletal muscle including membrane biogenesis and transport.

JP-2-knockout mice

JP-2 is expressed in skeletal, cardiac and smooth muscle cells. In embryonic cardiac myocytes antibody specific to JP-2 reacted with the cell periphery, where peripheral coupling between the plasma membrane and the developing SR is often detected by ultrastructural analysis, while JP-2 predominantly localized at the diad in mature cardiac myocytes.[121] The targeted disruption of the JP-2 gene induced embryonic lethality in the homozygous state, and the JP-2-knockout embryos exhibited cardiac arrest at ~E10.5. Electron-microscopic analysis demonstrated that mutant cardiac myocytes lacking JP-2 showed the deficiency of junctional membrane structures with ~12 nm gap sizes, assigned tentatively as functional peripheral coupling. In Ca^{2+}-imaging analysis, a large number of myocytes in knockout cardiac tubules showed irregular Ca^{2+} transients that were not synchronized with heartbeats and occurred randomly, although uniform and synchronized Ca^{2+} transients were definitely observed in myocytes of wild-type embryonic hearts. The abnormal Ca^{2+} transients in JP-2-knockout myocytes were probably due to unregulated RyR2 activation caused by the loss of functional communication between DHPR and RyR2.

JP-3-knockout mice

The subsurface cistern is a common junctional membrane structure between the plasma membrane and the ER in neurons of the central nervous system. Both JP-3 and JP-4 are co-expressed in the brain, and *in situ* hybridization analysis revealed that their overall regional distributions are similar. Knockout mice lacking JP-3 grew and reproduced normally, and did not show any morphological abnormalities in the brain.[515] In our several behavioral tests, the mutant mice showed impaired performance specifically in balance/ motor coordination tasks. No obvious abnormalities were detected in electrical transmission among cerebellar neurons in the mutant mice, and the cause of this motor discoordination is still unclear. It is interesting to note the possible linkage between motor discoordination in JP-3-knockout mice and in human disease named Huntington's disease-like 2 (HDL-2); triplet repeat expansions within the JP-3 gene are associated with HDL-2 patients. The collaborative contribution of JP-3 and JP-4 in the brain is proposed on the basis of their expression profiles, therefore, to know the physiological functions of JPs in the brain, we furthermore need to generate JP-4-knockout mice and double knockout mice lacking both JP subtypes.

CONCLUDING REMARKS

Knockout mice lacking RyRs defined the essential contribution of these subtypes to Ca^{2+} signaling in excitable cells. However, the functions of RyRs are not well characterized in smooth muscle cells or neurons. On the other hand, knockout mice lacking JP subtypes demonstrate that the functioning of RyR subtypes requires JP-mediated formation of junctional membrane structures. Although the significance of RyR and JP subtypes have been determined, many important issues are still in mystery, for example: physiological modulations, sorting into defined subcellular regions, or gene activations of RyR channels. Our knockout mice may be useful as *in vivo* experimental model systems for future analysis of the physiological roles of RyR subtypes.

Chapter 15

REGULATION OF RYANODINE RECEPTOR Ca^{2+} RELEASE BY MACROMOLECULAR COMPLEXES

Xander H.T. Wehrens, Stephan E. Lehnart, and Andrew R. Marks
Depts. of Physiology and Cellular Biophysics, and Medicine, Center for Molecular Cardiology, Columbia University College of Physicians and Surgeons, New York, NY

INTRODUCTION

Intracellular calcium (Ca^{2+}) release from the cardiac sarcoplasmic reticulum (SR) occurs through the process of Ca^{2+}-induced Ca^{2+} release (CICR). Preceding every muscle contraction, depolarization of the cell membrane causes a small Ca^{2+} flux into the cell via voltage-gated L-type Ca^{2+} channels (LTCC), this triggers the release of a much larger amount of Ca^{2+} from the SR via ryanodine receptors (RyR).[516,517] CICR increases the open probability (Po) of RyRs by the local elevation of the Ca^{2+} concentration in the vicinity of the Ca^{2+} release channels. Since the gain of intracellular Ca^{2+} release for a given LTCC Ca^{2+} influx can be increased or decreased, modulation of the Ca^{2+}-sensitivity of RyR is a fundamental mechanism to regulate excitation-contraction (EC) coupling (see also Chapters 7-8). Phosphorylation of RyR by cAMP-dependent protein kinase (PKA) or Ca^{2+}/calmodulin-dependent protein kinase II (CaMKII) can increase the Ca^{2+} sensitivity of RyR, thereby increasing the gain of EC coupling and augmenting muscle contraction.[247,298,350] In addition to phosphorylation, RyR activity is also modulated by accessory proteins, including calmodulin (Chapter 16), calstabin1 (FKBP12), calstabin2 (FKBP12.6), and sorcin. In this chapter, we describe the components of the RyR macromolecular complex, and the regulation of RyR channel activity by protein kinases and phosphatases.

RYANODINE RECEPTOR MACROMOLECULAR COMPLEX

RyRs are large homotetrameric ion channels comprised of four RyR monomers (each with a molecular mass of ~560 kDa). RyR monomers have a large cytoplasmic N-terminal domain, as well as transmembrane (TM) and pore-forming regions near the C-terminus (see Chapter 1).[3,4] The N-terminal region comprises 90% of the RyR sequence and forms a cytoplasmic domain that serves as a scaffold for proteins that modulate the channel function.[123,298,518-523]

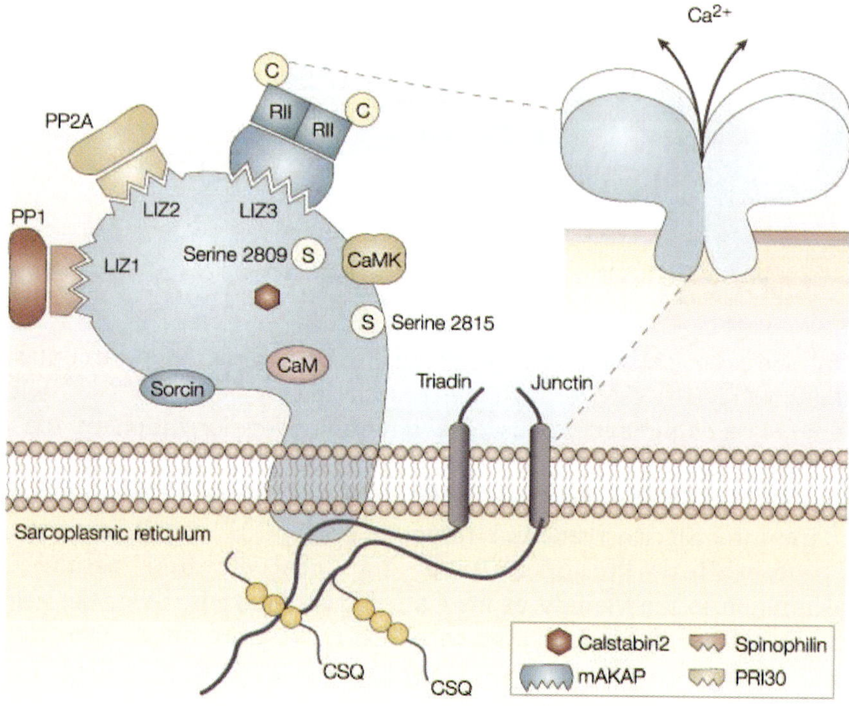

Figure 15-1. **RyR2 macromolecular complex.** Leucine/isoleucine zippers (LIZ) on RyR2 mediate binding of adaptor proteins that target protein phosphatases PP1 and PP2A, and protein kinase A (PKA) to the channel complex. PKA consists of two regulatory (RII) and two catalytic (C) subunits. Calstabin2 (FKBP12.6), calmodulin (CaM), CaMKII, and sorcin also bind to the cytoplasmic surface of RyR2. 'S' indicates the PKA (Ser 2809) and CaMKII (Ser 2815) phosphorylation sites on RyR2. Triadin and junctin have transmembrane domains and bind to the intraluminal SR domain of RyR2. Calsequestrin (CSQ) binds and unbinds to the triadin-junctin-RyR2 complex depending on the SR Ca^{2+} concentration during the EC coupling cycle. Reproduced, with permission, from Wehrens *et al.*[524]

Recent studies have revealed that protein kinases and phosphatases are targeted to the cytoplasmic scaffold domain of RyRs, and modulate their function in response to extracellular signals such as stress responses (Fig. 15-1).[5,6] Specific association between RyR and the associated regulatory proteins was demonstrated using co-immunoprecipitation experiments in which RyRs were solubilized in 0.25% Triton-X100, and each of the components of the RyR macromolecular complex were shown to co-sediment with RyR on sucrose gradients using CHAPS solubilized membranes.[5] The association of kinases and phosphatases with RyR allows for local regulation of the channel activity.[525,526] Highly conserved leucine/ isoleucine zipper (LIZ) motifs in RyR mediate binding to cognate LIZs in the targeting proteins for kinases and phosphatases.[6] This feature of ion channel macromolecular complexes is shared by both intracellular Ca^{2+} release channels (RyRs and IP_3Rs),[6,527] and by voltage-gated ion channels.[528,529] The catalytic subunit of PKA (C) as well as its regulatory subunit (RII) are bound to the anchoring protein mAKAP (AKAP6), which in turn is bound to RyR1/ RyR2 via LIZ motifs (Fig. 15-1).[5] The protein phosphatase 1 (PP1) is bound to RyR1/ RyR2 via spinophilin,[6,530] and protein phosphatase PP2A selectively associates with RyR2 through its adaptor protein PR130.[6] Finally, we as well as others have recently shown that the Ca^{2+}/calmodulin-dependent protein kinase II (CaMKII) binds to RyR2, although the binding site has not yet been identified.[298,523]

The Ca^{2+} channel-stabilizing proteins calstabin1 (also known as FKBP12) and calstabin2 (also known as FKBP12.6) associate with RyR1 and RyR2, respectively, such that one calstabin protein is bound to each RyR monomer.[10,148,299,531-533] Thus, there are four calstabin molecules bound to each RyR1 and RyR2 channel complex. RyR1 and RyR3 channels can bind calstabin1 and calstabin2, although the affinity for calstabin1 is higher.[532-534] Therefore, *in vivo*, RyR1 and RyR3 have calstabin1 bound because of its higher abundance in the cytosol.[532,533] RyR2 channels exhibit a relatively higher affinity for calstabin2, and bind calstabin2 *in vivo*.[533,535]

Cryo-electronmicroscopy studies of the RyR1 complex show that calstabin1 binds to RyR1 on the outer surface of the cytoplasmic domain (see Chapter 3).[111] Recent observations suggest that the binding site of calstabin2 on the three-dimensional structure of RyR2 is similar to that of calstabin1 on RyR1.[108] Valine 2461 (V2461) on RyR1 [corresponding to isoleucine 2427 (I2427) on RyR2] is critical for calstabin1 binding.[536] The bond formed by V2461 and proline 2462 (Pro2462) (or I2427-P2428 in RyR2) is likely constrained in a high energy, unstable twisted-amide transition state intermediate of a peptidyl-prolyl bond (unable to isomerize to either *cis* or *trans* due to presumed steric hindrances in the RyR structure)[148]. It is to this high energy, unstable twisted-amide that calstabin 1 and 2

(FKBP12, FKBP12.6) bind with high affinity.[536] This model is supported by the finding that introducing flexibility around this peptidyl-prolyl bond with the mutation of V2461 to a glycine residue abolishes binding of calstabin1 or calstabin2 to RyR1.[536] In this model, calstabin binds to RyR with high affinity and is only released when the channel is PKA phosphorylated which reduces the binding affinity for calstabin to the channel (see below). Since the target peptidyl-prolyl bond in RyR is constrained in the high energy transition-state intermediate between *cis* and *trans* isomerization cannot be completed, otherwise the calstabin would fall off the channel under physiological conditions. We have proposed that introduction of increased mobility around the peptidyl-prolyl bond by substituting a smaller amino acid, glycine, for either the valine or isoleucine allows for isomerization to proceed by reducing steric hindrance at that site and the binding affinity of calstabin to the channel is greatly reduced.[536] In support of this model Bultynck *et al.* recently concluded, based on molecular modeling studies, that the proline in the calstabin-binding region on RyR induces a bend in the alpha helix, which imposes a twisted amide transition state on the peptidyl-proline bond and enables calstabin to bind to this domain.[537]

In addition, it is likely that other regions on RyR are also involved in stabilizing the binding of calstabin to the channel since PKA phosphorylation of RyR2-2809 which is 347 residues away from the peptidyl-prolyl bond at 2461-2462 reduces the binding affinity by adding a negative charge resulting in electrostatic repulsion of calstabin2.[5] In agreement with this model, Masumiya *et al.* have proposed that other regions within the N-terminal domain of RyR2 are required for the binding of GST-calstabin2 to RyR2,[538] although they did not identify specific residues on RyR2 involved in calstabin2 binding.

Other proteins that bind to the cytoplasmic domain of RyR include calmodulin (CaM), a 16.7 kDa cytosolic protein that influences SR Ca^{2+} release (see Chapter 16),[539-541] and sorcin, a ubiquitous 22 kDa Ca^{2+}-binding protein reported to associate with both RyR2 and the LTCC (Fig. 15-1).[542,543] Sorcin may reduce RyR2 open probability, but this effect can be relieved by PKA phosphorylation of sorcin.[521] A functional role for sorcin in the RyR channel complex is less well defined.

RyR also binds proteins at the luminal SR surface (e.g., triadin, junctin, and calsequestrin; see Fig. 15-1). Junctin[227] and triadrin[128] are presumably involved in anchoring RyR to the SR membrane. Calsequestrin (CSQ) is a major Ca^{2+} binding protein in the SR, and provides high-capacity low-affinity intraluminal Ca^{2+}binding.[206,544] It has been suggested Ca^{2+}-dependent conformational changes in CSQ may modulate RyR channel activity,[545] although the exact nature of the CSQ-RyR modulation requires further investigations.[546-548]

REGULATION OF RYRs BY PHOSPHORYLATION/ DEPHOSPHORYLATION

PKA phosphorylation

Phosphorylation of RyR by PKA is physiologically important as it plays a role in augmenting SR Ca^{2+} release during stress in order to increase cardiac output.[294,346,350,549] Phosphorylation of RyR by PKA is the downstream event in a signaling pathway that begins with the activation of β-adrenergic receptors (β-AR), via stimulation of the sympathetic nervous system, which activates adenylyl cyclase (AC) via specific G-proteins, resulting in generation of the second messenger cyclic AMP (cAMP), which in turn activates PKA (Fig. 15-2). This evolutionarily conserved mechanism is part of the "fight-or-flight" response that allows for rapid enhancement of cardiac contractility and cardiac output during exercise or stress.[550,551]

Recent data also suggest that β-AR stimulation and PKA phosphorylation of RyR2 may increase cardiac chronotropy.[552] β-AR stimulation increases the likelihood for RyRs to open (i.e., more RyRs are recruited within a given T-tubule/ SR junction), augmenting the Ca^{2+} spark amplitude.[329] The fraction of T-tubule/SR junctions within a cardiomyocyte that fire in response to excitation is also increased by β-AR stimulation.[553] Thus, the overall enhanced SR Ca^{2+} release by RyRs following β-AR stimulation is characterized by synchronization and augmentation of RyR gating both within and among T-tubule/SR junctions.[329]

Phospho-peptide mapping has shown that PKA phosphorylates serine 2809 on RyR2.[345,554] These results have been confirmed in several studies using GST-fusion proteins, mutations in the full-length recombinant RyR2 channel, and a phospho-epitope specific antibody.[5,294,298,326,349] Similar studies have revealed that the homologous serine 2843 is the PKA phosphorylation site on RyR1.[555]

Several laboratories have examined the functional effects of exogenously applied PKA on single channel behavior of RyR2.[5,294,326,346,349,350,556] Most of these studies have demonstrated that phosphorylation by PKA increases the open probability (Po) of RyR2 by increasing the sensitivity of RyR2 to Ca^{2+}-dependent activation.[5,294,298,346] However, some studies have shown first an increase in RyR2 open probability followed by a slight decrease in the steady-state Po of RyR2 channels.[247] The role of RyR1 and RyR2 PKA phosphorylation has also been evaluated using phosphorylation-site mutants that mimic constitutively PKA phosphorylated or dephosphorylated channels converting serine to aspartatic acid (RyR1-S2843D, RyR2-S2809D) or an alanine (RyR1-S2843A, RyR2-S2809A) substitution. Our lab has shown that recombinant RyR1-S2843A or RyR2-S2809A mutant channels exhibit a sensitivity to Ca^{2+}-dependent activation similar to wild-type channels.[294,298,555] Mutant channels that mimic constitutively PKA phosphorylated channels, RyR1-S2843D and RyR2-S2809D, exhibit increased channel activity and Ca^{2+}-sensitivity, compared to wild-type channels.[294,298,555] In contrast, in using a heterologous expression system, Stange *et al.* reported that RyR2-S2809D channel function was similar to the wild-type channels, likely due to the presence of non-physiologically excessive levels of calstabin in these experiments, which overcomes of the effect of PKA phosphorylation.

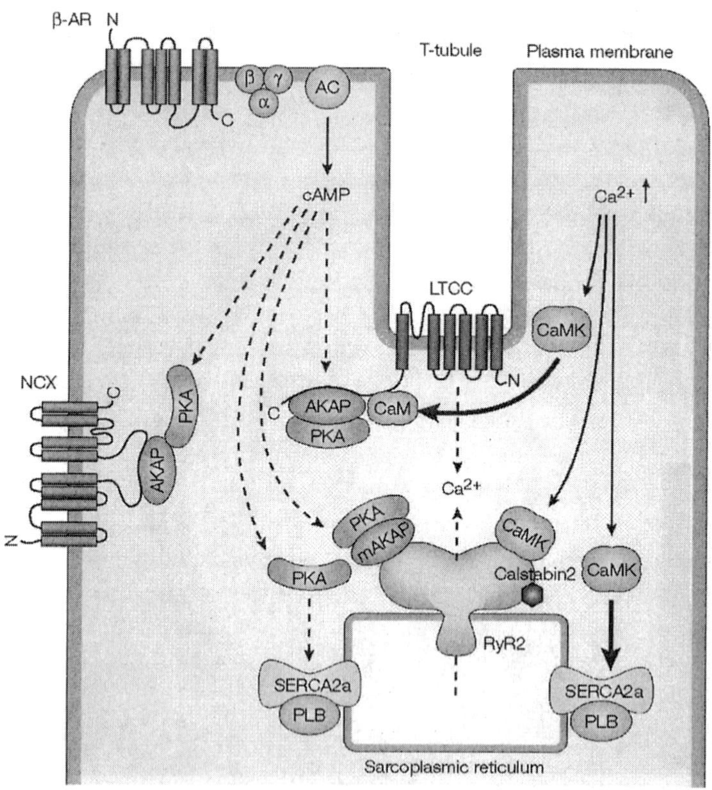

Figure 15-2. **Regulation of intracellular Ca^{2+} signaling in the heart.** Several intracellular signaling pathways can increase the gain of the EC-coupling system. Agonist-activation of the β-AR allows for activation of adenylate cyclase (AC) via G-proteins. The subsequent generation of cyclic AMP (cAMP) activates protein kinase A (PKA), which may be targeted to LTCC via an AKAP, and RyR2 and NCX via AKAPs as well. Faster heart rates increase the average cytosolic Ca^{2+} concentration, which activates CaMKII. CaMKII can phosphorylate LTCC, RyR2 (to which CaMKII is directly targeted), and PLB. Both PKA and CaMKII phosphorylation increase the RyR2 open probability. Reproduced with permission from Wehrens *et al.*[524]

In normal cardiomyocytes, PKA-phosphorylation of RyR2 does not increase the spontaneous Ca^{2+} spark frequency under conditions that simulate diastole in the heart, when RyR2 is expected to be tightly closed.[297] These data are consistent with the fact that healthy subjects or animals do not develop SR Ca^{2+} leak and arrhythmias during exercise.[294,299] On the other hand, recent data show that PKA-phosphorylation of RyR2 enhances RyR2 activity and increases EC coupling gain during the early phase of EC coupling when only a small number of LTCCs are open.[295,557] In addition, stimulation of β-AR receptors and increased intracellular PKA activity may augment the function of LTCCs, Na^{+}/Ca^{2+} exhanger (NCX), and the SR Ca^{2+}-ATPase (SERCA2a), which may contribute to enhanced EC coupling following exercise or stress (Fig. 15-2).[558]

PKA reduces calstabin binding to RyR

Of all the proteins that bind to the cytoplasmic/scaffold domain of the RyRs, the functional role for calstabins in the RyR macromolecular complex is one of the best understood. Calstabin1 was originally identified as KC7, a peptide that co-purifies with RyR1.[10,531] The functional role for calstabin1 in the RyR1 complex was first demonstrated using a heterologous co-expression system in which it was shown that calstabin1 stabilizes the open and closed states of the channel.[522] Similar findings were reported for calstabin2 in the RyR2 complex.[559]

PKA-phosphorylation of RyR2-S2809 reduces the binding affinity for calstabin2 resulting in the dissociation of calstabin2 from the macromolecular complex.[5,294,298] Similarly, PKA-phosphorylation of RyR1 can result in the dissociation of calstabin1 from RyR1 channels.[536] Some groups, however, have shown that calstabin2 may bind to PKA phosphorylated RyR2 under certain experimental conditions.[325,326,560] These apparent contradictory findings may be explained by the presence of relatively higher concentrations of calstabin2 (e.g., when calstabin2 is overexpressed with RyR2 under physiological conditions as in Stange *et al.*[325] and Xiao *et al.*[326], or added in excess amounts as in Xiao *et al.*[326]). The presence of excessive amounts of calstabin2 allows it to bind to PKA-phosphorylated RyR2 or RyR2-S2809D because it overwhelms the shift in binding-affinity induced by PKA-phosphorylation of RyR2-S2809.[298]

Since calstabin2 concentrations in mammalian hearts are in the range of 200-400 nmol/L, PKA phosphorylation during stress or exercise will result in the partial dissociation of calstabin2 from RyR2 because it decreases the affinity of calstabin2 binding to RyR2 to ~600 nM.[298,561] The partial depletion of calstabin2 from the RyR2 channel complex increases the Po of the channel resulting in increased intracellular Ca^{2+} release and augmented cardiac contractility under conditions of increased β-adrenergic signaling.[294] Calstabin2 is also critical to normal RyR2 channel operation in the heart under resting conditions.[5,559,562] Binding of calstabin2 stabilizes the RyR2 channel in the closed state during the resting phase of the cardiac contraction when the chambers refill with blood (diastole).[294,522] Maintaining RyR2 in the closed state during diastole is critically important for preventing aberrant diastolic SR Ca^{2+} release (leak) that can trigger cardiac arrhythmias.[294]

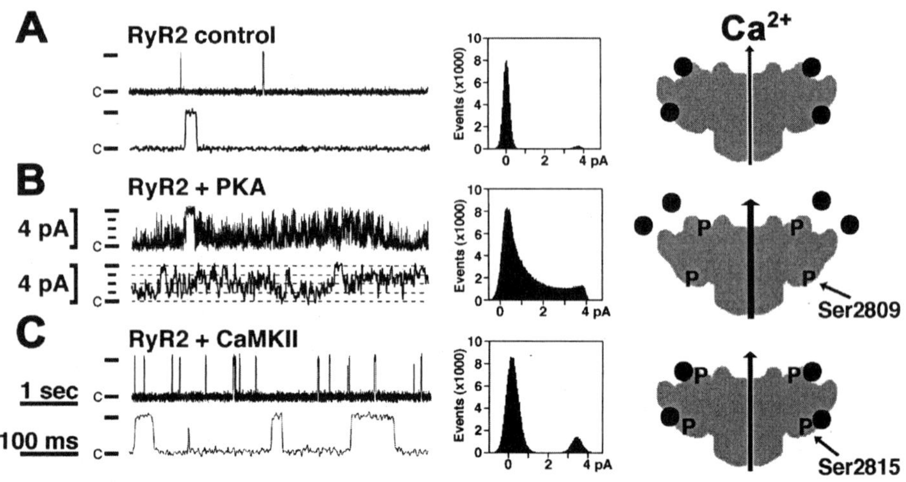

Figure 15-3. **Effects of PKA or CaMKII phosphorylation of RyR2 on channel function and composition of the macromolecular complex under diastolic conditions. A**. Non-phosphorylated RyR2 channel function under diastolic conditions. Amplitude histogram shows dominance of the closed state, on the right is shown the binding of four calstabin2 subunits to the non-phosphorylated RyR2 channel. **B**. Exercise and stress activate the β–adrenergic receptor signaling pathway and PKA. PKA phosphorylation of Ser^{2809} on RyR2 increases the open probability and decreases the binding affinity for the channel-stabilizing subunit calstabin2, resulting in partial channel openings (subconductance states). **C**. Increasing the heart rate activates Ca^{2+}/calmodulin-dependent protein kinase II (CaMKII). Autophosphorylation of CaMKII activates this enzyme resulting in phosphorylation of Ser^{2815} on RyR2 and increased open probability of the channel without dissociating calstabin2 (and without inducing subconductance states). Reproduced and adapted, with permission, from Wehrens *et al.*[298]

Dissociation of calstabin2 from the RyR2 channel complex due to PKA phosphorylation of the channel, or competing it off with the drug rapamycin results in subconductance states (Fig. 15-3).[5,522,559,563,564] Subconductance states are open events with less than the normal unitary current amplitude. Thus, calstabin increases the probability of full conductance openings of RyR channels. RyR channels are present on the terminal cisternae of the SR in a dense array such that the corners of each channel contact its neighbors in a checkerboard type of pattern. Calstabins also functionally couple groups of RyR channels to permit synchronous opening and closing (gating) of arrays of channels.[316,536] This phenomenon, called 'coupled gating', enables arrays of RyR channels to gate in unison, a process that enhances the efficiency of SR Ca^{2+} release and helps terminate SR Ca^{2+} release by inducing the closure of arrays of channels when the first channel in the group closes. This model is supported by experiments in which release events, known as Ca^{2+} sparks, are observed to have defective termination when calstabin2 is depleted from the RyR2 macromolecular complex.[287,565]

Phosphorylation by CaMKII

Ca^{2+}/calmodulin-dependent kinase II plays an important role in regulating EC coupling in the normal heart.[566] CaMKII activity increases at higher heart rates. We have proposed that CaMKII mediates increased SR Ca^{2+} release leading to enhanced contractile force in the heart in a heart rate dependent manner.[298] This phenomenon is known as the 'positive force-frequency relationship'.[567] CaMKII phosphorylation of several key Ca^{2+} handling proteins leads to increased SR Ca^{2+} release and improved Ca^{2+} removal from the cytoplasm. This function is important because it allows for more efficient contraction and relaxation of the heart required to support cardiac output at increased heart rates (Fig. 15-2).[298,355,566]

Recent studies have revealed that CaMKII-delta associates with and regulates the activity of RyR2 in the heart.[298,338,523] Based on phospho-peptide mapping, it was proposed that CaMKII phosphorylates the same residue on RyR2 as PKA (serine 2809).[345,349,554] However, using site directed mutational analyses that were not previously conducted we recently demonstrated that CaMKII phosphorylates serine 2815.[298] The CaMKII phosphorylation site in RyR2, S2815, is 6 residues away from the site originally proposed as the CaMKII site, and is contained in the phosphorylated peptide that was identified as both the PKA and CaMKII site. however, these earlier studies did not recognize that two distinct phosphorylation sites, the PKA site at S2809 and the CaMKII site at S2815, were both contained in the same phoshorylated peptide. [345,349,554] We showed that mutating Ser2815 to alanine in full-length recombinant RyR2 channels abolishes CaMKII phosphorylation.[298] Identification of the CaMKII phosphorylation site on RyR2, which was also confirmed using a phospho-epitope specific antibody, has facilitated the elucidation of the functional effects of CaMKII phosphorylation of RyR2.[296,298,338,346,350,554,568] Single channel studies of CaMKII phosphorylated wild-type RyR2 channels, and RyR2-S2815D mutant channels, that mimic constitutively CaMKII-phosphorylated RyR2, have shown that CaMKII phosphorylation of RyR2-S2815 increases the open probability of the channel by augmenting the sensitivity to Ca^{2+}-dependent activation (Fig. 15-3).[296,298,338] In contrast to phosphorylation by PKA, CaMKII-phosphorylation does not dissociate calstabin2 from the RyR2 channel because the binding affinity for calstabin2 is not reduced (Fig. 15-3).[298]

In ventricular myocytes, CaMKII phosphorylation of RyR2 causes an increase in Ca^{2+} spark frequency, which can be blocked by the CaMKII-inhibitor KN-93.[296] These data are consistent with an increase in RyR2 open probability following CaMKII phosphorylation.[298] Therefore, it is likely that activation of CaMKII during increased heart rates causes faster and increased SR Ca^{2+} release via CaMKII-phosphorylated RyR2,[298,351] thereby contributing to the "positive force-frequency response" in order to maintain and enhance cardiac output despite shorter cycle lengths.

Dephosphorylation by phosphatases

The activity of RyR2 is also regulated by protein phosphatases PP1 and PP2A, which are targeted to the macromolecular channel complex (Fig. 15-1).[6,350,569] Terentyev *et al.* have reported that protein phosphatase 1 (PP1) may increase RyR2 activity, although this study is in contrast with several other studies that reported that PP1 decreases RyR2 activity,[357,358,556,570-572] and that PKA/ CaMKII phosphorylation increases RyR2 activity.[5,296,298,346]

Interaction between phosphorylation and calcium activation

It has been proposed that PKA phosphorylation of RyR2 channels increases the sensitivity for Ca^{2+} dependent activation,[5] and these observations were recently confirmed using recombinant RyR2 channels.[294] Interestingly, RyR2 missense mutations which are linked to genetic forms of sudden cardiac death (SCD)[53,54] decrease the calstabin2 binding affinity in RyR2 and induce a leftward shift in Ca^{2+} dependent RyR2 activation.[294,573] In other words, these mutant RyR2 channels show a higher open probability for any given cytosolic Ca^{2+} concentration following PKA phosphorylation. We have proposed that during diastole when cytosolic Ca^{2+} concentrations are very low (~100 nM) in order to permit relaxation of cardiac muscle, spontaneous diastolic activation of mutant RyR2 channels occurs more frequently in SCD-linked mutant RyR2 compared with wild-type RyR2, during stress (exercise) due to PKA phosphorylation of the channel.[297]

In addition to calstabin2, millimolar Mg^{2+} concentrations, which inhibit RyR2 activity, likely help maintain RyR2 in the closed state during diastole.[574] The EC_{50} for Mg^{2+} sensitivity of maximally activated RyR channels is in the low millimolar range.[574,575] Since gating of RyR depends on both Ca^{2+} activation and Mg^{2+} inhibition, regulation of the channel by these two cations has been proposed to be competitive.[574,576] However, the exact molecular mechanisms of Ca^{2+} activation and Mg^{2+} inhibition are not well understood, as Ca^{2+} activating and inhibitory sites have not yet been precisely identified on RyR2.[577,578]

Ca^{2+} spark rates in skeletal muscles are also regulated by cytosolic Mg^{2+} concentrations.[579] Experiments using single RyR1 channels showed that free Mg^{2+} (1 mM) does not block activation of the channel in the presence of maximal PKA phosphorylation. However, Mg^{2+} blocked RyR1 activation in the dephosphorylated state.[556] Enhanced SR Ca^{2+} release may also occur during altered conditions that favor increased PKA phosphorylation of RyR2 in the setting of decreased Mg^{2+} concentrations, such as hypoxia, ischemia, or fatigue.[272] Under these conditions, diastolic SR Ca^{2+} leak would be enhanced. Indeed, decreased Mg^{2+} sensitivity of RyR has been demonstrated to be an important mechanism of SR Ca^{2+} leak in malignant hyperthermia[580], and in catecholaminergic ventricular arrhythmias.[573] Future studies will be required to characterize the exact nature of Ca^{2+} and Mg^{2+} dependent regulation of PKA phosphorylated RyRs *in vivo*.

CONCLUDING REMARKS

The cytoplasmic domain of the RyR/ intracellular Ca^{2+} release channel serves as a scaffold for accessory proteins that modulate channel activity. The association of protein kinases and phosphatases allows for local regulation of RyR activity. In non-diseased muscle, during the classic "fight or flight" stress response, PKA phosphorylation of RyR increases systolic SR Ca^{2+} release by increasing EC coupling gain. PKA phosphorylation of phospholamban and the SR Ca^{2+}-ATPase also enhances SR Ca^{2+} uptake. Thus, both SR Ca^{2+} uptake and release are augmented resulting in increased Ca^{2+} transients and enhanced muscle contration. In part this is achieved by enhancing Ca^{2+}-dependent activation of RyRs via PKA-phosphorylation of RyR1/ RyR2 which reduces the binding affinity of the channel-stabilizing protein calstabin1 (FKBP12)/ calstabin2 (FKBP12.6), respectively. Calstabin stabilizes the closed state of RyRs, thereby reducing RyR open probability and preventing aberrant calcium (Ca^{2+}) release in resting muscles. In response to an increase in heart rate, activation of CaMKII increases RyR2 activity leading to augmented SR Ca^{2+} release. Thus, regulation of RyR2 open probability via phosphorylation/dephosphorylation contributes to the dynamic modulation of EC coupling in skeletal and cardiac muscles.

Chapter 16

RYR1 MODULATION BY CALMODULIN

Effects of protein-protein interaction and redox modification

Paula Aracena[1,2], Cecilia Hidalgo[2], and Susan L. Hamilton[1]
[1] *Molecular Physiology and Biophysics Department, Baylor College of Medicine, Houston, TX;* [2] *FONDAP Center for Molecular Studies of the Cell, Facultad de Medicina, Universidad de Chile, Santiago, Chile*

INTRODUCTION

Ryanodine receptor regulation is both complex and extensive. In addition to its modulation by ions and small molecules,[210] this channel is also regulated by interactions with a wide array of proteins.[344,581] In this chapter, we will focus on the regulation of type-1 ryanodine receptors (RyR1) by calmodulin. In particular, we discuss how this specific interaction is modulated by other protein-protein interactions and cysteine redox modification in the context of EC coupling.

CALMODULIN STRUCTURE, FUNCTION AND INTERACTION WITH RYR1

Calmodulin is a Ca^{2+}-binding protein ubiquitously present in the cytoplasm of eukaryotic cells. Changes in its three-dimensional structure that occur upon Ca^{2+} binding allow calmodulin to function as a Ca^{2+} sensor and to differentially regulate downstream signaling pathways. Calmodulin has a number of target molecules including kinases, phosphatases, and ion channels. In skeletal muscle both of the major channels that participate in excitation-contraction coupling, the sarcoplasmic reticulum Ca^{2+} release channel or ryanodine receptor and the T-tubule L-type voltage-dependent Ca^{2+}-channel/ dihydropyridine receptor (DHPR) are modulated by calmodulin. In this review chapter we concentrate on the regulation of these two channels by calmodulin. The reader is directed to selected recent reviews for in-depth discussions of other calmodulin targets.[582-585]

Structure

Calmodulin is a 17-kDa protein composed of 148 amino acid residues arranged in two globular, helix loop helix, domains or lobes linked by a single helix. Like many cytosolic Ca^{2+}-binding proteins, the Ca^{2+} binding EF-hand motifs are arranged in pairs: one pair per each lobe termed I and II for the N-terminal lobe and III and IV for the C-terminal lobe (for review, see Hoeflich *et al.*[583])

The Ca^{2+}-free and Ca^{2+}-bound forms of calmodulin are termed apocalmodulin (apoCaM) and Ca^{2+}/calmodulin (CaCaM). The two forms share some features in their three-dimensional structures;[586,587] but the binding of Ca^{2+} to apoCaM changes its interhelical angles, leading to the exposure of its lobe-hydrophobic cores, thus allowing CaCaM to interact with different downstream targets.[588] Several types of calmodulin binding motifs have been identified (for review see Roads *et al.*[589]). One of CaM binding sequences is designated an IQ-motif, which is a basic amphipathic helix consisting of approximately 20 amino acid residues with a consensus sequence of IQXXXRGXXXR, where the first position can be Ile, Leu or Val (for review, see Bahler *et al.*[582]).

CaM has no tryptophan residues in its amino acid sequence, precluding the analysis of changes in tryptophan fluorescence to assess conformational changes in the protein upon binding Ca^{2+} or interacting with a target site. Mutation of phenlyalanine residues at positions 19 and 92, however, has allowed the assessment of the affinity of the N and C-lobes, respectively, of CaM for Ca^{2+}.[590,591] Using these mutants, it has been shown that both calmodulin lobes display cooperativity in Ca^{2+}-binding. The apparent dissociation constants for Ca^{2+} binding to the E-F hands in the N-terminal lobe of unbound CaM were calculated as 4.45 ± 0.1 and 1.0 ± 0.1 μM, whereas a single value of 14.0 ± 2.4 μM was calculated for the C-terminal lobe.[590,591]

Functional effects on RYR1 activity

ApoCaM enhances channel activity while CaCaM inhibits it.[592,593] Since both CaM and RyR1 are Ca^{2+} binding proteins the question naturally arises as to whether the Ca^{2+} dependence of the functional effects of CaM arises from Ca^{2+} binding to CaM, RyR1 or both. In the absence of CaM, native (as opposed to oxidized or reduced) RyR1 activity shows a bell shaped dependence on Ca^{2+} concentration: At 1 to 10 μM concentrations, Ca^{2+} binds to a putative high affinity site on RyR1 and enhances its activity while at concentrations above 0.1 mM concentrations, Ca^{2+} binds to a low affinity site and inhibits channel activity. In the presence of CaM, the channel is activated at lower Ca^{2+} concentrations, partially inhibited at intermediate Ca^{2+} concentrations and inhibited further at Ca^{2+} concentrations above 0.1mM.[594] To differentiate between events arising from Ca^{2+} binding to CaM from those arising from Ca^{2+} binding to RyR1, we examined the effects of a Ca^{2+} binding site mutant of CaM, E1234Q[595-597] on the activity of RyR1 at different Ca^{2+} concentrations. We found that this CaM which is unable to bind Ca^{2+} was an activator of RyR1 at all Ca^{2+} concentrations, suggesting that it is Ca^{2+} binding to CaM that converts it from an activator to an inhibitor of the channel.[598] Furthermore, we have shown that Ca^{2+} binding to the C-terminal lobe of calmodulin is sufficient for the switch in calmodulin function.[598]

Interaction with RYR1 and Ca^{2+}

To identify the location of the CaM binding site on RyR1, we first used the ability of CaM to protect sites on RyR1 from tryptic digestion.[540] We found that CaCaM could protect sites after amino acids 3620 and 3627 from tryptic cleavage[540] while apoCaM could protect both these same two sites (3620 and 3627) as well as two new sites after amino acids 1983 and 1999.[541] The distance between these two sites in the primary sequence suggests that: 1) there are two discreet apoCaM binding sites on RyR1, 2) two regions of the protein (amino acids 1983-1999 and 3620-3627) come together in the quaternary structure of RyR1 (either inter or intramolecularly) or 3) CaM binding to RyR1 allosterically alters the conformation of one or both of these regions moving them to locations inaccessible to proteases. We have shown that each subunit of RyR1 binds only one molecule of apoCaM or one molecule of CaCaM,[594] eliminating the first interpretation. In addition, since apoCaM and CaCaM have opposite functional effects it seems unlikely that the protection of the cleavage sites at 3620 and 3627 arises from allosteric burying of these regions. We have also shown that E1234Q CaM (an activator of the channel at all Ca^{2+}concentrations) and a mutant CaM with 3 additional amino acids (a competitive antagonist of apoCaM at low Ca^{2+}) protect the sites after amino acids 1983 and 1999 at high and low Ca^{2+}, respectively. Since the sites after amino acids 1983 and 1999 are protected from tryptic digestion when the channel is presumably in different functional states it again seems unlikely that the protection is due to an allosteric burying of these sites. Furthermore, peptides corresponding to amino acids 3614-43 and to 1975-1999 have been shown to bind both CaCaM and apoCaM.[599,600] These findings, taken together, suggest that the CaM binding site on RyR1 is noncontiguous and is formed by amino acids at both 3614-43 and 1975-1999. The contributions of these two sequences to the CaM binding site raises the question of whether these sequences come together within a subunit or between two adjacent subunits. As will be discussed below, our data support an intersubunit binding site for CaM in the RyR1 tetramer. Yamaguchi *et al.*[601] confirmed the contribution of the sequence from 3614-43 to the CaM binding site by creating RyR1 mutations within this region (W3620A and L3624D) and showing that these mutations decreased the affinity of RyR1 for calmodulin, particularly at low Ca^{2+}.[601]

All of our data have suggested that both apoCaM and CaCaM are binding to these same two regions of RyR1. This is somewhat surprising since Wagenknecht and coworkers[113] showed a 33Å center to center displacement of CaM in the 3D structure of RyR1 at high versus low Ca^{2+} concentrations. Also, considering the major conformational change that takes place in CaM upon binding Ca^{2+}, it is difficult to see how these two forms of CaM could bind to the same site. We have shown that, upon binding Ca^{2+}, CaM appears to shift N-terminally within the 3614-43 sequence, suggesting that different determinants within this sequence are required for CaCaM and apoCaM binding. However, it seems unlikely that this shift would account for the 33 Å displacement seen in the 3D structure and it is possible that the location of these sequences that constitute the CaM binding site in the 3D structure is dependent on the functional state of the channel. It is important to keep in mind with mapping of the sites in the 3D state that apoCaM is an activator of the Ca^{2+} free channel and CaCaM is an inhibitor of the Ca^{2+} bound channel. The addition of Ca^{2+} to the apoCaM bound channel will lead to binding of Ca^{2+} to both CaM and RyR1. The combined changes in the structure of CaM and RyR1 may together account for the 33Å displacement.

A RELATIONSHIP BETWEEN CALMODULIN AND REDOX MODULATION OF RYR1

Another feature of CaM binding to RyR1 is its redox sensitivity. Oxidation of the channel abolishes both apoCaM and CaCaM binding while treatment of RyR1 with N-ethyl maleimide under conditions that lead to alkylation of less than 2% of the total cysteines on the channel abolishes apoCaM but not CaCaM binding. Conversely, oxidation of RyR1 produces an intersubunit disulfide bond and this oxidation can be prevented by bound CaM. These findings suggest that there might be a redox sensitive, hyper-reactive cysteine close to the CaM binding site. Using [^{14}C]-NEM labeling, proteolysis, and N-terminal sequencing of fragments we showed that one of the cysteines involved in the intersubunit disulfide bond and whose alkylation could block apoCaM binding was C3635.[602,603]

REDOX MODIFICATION OF RYR1

During the last 15 years, increasing evidence has accumulated supporting the redox modulation of RyR channels.[484,604,605] It has been shown that a small number of hyper reactive sulfhydryls on RyR1 are susceptible to oxidation,[606-610] S-nitrosylation,[611,612] and S-glutathionylation[613] by a number of endogenous redox-active agents (such as superoxide anion, hydrogen peroxide, nitric oxide, glutathione disulfide, and S-nitrosoglutathione). Typically, exposure of RyR1 to these agents increases its sensitivity towards activators and/or decreases its sensitivity towards inhibitors[613-615] As mentioned above, at the molecular level, oxidation of RyR1 leads to disulfide cross-linking of neighboring subunits.[606] RyR1 Cys3635 appears to be central to the modulation of RyR1 by nitric oxide, as demonstrated by studies from Gerhard Meissner and colleagues using a RyR1 Cys3635Ala mutant. They demonstrated that S-nitrosylation of RyR1 by nitric oxide takes place on this residue alone.[616] However, they have shown that mutation of this residue does not alter calmodulin binding[601,616] and that NO treatment of vesicles does not alter calmodulin binding.[612] One possible conclusion from these and our studies is that Cys3635 may not be crucial for calmodulin binding, but alkylation of this residue by NEM may sterically inhibit apoCaM binding while oxidation to produce an intersubunit disulfide may limit the access of both apoCaM and CaCaM to the CaM binding site between 3614-43. Additional studies have shown that exposure of RyR1 to S-nitrosoglutathione elicits S-nitrosylation of 2-3 RyR1 cysteine residues, none of which corresponds to Cys3635.[617] It is not yet known whether these treatments alter CaM binding.

We have recently shown that RyR1 cysteine residues can form glutathione adducts through S-glutathionylation upon treatment with S-nitrosoglutathione;[613] since this agent also leads to S-nitrosylation of the channel protein, we are currently working to discriminate whether S-glutathionylation of RyR1 changes its interaction with calmodulin.

CALMODULIN MODULATION OF EC COUPLING

Three regions of the C-terminal tail of the DHPR α1-subunit have been implicated in calmodulin binding to this channel: A, CB and IQ.[599,618,619] We have shown that a peptide representing the CB region of DHPR is able to inhibit RyR1 activity.[599] Furthermore, a RyR1 peptide representing the 3609-43 sequence is able to strongly interact with DHPR α1-subunit from detergent-solubilized transverse-tubule membranes.[620] We suggested that coupled DHPR and RyR1 in triads may interact through these calmodulin-binding motifs, precluding calmodulin binding to both sequences. Calmodulin would bind to these regions when DHPR and RyR1 are not coupled. In addition to the implication that calmodulin-binding motifs may be used to bind proteins other than calmodulin itself, these observations suggest that calmodulin may participate in the molecular control of EC-coupling.[620]

CONCLUDING REMARKS

The 3614-43 CaM-binding motif on RyR1 appears to represent a more general protein-protein interaction motif since it can also interact with a determinant in the carboxyterminal tail of the L-type Ca^{2+} channel.[620] This finding raises important questions about the role of calmodulin in mechanical excitation-contraction coupling in skeletal muscle. A recent study by O'Connell *et al.*[621] has suggested that mutations that destroy CaM binding to RyR1 have little effect on mechanical E-C coupling. This suggests that CaM is either not involved in mechanical E-C coupling, or it can compete at this one site of interaction between the two proteins but does not greatly alter coupling. ApoCaM binding to RyR1 increases the affinity of the Ca^{2+} activating site on RyR1 for Ca^{2+}.[594] One possibility is that the primary role of CaM-RyR1 interaction is to modulate the behavior of channels that are not mechanically gated by the DHPR. We propose that apoCaM increases RyR sensitivity to Ca^{2+}, thereby facilitating CICR, while Ca^{2+}-CaM may help the channels to close or control the number of channels that are open at any one time.

Chapter 17

RYANODINE RECEPTOR FUNCTION IN INFLAMMATION

Edmond D. Buck[1,3] and Barbara E. Ehrlich[1,2]
Depts. of Pharmacology[1] and Cellular & Molecular Physiology[2], Yale University, New Haven, CT; and Warner Instruments[3], Hamden, CT

INTRODUCTION

The role of ryanodine receptors as an integral component in the inflammation response is currently unexplored. A survey of the literature, however, provides indication that ryanodine receptors participate directly with, or are modulated by elements of several metabolic pathways critical to the inflammatory response. In this chapter we outline and discuss the involvement of ryanodine receptor activity within the context of inflammation.

A BRIEF REVIEW OF INFLAMMATION

The inflammation response is intimately associated with the immune system and functions as a protective mechanism of vascularized tissue to invasion, injury or insult. The main features of the inflammatory response are vasodilation, increased vascular permeability, cellular infiltration, and activation of the immune system.[622] In general, inflammation is described as being either acute or chronic in nature. However, the distinction is often blurred and there is much overlap between the two categories.

Acute inflammation is characterized by neutrophil infiltration and edema.[622-625] It is sudden in onset, of short duration and usually leads directly to healing. It occurs in response to physical insult (e.g., mechanical injury, temperature extremes, and infrared, microwave or ultraviolet radiation), chemical agents (e.g., caustics, poisons, and venoms), biological agents (e.g., viruses, microorganisms and parasites), as well as to antigens. In addition, metabolic byproducts of ischemia and the oxidative burst following reperfusion can induce acute inflammation through the action of reactive oxygen species (ROS).[626,627] Regardless of the inducing mechanism, the acute inflammation response is characterized by a sequence of cellular events indicating a convergence to a common set of activated metabolic pathways.

Chronic inflammation, on the other hand, is characterized by infiltration of mononuclear phagocytes and lymphocytes into the affected area.[622,624] These cells are recruited by the release of chemotactic factors from mast cells and neutrophils.[623,628] The chronic response is distinguished from the acute response because of its delayed onset, slower progression, and it involves a greater proliferation of cellular and chemical mediators.

The process leading from acute to chronic inflammation is often normal but can become pathological when the inducing agent cannot be effectively removed. Examples of this principal include pathologies resulting from exposure to the tuberculosis bacterium (Mycobacterium tuberculosis)[629] and to asbestos.[630] Alternatively, chronic inflammation can be primary in origin, skipping the acute phase entirely, as is seen in various viral infections, autoimmune diseases, parasitic infections, and malignant tumors. Furthermore, chronic inflammation does not always lead to healing, and prolonged inflammation can lead to persistent and often irreversible conditions such as diabetes, arteriosclerosis, Alzheimer's disease, cancer and arthritis.[631]

RYANODINE RECEPTORS AND CHEMICAL MEDIATORS OF INFLAMMATION

Inflammatory signaling molecules are produced by many cell types, including endothelial cells, neural cells, neutrophils, macrophages, and mast cells.[624,631] Chemical mediators used by these cells include histamine, nitric oxide, bradykinin, and the eicosanoids.[624] Although the traditional view is that these signaling molecules primarily stimulate the phosphoinositide pathway, additional cellular pathways are also invoked. Interestingly, each of the above described cells involved in the inflammatory response possesses functional ryanodine receptors.[632-635]

Many signaling molecules recruit the ryanodine receptor pathway to shape the spatio-temporal response of inflammation. An inflammatory response can also be directly initiated by the ryanodine receptor pathway.

The interaction between ryanodine receptors and several mediators of inflammation is highlighted here.

Histamine

Histamine is one of two principal agents producing the commonly observed effects of inflammation and hypersensitivity. These effects include vasodilation, vascular permeability, and smooth muscle contraction.[636] Histamine is released from mast cells and basophils, both of which are present throughout the body. Resting mast cells can be found in connective tissue and in the bloodstream, whereas basophils infiltrate tissue from the bloodstream only after activation.[628,637] Mast cell and basophil bodies contain a large number of storage granules containing histamine, heparin and various proteases.[638] Upon stimulation, these cells degranulate, releasing their contents into the extracellular space.

Following degranulation, activated mast cells produce numerous inflammatory signaling molecules, including nitric oxide (NO), leukotrienes (LT), and prostaglandins (PG).[638,639] Histamine released from mast cells further stimulates the production of NO, LT and PG in other tissues, producing the positive feedback which is a hallmark of the inflammatory process. Leukocytes, brought into the inflamed area by chemotactic factors, rapidly degrade histamine which limits its distribution and metabolic half-life.

The H1, H2 and H3 receptors are three receptor subtypes which mediate the biological activity of histamine.[640,641] H1 receptors are G-protein coupled receptors[641,642] linked to signal transduction systems that, in turn, initiate a variety of functions. H1 receptors are located in human bronchial muscle, smooth muscle, and endothelial cells[641,642] They upregulate $InsP_3$ production, leading to increased intracellular calcium release and smooth muscle contraction. While distributed elsewhere, H2 receptors are primarily located in the lining of the stomach and in heart muscle.[643] H2 receptors of the stomach lining are a popular pharmaceutical target since over-stimulation of these receptors leads to elevated gastric acid secretion and gastroesophageal reflux disease (GERD).[644] In addition, H2 receptor stimulation leads to activation of adenylate cyclase and increased production of cyclic AMP,[645] which is the crucial co-factor for numerous cellular processes including cyclic AMP-dependent kinase (PKC), a regulator of the ryanodine receptor.[471] Stimulation of H3 receptors, found predominately in neural tissue, results in inhibition of neurotransmitter release,[636] presumably by altering intracellular calcium signaling.

Several studies have shown an interaction between histamine stimulated increases in intracellular calcium and ryanodine receptor function. Histamine challenge stimulated increases in both $InsP_3$ and intracellular calcium concentrations in rat cerebellar granule cells. Interestingly, preincubation with 10 μM ryanodine attenuated the histamine stimulated increase in calcium by 57% with no effect on InsP3 levels.[646] In porcine urinary bladder, activation of H1 histamine receptors resulted in an increase in $InsP_3$ concentration and a commensurate rise in intracellular calcium.[647] These histamine-stimulated increases in calcium were blocked by depletion of stores with thapsigargin or by 10 μM ryanodine.

When membrane potential and isomeric force in rabbit middle coronary artery was examined, exposure to caffeine stimulated a transient contraction and a sustained membrane depolarization, both of which were blocked by ryanodine.[643] Similar to caffeine, histamine also induced a transient increase in contraction and sustained depolarization. However, pre-exposure with ryanodine or depletion of stores by caffeine abolished muscle contraction and attenuated membrane depolarization.[643] Taken together, these findings indicate that histamine interacts indirectly on ryanodine receptors.

Nitric oxide

Nitric oxide (NO) is a highly diffusible signaling molecule with a short half-life. It is synthesized during the conversion of L-arginine to citrulline by members of the family of nitric oxide synthases (NOS) in a process utilizing NADPH.[648] Chemically, NO is highly reactive with oxygen, superoxide anion, and various cellular components.[649] Consequently, it acts close to its site of production without the need for specialized storage structures. NO is an endogenous modulator of many cellular functions.[650]

There are three members of the NOS family: neuronal NOS (nNOS or NOS-1), inducible NOS (iNOS or NOS-2) and endothelial NOS (eNOS or NOS-3). nNOS and eNOS are constitutively expressed; the expression of iNOS is dynamic. As implied, nNos and eNOS are found in neuronal and muscle cells, and in endothelial cells, respectively. iNOS, originally described in mouse macrophages,[651] is the major enzyme for NO synthesis in immunity and inflammation.[652-654]

NO compromises muscle function in inflammation. iNOS, present in macrophages, is plentiful in skeletal[649,655] and cardiac[649,655,656] muscle. In addition, mast cells in inflamed muscle can act both as a source of NO production and as a downstream target.[657,658] NO has been shown to reduce muscle contractility[659] and ryanodine receptor function.[612,660,661] It is therefore likely that mast cell mediated NO release contributes to the pathophysiology of inflamed muscle by a direct action of NO on ryanodine receptors.

Synaptic plasticity in long term potentiation (LTP) depends on calcium release in both presynaptic and postsynaptic neurons.[662,663] NO has been shown to act as a transsynaptic messenger during hippocampal LTP.[663] In Aplysia motor neurons, classical LTP is blocked by NOS inhibition and intracellular calcium release from ryanodine sensitive stores in the presynaptic neuron is required for LTP.[664] These results suggest that NO acts on presynaptic ryanodine receptors during LTP.

Bradykinin

Bradykinin is the second of two principal agents (the other being histamine) producing the commonly observed effects of inflammation and hyper-sensitivity. Bradykinin acts as a primary mediator of nociception (the perception of pain) during inflammation and has been shown to stimulate nociceptive neurons in skin,[665] muscle,[666,667] joints[668] and viscera.[669] It is a powerful regulator of the general inflammation response and can, by itself, induce the full complement of inflammation symptoms, including fever, redness, edema and pain.[670] Bradykinin and related peptides (kinins) have been shown to regulate or induce changes in hyperalgesia (increased sensitivity to pain), blood pressure, cell migration, and smooth muscle contraction and relaxation.[671,672] Kinins have also been implicated in various pathologies including asthma, allergy, arthritis, hypertension, Alzheimer's disease and endotoxic shock.[672-674]

Kinins can be generated by contact activation or through a tissue pathway.[673] Contact activation requires the presence of three plasma proteins, namely, coagulation factor XII (Hageman factor), prekallikrien, and kininogen.[673] First, pre-Hageman factor is activated by contact with a foreign surface or by enzymatic activity. Activated Hageman factor then cleaves prekallikrien into kallikrien. Kallikrien, in turn, forms bradykinin from kininogen.[674] To halt the process, kinins are inactivated by kininases,[674] allowing exquisite control of the formation of bradykinin.

Kinins act via B1 and B2 receptors. Although B2 receptors are constitutively expressed, B1 receptors are induced by tissue injury. Upregulation of B1 receptors have been observed in the heart following ischemia[675] and inflammation.[676] Although there is a well-established connection between bradykinin receptors and $InsP_3R$ signaling, no direct connection between bradykinin receptor function and ryanodine receptor function has yet been determined. However, the observation that activation of B1 receptors stimulates contraction of rabbit aorta suggests a link between increases in bradykinin and ryanodine receptor activation.[677]

Bradykinin is associated with nociceptive processes, in part via production of NO, which is released by neural cells, and leads to the production of cGMP.[671,672] In cultured rat dorsal root ganglion neurons, bradykinin increased excitability and this effect was significantly reduced by pre-exposure to ryanodine.[678] Similarly, in a hybrid (neuroblastoma x glial) cell line, bradykinin-induced changes in intracellular calcium release was reduced 72% by prior emptying of the ryanodine sensitive calcium store with caffeine.[679] The interpretation of the effect of caffeine is complicated by its ability to inhibit the $InsP_3R$ directly. Nonetheless, the inhibition by ryanodine supports the inclusion of ryanodine receptors as a contributor to bradykinin responses in cells.

Eicosanoids

The eicosanoids are a family of metabolically active molecules derived from arachidonic acid. The major members are the prostiniods, which include the prostaglandins, prostacyclins and thromboxanes and are products of the cyclooxygenase pathway, and the leukotrienes, which derive from the lipoxygenase pathway. The activation of phospholipase A2 catalyzes the release of arachidonic acid from phospholipids of the plasma membrane, which then enters into either the cyclooxygenase or lipoxygenase pathway.

The synthesis of prostiniods in the cyclooxygenase pathway starts with the release of arachidonic acid by the action of PLA_2. Arachidonic acid is converted to prostaglandin G_2, or PGG_2, the substrate for a glutathione-dependent hydroperoxidase, which yields PGH_2. In turn, PGH_2 is the substrate for subsequent enzymatic modifications (e.g., thromboxane synthase, prostacyclin synthase) leading to the various prostaglandins (PGD_2, PGE_2, PGF2α), prostacyclin (PGI_2) and thromboxanes (TXA_2, TXB_2). Arachidonic acid itself activates a calcium influx pathway[680,681] and directly inhibits the $InsP_3R$,[682] but the role of the other metabolites in this pathway, with respect to calcium signaling, has yet to be determined.

The synthesis of the leukotrienes in the lipoxygenase pathway also starts with the release of arachidonic acid by the action of PLA_2. The first step is the co-localization of 5-lipoxygenase (5-LOX) with '5-LOX activating protein' (FLAP) in the cell membrane[683,684] to form an active complex. Arachidonic acid binds to the activated FLAP protein complex and is converted into 5-HPETE by 5-LOX.[685] Using 5-HPETE as a substrate, 5-LOX further catalyses the formation of leukotriene A_4 (LTA_4) which is released into the cytosol.[686] Leukotriene B_4 (LTB_4) is biosynthesized from LTA_4 by the action of LTA_4 hydrolase.[687] There are two classes of leukotrienes, one comprising LTB_4 and the other including the cysteinyl containing sulfidopeptide leukotrienes (CysLTs) LTC_4, LTD_4, and LTE_4.[688] The CysLTs are potent proinflammatory mediators[689] produced by mast cells, eosinophils, basophils and macrophages.[690] The primary cellular function of LTB_4 is to act as a powerful chemoattractant of neutrophils.[691]

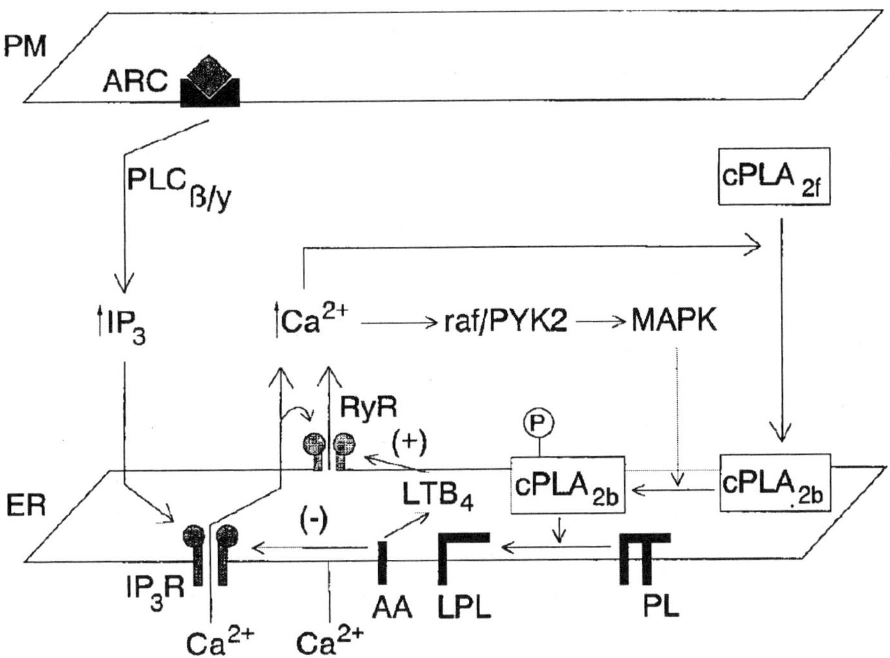

Figure 17-1. **Proposed mechanism for the regulation of IP_3R activity by arachidonic acid.** Ca^{2+} released from the endoplasmic reticulum (ER) through the IP_3R induces the translocation of the inactive free form of $cPLA_2$ ($cPLA_{2f}$) from the cytosol to the ER ($cPLA_{2b}$). Ca^{2+} can also stimulate the MAP kinase (MAPK) pathway raf and/or protein tyrosine kinase 2 (PYK_2). The combination of translocation and phosphorylation by MAP kinase results in the activation of $cPLA_2$. Subsequently, arachidonic acid (AA) is released from membrane phospholipids (PL) that can be utilized for the production of eicosanoids. AA also inhibits the IP_3R. Thus, the cytosolic Ca^{2+} concentration will decrease and phosphorylation as well as membrane binding of $cPLA_2$ can no longer be maintained. This, in turn, causes inactivation of $cPLA_2$. Note that the release of arachidonic acid is not necessarily linked to the production of LTB_4. However, if synthesized, LTB_4 could activate Ca^{2+} release from the same or a distinct pool containing the RyR. ARC, agonist receptor complex; PM, plasma membrane; PLC, phospholipase C, LPL, lysophospholipid. Activating and inhibitory effects are indicated as (+) and (-), respectively. With permission from Striggow *et al.*[682]

Several studies have shown a role for leukotriene regulation of ryanodine receptors. LTB_4, at a concentration of 100 nM, stimulated single channel activity of the ryanodine receptor from canine cerebellar preparations.[682] The $InsP_3$-gated channel from these same preparations was refractory to the leukotrienes. Interestingly, the $InsP_3$-gated channel was inhibited by nanomolar concentrations of arachidonic acid, but 10 μM arachidonic acid had no effect on ryanodine receptor channel activity.[682] In another study, the cysteinyl-leukotriene D_4 (LTD_4) was shown to stimulate an increase in intracellular calcium in human detrusor muscle.[692] The authors concluded that the bulk of the stimulated rise in calcium was from $InsP_3$-mediated intracellular stores, but they also observed that 10 μM ryanodine attenuated the amplitude of the calcium signal. This observation strongly suggests that ryanodine receptors may be important in the LTD_4-dependent release of calcium from intracellular stores in this muscle.

The effect of capsaicin on intracellular calcium stores in dorsal root ganglion cells appears to use the cyclooxygenase pathway. First, a brief application of capsaicin (10 μM) stimulated increased intracellular calcium levels in calcium-free solution.[693] This calcium release was inhibited by ruthenium red and dantrolene, antagonists of the ryanodine receptor, as well as by pre-emptying stores with caffeine.[693] $InsP_3$ receptor agonists were without effect on the capsaicin-induced calcium release in these cells, suggesting that intracellular calcium release is mediated through a ryanodine sensitive store. Direct activation of the VR1 capsaicin receptor by HPETE and LTB_4 was reported using patch clamp studies in native dorsal root ganglion.[694] HPETE and LTB_4 also activated the cloned VR1 capsaicin receptor expressed in HEK cells while prostaglandins and unsaturated fatty acids failed to activate the channel.[694] Taken together these findings show that intracellular calcium release is part of the capsaicin response and further supports the hypothesis that LTB_4 acts directly on the ryanodine receptor in dorsal root ganglion.

CD38

CD38 is a 45 kDa homodimeric cell surface protein found in numerous cell types, including neutrophils,[633] neural tissue[695] and muscle.[696] CD38 catalyzes the production of cyclic ADP-ribose (cADPR) from NAD^+.[695,697] cADPR stimulated calcium release from ryanodine sensitive stores, first described for sea urchin egg homogenates,[698] has been observed in numerous cell types and tissues, including neurons, cardiac muscle, skeletal muscle, smooth muscle, non-excitable cells, and lymphomas. As a consequence, cADPR is well established as a ryanodine receptor agonist.[699]

A defining characteristic of asthma is smooth muscle spasm.[700] Smooth muscle spasms leading to airway constriction are mediated by an exaggerated immune response to antigens binding to mast cells present in the epithelial lining of the lung.[700] The cellular pathways activated to induce these spasms are complex because calcium regulation in smooth muscle is mediated by both ryanodine- and $InsP_3$-sensitive stores.[632,647,701] Recently,

CD38 expression and cADPR activity was shown to be increased in airway smooth muscle following exposure to cytokines.[696] Increased expression of CD38 in these cells resulted in an amplification of bradykinin-stimulated calcium release from intracellular stores which was blocked by exposure to cADPR antagonists.[702] Furthermore, smooth muscle relaxants have been shown to shift intracellular calcium release to subplasmalemmal stores, rather than from stores located in the center of the cell.[703] These results suggest that amplified smooth muscle contractions seen in asthma result from cADPR acting on ryanodine receptors located in deep cytosolic stores.

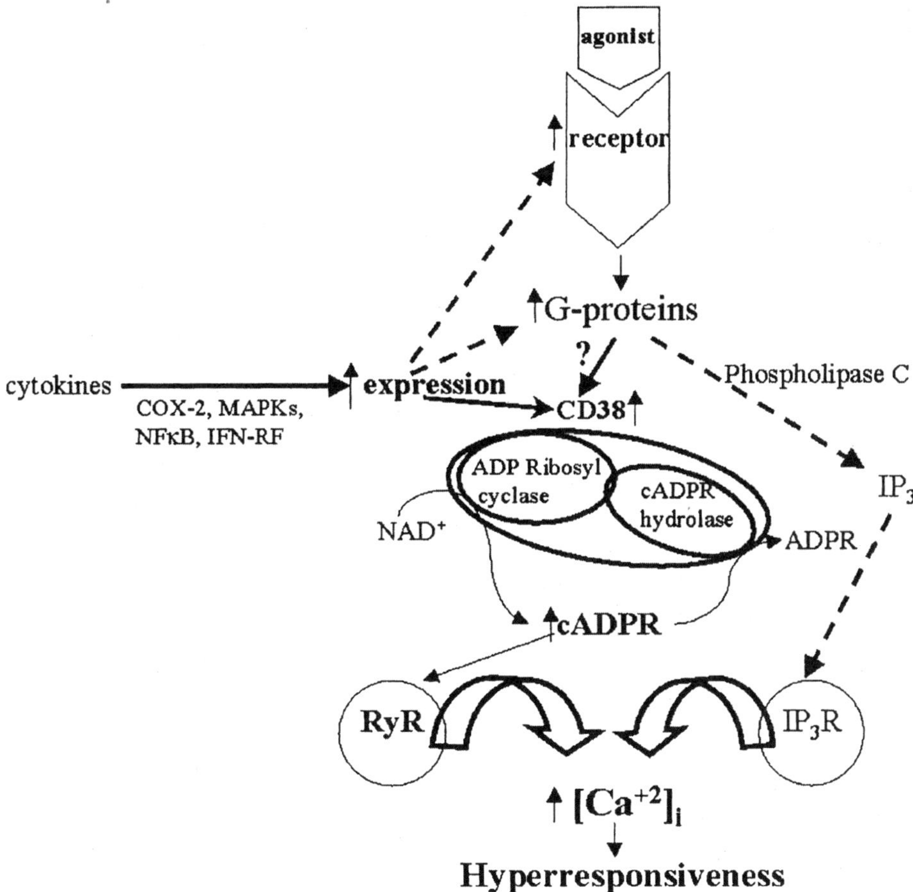

Figure 17-2. **A model describing the mechanisms of cytokine-induced ASM hyperresponsiveness.** Cytokines up-regulate expression of a multitude of genes including that of CD38 through multiple signal transduction mechanisms (MAPKs, NF-kB, etc.). The increased second messengers (cADPR, IP_3) result in augmented calcium release through intracellular calcium channels. Dotted arrows represent previously described findings. Taken with permission from Deshpande *et al.*[696]

A recent report using CD38 knockout (CD38-/-) mice has demonstrated the importance of cADPR as a mediator of resistance to bacterial infection. CD38-/- mice were infected with *Streptococcus* pneumoniae and survival was assessed. CD38-/- mice were 10-fold more susceptible to infection than wild-type controls as a result of inhibited neutrophil chemotaxis.[633] In wild-type neutrophils, intracellular calcium release was stimulated by ryanodine and cADPR and ryanodine-stimulated calcium release was blocked by ruthenium red.[633] No calcium release was seen in wild-type neutrophils when cADPR was hydrolyzed by heat inactivation,[704] or in the presence of the inactive cADPR analog, 8-Br-cADPR.[705] In the presence of fMLP, a potent chemotactic agent for neutrophils,[706] CD38-/- neutrophils did not chemotax.[633] These data show that neutrophil chemotaxis towards fMLP is controlled by cADPR stimulated calcium release from ryanodine sensitive intracellular stores.

CONCLUDING REMARKS

Inflammation is vital to the survival of animals and plays an important role in both health and disease. This highly regulated and complex process interacts with many systems throughout the body to maintain wellness. Pathologies associated with chronic inflammation, or metabolic disregulation of inflammation, result in the expression of many disease states. Intracellular calcium channels, such as the ryanodine and $InsP_3$ receptors, are known to modulate the function of numerous biochemical pathways by integrating inputs from many signaling cascades. This sensitive response leads to exquisite control of the processes involved. The ability of ryanodine receptors to react to chemical mediators of inflammation, coupled with the presence of ryanodine receptors in many cells crucial to the inflammatory response, underlies the importance of calcium in regulating the physiology of inflammation.

Chapter 18

RYANOIDS, RECEPTOR AFFINITY AND RYR CHANNEL SUBCONDUCTANCE

Why the discordance?

Henry R. Besch Jr.[1], Chun Hong Shao[2], and Keshore R. Bidasee[2]
[1]*Dept. of Pharmacology and Toxicology, Indiana University School of Medicine, Indianapolis, IN;* [2]*Dept. of Pharmacology, University of Nebraska Medical Center, Omaha, NE*

INTRODUCTION

For almost half a century, secondary metabolites of the rain forest shrub *Ryania speciosa* Vahl have intrigued biologists with their complex pharmacology. The first compound identified from *R. speciosa* was ryanodine, the development history of which is fascinating.[707] Early studies with ryanodine (actually a co-crystal of a ~40:60 mixture of ryanodine and dehydroryanodine) using a muscle homogenate sediment fraction showed a temporally biphasic effect on heavy microsomal sediments. Later studies using striated muscle microsomes enriched in junctional membranes established that ryanodine is without direct effects on the sarcoplasmic reticular Ca^{2+} pump, thereby suggesting a hypothetical pathway by which Ca^{2+} exits the intravesicular compartment.[708] With [^{3}H]ryanodine, this calcium release channel (CRC) was subsequently cloned and then shown to be identical with the sarcoplasmic reticulum foot protein previously described by Franzini-Armstrong and colleagues. Details of this era are well described in comprehensive reviews on ryanodine receptors/ (RyR) (see, e.g. Sutko *et al.*,[109] from among PubMed's retrieval of 360 ryanodine receptor reviews since 1988) and elsewhere throughout this book.

MULTIPLE RYANOID EFFECTS

Mechanistic studies with single RyR incorporated into planar lipid bilayers explained the biphasic effect noted throughout the early literature: nM [ryanodine] opens the Ca^{2+} efflux pathway whereas μM [ryanodine] closes it. This curious (antithetical) dual concentration-effect curve remains to be fully understood. The early explanation that ligand activation and deactivation of the CRC represents binding to a single high affinity and a single low affinity site, respectively, becomes ever less explanatory as mechanistic studies progress with secondary metabolites of *R. speciosa*, their chemical derivatives and certain toxins. Nevertheless, it is instructive to begin with the most parsimonious model of ryanoid action, namely a simple two-site binding assumption.

The channel activating effect of ryanodine is well supported by numerous studies which have clearly established that nM [ryanodine] interacts with high affinity on RyR (at one site, kinetically). As a result of this binding, ryanodine induces a subconductance state that: (i) is ~*half* of full unitary conductance, (ii) invariantly evidences a single *unique* subconductance value and (iii) has a duration half time of at least several *hours* (essentially irreversible on the time scale of bilayer experiments). When the [ryanodine] is raised to upper μM, the channel becomes silenced irreversibly in the closed state, a mode termed "shut" to distinguish it from brief closed intervals entered during normal channel activity.[709]

These three characteristics of ryanodine are canonical. However, derivatives of ryanodine, collectively termed ryanoids, are now known which violate each of them. The ever-expanding class of ryanodine congeners includes many examples of ryanoid actions that do not conform to the ryanodine dogma. First, some ryanoids can induce prolonged subconductance amplitude far different from *half*-open. Subconductances from as small as 6% to as high as 75% (or more) of fully open have been reported. Apparently RyR subconductance states can take virtually any value, although many cluster in the ~ half-open range. Early ryanoid single channel studies demonstrated a range of unique stable subconductances induced by newly available ryanoids.[710] Additional discrete, repeatable RyR subconductances due to other ryanoids now number in the dozens. Thus, point (i) above clearly cannot be taken as characteristic of ryanoids in general. The logical conclusion from this essentially rheostatic subconductance behavior of RyR CRC is that ryanoids probably do not induce stabilization of a particular few preferred conformations of the native RyR. This argues against the notion that induction of the ryanoid subconductance state occurs principally by allosteric mechanisms. It does not, however, establish that more than one activating binding site might be involved. Secondly, from recent reports it has become clear that a ryanoid is not limited to producing a single subconductance amplitude. Indeed, several ryanoids each reproducibly effect multiple (≥3) distinct subconductance states. Thus, point (ii) above cannot be taken as characteristic of ryanoids in general.

Third, regarding subconductance persistence (or the "irreversibility") of ryanoids, it has become clear that subconductance duration varies widely among ryanoids. Indeed, C_{10}-O_{eq} succinyl ryanoids interact weakly with RyR[711] and in recent single channel studies were shown to produce some subconductances so fleetingly brief as to challenge resolution by current single channel recording technology.[166] Even for ryanodine per se, persistence of the subconductance is not invariant. In early studies, low nM [ryanodine] were shown to be readily reversible[712] and this seems confirmed more recently in intact fibers,[713,714] and in bilayers (unpublished observations). In fact, it has been clear for some time from microsomal binding studies that [^{3}H]ryanodine dissociation half time is an order of magnitude shorter at nM than at μM [ryanodine].[715] Thus, point (iii) above cannot be taken as characteristic of ryanoids in general. Furthermore, the latter results suggest involvement of at least two ryanoid binding sites being engaged within the activation portion of the concentration-effect curve, since the dissociation-slowing effect began within the nM [ryanodine] range. This argues -- but again does not prove -- that more than one ryanodine molecule becomes bound before induction of the RyR shut mode by a final binding. If so, then binding of at least three ryanoid molecules underlies the complete concentration-effect curve. Ryanoids having more discriminate effects confirm the latter.

RYANOID RECEPTOR AFFINITY DISCORDANCE

Ryanoid binding data fail to provide a satisfactory basis to explain these discriminant functional effects of ryanoids. Binding studies based on competitive displacement studies using [^{3}H]ryanodine as the signal ligand, routinely show only a single high affinity K_d and a single low affinity K_d by usual Scatchard analyses.

However, recent studies with pyridyl ryanodine (PdRy) began to functionally challenge the single high affinity assumption.[709] The potency of PdRy's primary functional effect (activation) is equivalent to ryanodine's (EC_{50act} of 2.5 and 3.4μM, respectively) (Fig. 18-1 B), in the face of its 100-fold loss in affinity (Fig. 18-1 A). PdRy thereby definitively separated ryanoid functional effects from high affinity binding.[709] These data imply the surprising conclusion that PdRy can half-activate RyR at fractional receptor occupancy of 0.011 (based on their respective K_d values of 109nM and 1.2nM). This disparity showed clearly for the first time with a single ryanoid that activation potency can be high while apparent binding affinity is low.

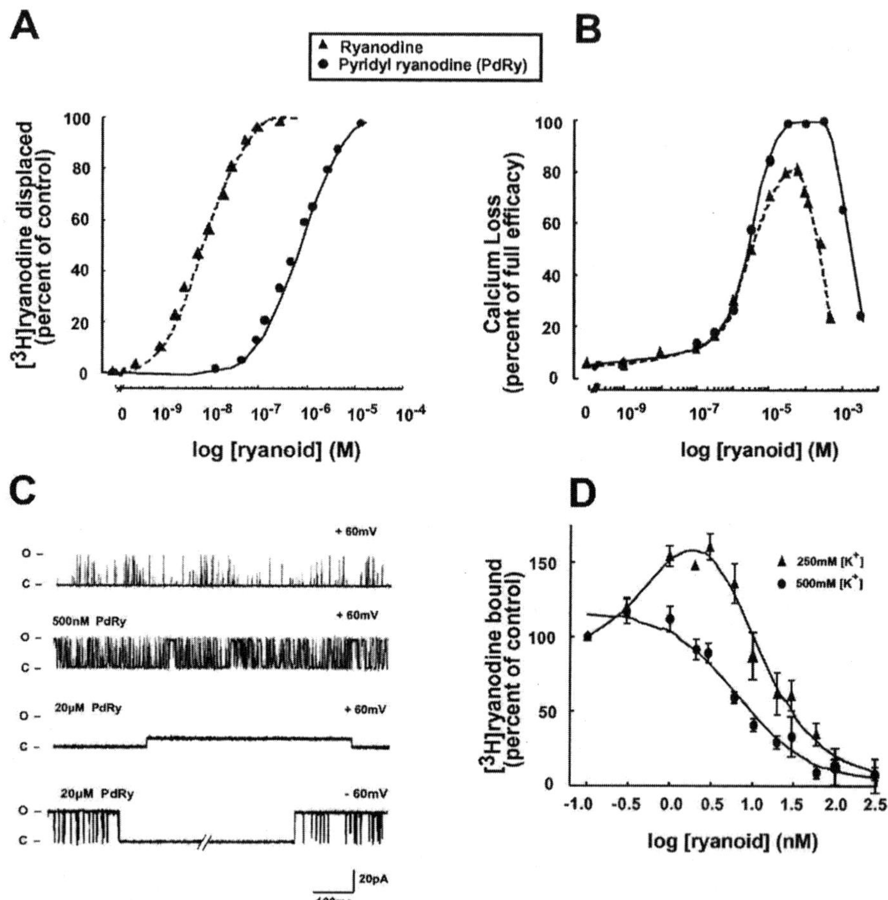

Figure 18-1. **A small fraction of highest affinity ryanoid binding sites initiates ryanoid threshold activation. A.** and **B.** show that the K_d of PdRy is ~100-fold less than ryanodine's but its channel activation potency is equivalent. **C.** Concentration effect relationship for PdRy in single channels reveals that activation occurs in at least two steps, only the second of which involves induction of the ryanoid subconductance. **D.** shows that a small fraction of ryanodine binding sites becomes evident at lowered ionic strength of the buffer. At 250mM [K^+], the binding curve fit significantly better to a two site model than to a one site model (p = 0.001), with K_{d1} = 1.3nM (4.7% of total sites) and K_{d2} = 5.7nM. Both curves shown in **D** are nonlinear regression fits via Prism 3.0 (GraphPad Software, San Diego). At the usual [K^+] of 500mM, K_d was 3.4nM. Methods previously published.[709,711,716,717]

A physical basis for the high activation potency of PdRy was revealed in single channel studies.[716] At nM [PdRy], only the RyR2 gating frequency was increased, without induction of the subconductance usually assumed to underlie CRC activation (Fig. 18-1 C, second panel). The increased gating frequency provides an increased integral channel open time, thereby enhancing time-averaged Ca^{2+} efflux. Thus PdRy activates RyR2 in two steps. A slightly higher [PdRy] can readily induce the subconductance and from there, the shut state (Fig. 18-1 C, third panel), returning thereafter to the subconductance. The first step is distinct from the second in (i) its concentration dependence and also (ii) in that it is *not* enhanced by a positive transbilayer holding potential.[716] This latter feature allows exploitation of an experimental tact to forestall induction of the subconductance with advancing [ryanoid], since induction of the subconductance is disfavored by negative holding potential but strongly promoted by positive holding potential. Reliably, at negative holding potential (Fig. 18-1 C, bottom panel) (and occasionally at positive holding potential) PdRy can shut RyR *directly* from the high frequency gating state. Notably, when shut from the high frequency gating state, the channel always returns directly to that state whereas when shut from the subconductance, it always returns to the subconductance (cf. Fig. 18-1 C, third panel). Clearly, the RyR can shut without a ryanoid positioned to effect a subconductance or alternately, even around a ryanoid that has induced its subconductance. Shutting is virtually independent of subconductance. These results strongly imply that the affinity of the ryanoid binding site that effects shutting by PdRy, while distinct from that responsible for the subconductance, is substantially equivalent to (perhaps even lower than) the affinity of the binding site responsible for the subconductance. It is predictable that this near equivalent affinity between them will have eluded detection in prior competitive displacement studies based on site-indiscriminant [^{3}H]ryanodine.

Further insights into the curious properties induced by the pyridyl in place of the pyrrole –the single difference between ryanodine and PdRy– were afforded by derivatizing PdRy to increase its backbone flexibility, so as to produce a more readily reversible ryanoid, namely C_4, C_{12}-diketopyridyl-ryanodine (dkPdRy).[716] dkPdRy provides a prototype reversible ryanoid that, like its parent, effects two concentration-dependent, voltage independent functional consequences at levels below those inducing the voltage dependent subconductance, and Hill coefficients ~ 3, consistent with more than one high affinity ryanoid binding site. This projection was realized in binding displacement assays with dkPdRy, which discriminated a second K_d value within the high affinity range.[716]

Because the channel activating steps with PdRy and dkPdRy were more readily discerned at low [ryanoid] and low single channel P_o, we reasoned that less than optimal initial binding conditions in vesicles might foster discernment of an otherwise masked high affinity binding site. The simple tact of lowering buffer ionic strength did so, even for ryanodine per se (Fig. 18-1 D). At 250mM [KCl], over the range of 0.1 to 2nM, unlabeled ryanodine did not displace but rather augmented [^{3}H]ryanodine binding. This is consistent with the prior results, indicating increased binding from an increased channel gating frequency that exposed a higher affinity site, namely that responsible for the subconductance.

These separate lines of evidence raise fundamental questions about the simple two-site binding hypothesis. A model based on only one high affinity and one low affinity site becomes inordinately stretched to accommodate ryanoid results showing up to four functional states of the channel and at least three ryanoid binding sites on it. It is of interest that imperatoxin A[718] and suramin[719] also evince multiple binding and effector sites on RyR.

RYR CHANNEL SUBCONDUCTANCE AMPLITUDES

A substantial body of evidence has established the unique targeting of ryanoids to the RyR, even at near saturating [ryanoid]. A logical expectation from this specificity is that the affinity of ryanoids for the receptor should dictate their effects on it. This is precisely what was found in early binding affinity and single channel conductance data: a highly significant correlation between them ($r^2 = 0.983$) (Fig. 18-2 A).[710,711] When the ryanoid molecule is settled into a common position creating a single near nexus between the molecule and a pore RyR wall helix, this results in an ion-flow stricture, a primary component of that stricture seems to be the C_{10}-O_{eq} position. The lengths of the extended C_{10}-O_{eq} side chains were estimated from MOPAC software in ChemOffice (CambridgeSoft Corp, Cambridge). The linear correlation between ryanoid K_d and length interestingly extrapolated to zero conductance at 7.7 angstroms. Such a stricture may apply with lower affinity ryanoids when suitably positioned by a C_{10}-O_{eq} side chain as in the case of ß-alanyl ryanodol, which produces a subconductance equal to that of ß-alanyl ryanodine.[720]

A less strict correlation ($r^2 = 0.278$) obtains when diverse derivatives are included (Fig. 18-2 B), but importantly, comparative molecular field analysis permitted identification of structural loci having major influence on ligand interactions.[721]

An extensive, classic SAR investigation of ryanoid potency, efficacy and K_d values included five dozen newly derived ryanoids (without each index for each ryanoid).[722,723] From all the A-ring and C-ring derived ryanoids of this series, **both** functional effects in rat right ventricular muscle strips and respective ryanoid K_d values were given for 15 of them. Plotted, so as to facilitate comparisons with Fig. 18-1 A and 18-1 B, these data showed a trend toward dependence but due to numerous outliers the correlation was less than robust ($r^2 = 0.217$) (Fig. 18-2 C). (Note that Jefferies *et al.*[723] illustrated in a log-log plot (their Fig. 5) a subset of C-ring derivatives, among which an $r^2 = 0.85$ was reported).

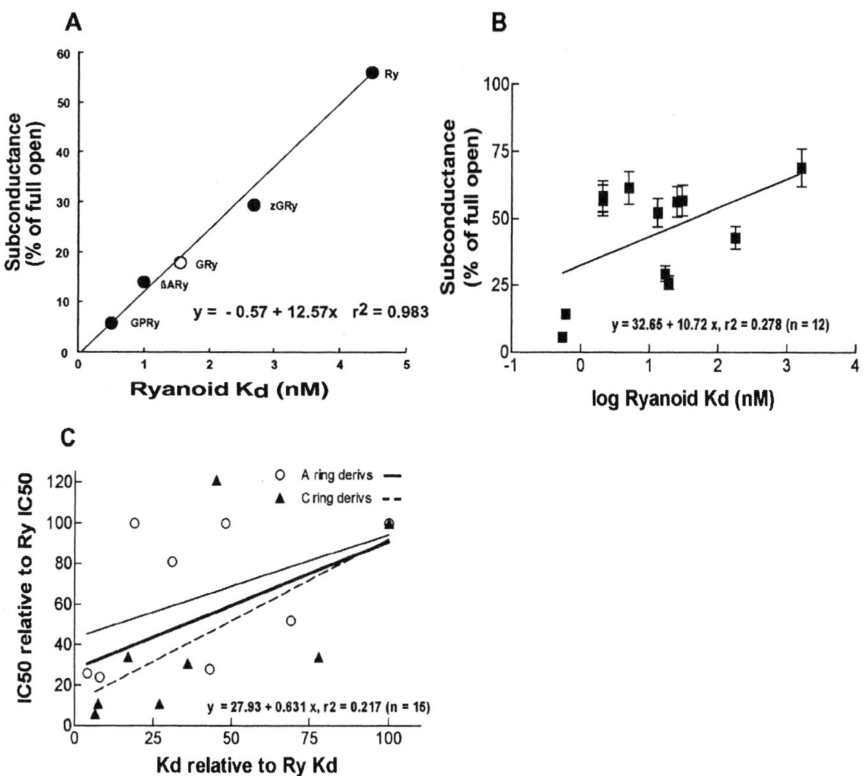

Figure 18-2. **Example affinity-function correlations among ryanoids. A**. Linear relationship between K_d and subconductance for five high affinity ryanodine homologs. The four C_{10}-O_{eq} ryanodine derivatives bear a basic N-terminus extending ever further from the C_{10}. K_d values from Humerickhouse *et al.*,[711] sub-conductance values from Tinker *et al.*,[710] (for the filled circles) and Hui *et al.*[714] (open circle). Abbreviations, (K_d and major subconductance): GPRy, guanidino-propionyl Ry (0.6nM, 5.8%); βARy, βalanyl Ry (1.0nM, 14.3%); GRy, glycyl Ry (1.6nM, 16.3%); zGRy, CBZ-alanyl Ry (2.7nM, 29.4%); Ry, ryanodine (4.4nM, 56.8%). SEM bars lie within the symbols. **B**. Correlation diminishes when even a few more diverse ryanodine derivatives are included (all data from Jefferies *et al.*[722], Table 18-1). C. Correlation between K_d and IC_{50} on rat ventricular strips; values relative to ryanodine, set at 100.[722,723]

The above brief samples of some of the best available ryanoid structure-function data raise intriguing questions regarding the relationship between bulk ryanoid binding and functional ryanoid effects. The correlations between ryanoid affinity and ryanoid effect should be much stronger consistently if there were only one high affinity ryanoid binding site. The collective data strengthen the results from dkPrRy[716] and other data summarized above suggesting binding and effect at more than one high affinity ryanoid binding site. In summary, when a wide array of ryanoids are taken altogether, less than robust correlations become apparent. Affinity assessments fail to predict subconductance amplitude.

Why the discordance? It is tempting to speculate that at the ≥ two high affinity binding and effector sites, different ryanoids interact with unequal emphasis, as was implied earlier from functional studies with the ryanoid secondary metabolites Esters E and F.[717] Binding to the first high affinity site (that increases channel gating frequency) could distort binding displacement assays and might, for example, underlie the major orienting role of the pyrrole in ryanoid binding[724] without informing the subconductance. Based on this speculation, we synthesized a pyrrole derivative (RSA1) that in single channel studies produces a high gating frequency ($P_O \sim 0.9$) but never a subconductance. RSA1 increased "maximal" control [^{3}H]ryanodine binding by ~3-fold.[725]

The elegant elucidation of the crystal structure of KcsA has ushered in a more fundamental understanding of membrane channel substructure (the teepee model).[9] Recent decisive mutation studies[37,74,77,167] confirm that a pore-region binding site directly effects ryanoid subconductance. A clever extrapolation of the teepee model to RyR provides a physical construct.[726] Since the subconductance-inducing effect can now be ascribed to the pore ryanoid binding site, this promotes the feasibility of other binding sites outside the voltage sensitivity of the RyR to explain the low correlation between apparent affinity and ryanoid effects.

We recently summarized ryanoid effects in a brief diagram, based on the range of effects of PdRy and dkPdRy on the single channel.[716] In an expansion of that diagram and incorporating the multiple considerations above, a simple summary cartoon of ryanoid binding and resultant altered gating (the symprosic model) is proposed (Fig. 18-3). It assumes the convenience of symmetry and only that the closed state of RyR is stabilized by some as yet unidentified interdomain interactions, which harbor affinity for some component of ryanoid molecules. When the RyR is destabilized by ryanoid interaction at one of initially equivalent interdomain sites, the ryanoid becomes enabled to bind within the pore region and effect the subconductance.[134,210,518]

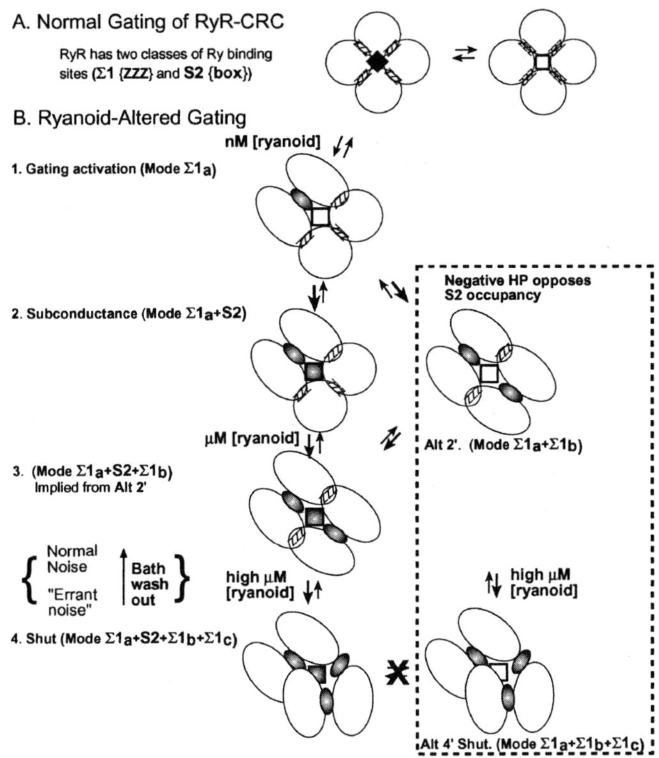

Figure 18-3. **Putative symprosic model of ryanoid binding to RyR resulting in gating and conductance changes. A**. Normal gating of RyR/ CRC. **B**. Ryanoid-altered gating. Interdomain clefts define putative interaction sites involved in stabilizing (zipping) the closed configuration of RyR and these provide a motif for a ryanoid binding site class ($\sum 1_{a,b,c}$) marked **zzz**) outside the transmembrane ion conduction path while a second distinct binding site (S2) resides within the pore (behind **solid square**). For simplicity, the holding potential insensitive binding sites are depicted as though they are in close proximity to the pore site but may or may not be physically adjacent. $\sum 1$ sites are (but the S2 site is not) available on the closed channel. Hill slope values ~ 3 are implicit.[716] **1.** Low [ryanoid] induces occupancy (depicted as shaded ellipse) of $\sum 1_a$ site, destabilizing the closed channel configuration. From 5% (with ryanodine) up to as high as 21% (with dkPdRy) of the total binding sites initiate activation. This activation increases gating (decreasing T_C, and thereby increases integral P_O). **2**. Opened channel (open square) reveals high affinity site within pore, allowing voltage-dependent binding to S2 to produce step-change to stabilized, partially-open channel subconductance mode. **3.** Occupancy of $\sum 1_b$ further destabilizes the closed configuration now increasing T_O, as well as decreasing T_C, producing errant noise in single channels. **4.** High µM - low mM [ryanoid] binds to site $\sum 1_c$, inducing global conformational changes to produce the long-duration closed (i.e., the "shut") state, confining the S2 site, regardless of its occupancy. Negative HP reveals functional effects shown in dashed box, readily observed with reversible ryanoids. When ryanoid dissociates from $\sum 1_c$, the channel always returns to the conductance it had prior to becoming shut. Note that sites $\sum 1_a$ and $\sum 1_b$ may be poorly discernable when bathing conditions dictate a high basal channel gating frequency. RyR-CRC, ryanodine receptor calcium release channel; HP, transmembrane holding potential.

At a similar [ryanoid], binding to a second interdomain site occurs, further destabilizing the RyR closed state and promoting further increased gating, in a sense, auto-catalytically. Extended distortion by a second molecule substantially diminishes affinity at the third interdomain site, accounting for the low affinity of the shutting ryanoid binding site. Importantly, only the subconductance site is strongly influenced by transmembrane holding potential, the effects of which are depicted here within the dashed box. For illustrative convenience, interactive domains are depicted adjacent to the subconductance-inducing site but the envisioned domains may not be proximal to the latter. It is clear that long range interdomain interactions are important to stabilizing the RyR in a closed configuration.[180,727]

POTENTIAL CLINICAL APPLICATION

Why do subtleties of subsite on RyR matter? If a ryanodine derivative is to become clinically useful in heart failure, perhaps akin to effects of JTV519,[728] ryanoids with RyR subsite selectivity, low subconductance and ready reversibility will be necessary. Even then, therapeutic success will require physiologic participation, namely use-dependence, as does antiarrhythmics.[729] An immediate target compound is C_{10}-O_{eq} guanidinopropionyl, diketo pyridyl ryanodine (or other reversible congener). Such studies are currently underway.

CONCLUDING REMARKS

Ryanodine and its congeners (ryanoids) target the sarco(endo)plasmic calcium release channel (CRC) with near absolute specificity. Among the subset of ryanoids having a higher affinity than ryanodine, K_d accurately predicts the subconductance amplitude that they induce in the CRC/ryanodine receptor (RyR.) in single channel studies, with a correlation coefficient approaching one. However, most chemical derivatives of ryanodine have lower binding affinity than ryanodine and among this array of ryanoids, the correlation between K_d and subconductance is less robust. Recent studies with pyridyl ryanodine and its more reversible congener diketo pyridyl ryanodine have begun to explain the discordance. These studies suggest that a high affinity ryanoid binding site(s) effects increased channel gating while another high affinity site, probably in close proximity of the channel pore, effects the subconductance. The latter site experiences the transmembrane holding potential whereas the former does (do) not.

Shutting of the channel requires yet another ryanoid binding, which also is not influenced by transmembrane holding potential. These results portend the potential of development a therapeutic ryanoid.

ACKNOWLEDGMENTS

This work was supported in part by grants from the Ralph W. and Grace M. Showalter Foundation (HRB) and the National Institutes of Health (KRB).

Chapter 19

SCORPION PEPTIDES AS HIGH-AFFINITY PROBES OF RYANODINE RECEPTOR FUNCTION

Georgina B. Gurrola, Xinsheng Zhu, and Héctor H. Valdivia
Dept. of Physiology, University of Wisconsin Medical School, Madison, WI

INTRODUCTION

A variety of peptide toxins in scorpion venoms interact with ionic channels with high affinity and exquisite selectivity. Distinct toxins recognize specifically voltage-dependent Na^+ channels,[730] several subclasses of K^+ channels,[730] and at least one subclass of Cl^- channels.[731] These scorpion peptides have become useful tools in the identification, purification and structural mapping of ionic channels.[732]

A subclass of scorpion peptides with high affinity for the Ca^{2+} release channel/ryanodine receptors (RyR) was reported for the first time in 1991.[733] Toxins from the venom of the African scorpion *Buthotus hottentota* induced a rapid, specific and reversible activation of RyR1, the RyR isoform that is mostly expressed in skeletal muscle. The finding was surprising because RyRs are intracellular Ca^{2+} channels that are supposedly inaccessible to the bulk of scorpion toxins, which are membrane-impermeable, ionized peptides targeted against external receptors. However, the ingenuity of nature is immense, and as we will see later, several mechanisms may account for penetration of these basic peptides into intracellular environments. Another peculiar finding was that these peptides *activated*, rather than blocked, RyRs by inducing the appearance of a long-lived subconducting state.[733] While this effect resembled the mechanism of action of the classical ligand ryanodine, the vast majority of scorpion toxins paralyze excitable tissues by antagonizing ion conduction.[730]

The first scorpion peptides purified to homogeneity that act on RyRs with nanomolar affinity were the *imperatoxins,* so called because they are derived from the scorpion *Pandinus imperator.*[734] Imperatoxin I ($IpTx_i$) is a ~15 kDa heterodimeric protein with phospholipase A_2 activity that indirectly inhibits RyRs by releasing unsaturated fatty acids from membrane phospholipids.[735] Imperatoxin A ($IpTx_a$), on the other hand, is a 3.7 kDa basic peptide that specifically increases [^{3}H]ryanodine binding to RyR1 (but not to RyR2, the cardiac isoform) by direct ligand-receptor interaction.[736] More recently, two peptides from the venom of the scorpion *Buthus martensis* (BmK AS and BmK AS-1), each having a rather unusual number (4) of disulfide bridges and long chain (66 amino acid residues), were found to activate [^{3}H]ryanodine binding to RyR1.[737] From *Scorpio maurus palmatus* venom was purified Maurocalcin (MCa), a 33-amino acid basic peptide that shares 82% homology with $IpTx_a$ and also exerts many of $IpTx_a$'s functional effects.[738] A novel subclass of scorpion peptides from *Buthotus judaicus* venom with activity against RyRs but with lower affinity than $IpTx_a$ or MCa was recently purified and sequenced.[739] Thus, a diverse group of scorpion peptides with distinct specificity and different affinity for RyRs is emerging. Here, we will discuss the most prominent structural and functional characteristics of $IpTx_a$, a representative example of this group of peptides.

STRUCTURAL FEATURES

$IpTx_a$ is a 33-amino acid basic peptide with molecular weight = 3,759 Da.[740] It is a thermostable and globular peptide due to 3 disulfide bridges that condense its backbone and stabilize its structure.[740] This peptide does not display the cisteine pattern necessary to maintain the classical α/β structure common to scorpion toxins that block Na^+, K^+, or Cl^- channels.[741,742] Rather, $IpTx_a$ displays a cisteine arrangement corresponding to the "inhibitor cisteine knot" found in μ-agatoxins and ω-conotoxins, a subclass of spider and marine snail toxins, respectively, that block voltage-dependent Ca^{2+} channels.[743,744] $IpTx_a$, therefore, conforms structurally with more fidelity to spider and snail toxins that block Ca^{2+} channels than to scorpion toxins that block Na^+ or K^+ channels.

Recently, the three-dimensional structure of $IpTx_a$[745] and MCa[746] were solved by NMR. Owing to their high degree of homology and distinctive cisteine pattern, both peptides display the "inhibitor cisteine knot" fold, in which the disulfide bond between C16 and C32 penetrates through a 13-residue ring formed by the peptide backbone and the other two disulfide bonds (Fig. 19-1). The structure of $IpTx_a$ consists of two antiparallel β-strands formed by residues K20-K23 (β-strand I) and K30-R33 (β-strand II), connected by four reverse chains.[745] The structure of MCa consists of three β-strands and four reverse chains.[746] Both toxins display a surface rich in basic residues (K19-R24, R33) and an opposite surface rich in acidic residues (D2, D13-D15, E29). The main structural differences between $IpTx_a$ and MCa are found near the amino-terminal region, where residues 9-11 of MCa form an additional peripheral β-strand (Fig. 19-1).

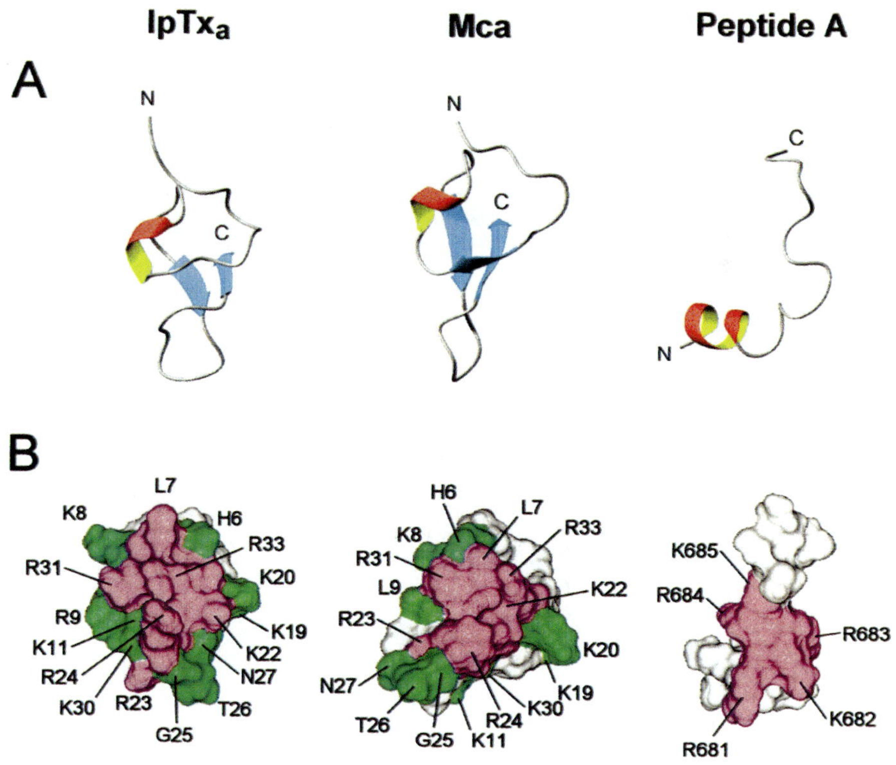

Figure 19-1. **Three-dimensional structures of $IpTx_a$, MCa, and Peptide A.** (**A**) Backbone alone, and (**B**) CPK representation, highlighting amino acids that participate in binding to RyR1. Taken, with permission, from Lee *et al.*[745]

Functional analogy between $IpTx_a$ and a segment of the II-III loop of the DHPR

Using synthetic peptides corresponding to different segments of the II-III loop of the α_1 subunit of the skeletal dihydropyridine receptor (DHPR), Ikemoto's group[747] found that the amino-terminal region (peptide A, T671-L690) activates RyR1. Gurrola *et al.*[748] noted that $IpTx_a$ shares structural similarities with peptide A (Fig. 19-2). Both peptides display a cluster of basic amino acids (rectangle) followed by a hydroxylated residue (circle) (^{19}KKCKRR-x-T^{26} in $IpTx_a$ and ^{681}RKRRK-x-S^{687} in peptide A). Based on this observation, it was proposed that $IpTx_a$ acts as a peptide mimetic of an endogenous activator of RyR1.[748]

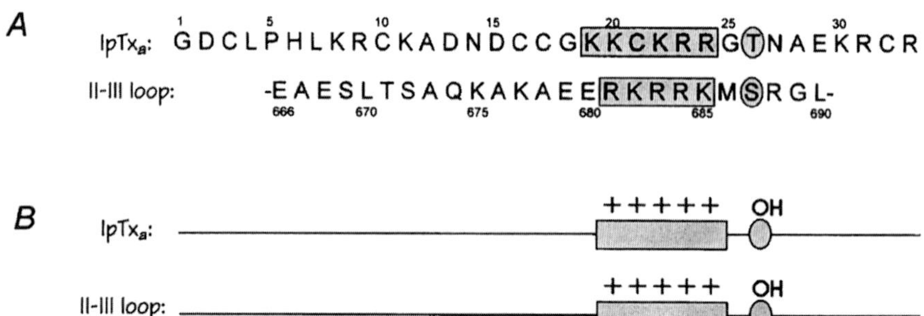

Figure 19-2. **Proposed homology between $IpTx_a$ and Peptide A of the II-III loop of the DHPR.** Taken, with permission, from Gurrola *et al.*[748]

To probe for $IpTx_a$'s active site, amino acid substitutions were performed using solid-phase peptide synthesis. Substitution of R23 (R23E) or T26 (T26A and T26E) in $IpTx_a$ substantially decreased the capacity of this peptide to activate RyR1.[748] Since substitution of K14 (K14E), another basic amino acid not encompassed in the aforementioned cluster, had no major effect, it was concluded that the structural domain cluster-hydroxylated residue was involved in the binding of $IpTx_a$ to RyR1. Gurrola *et al.*[748] also found that $IpTx_a$ and peptide A likely activate RyR1 by a similar mechanism and appear to compete for the same binding site on RyR1.

A similar work involving MCa identified R24 as a critical amino acid in the toxin's binding site.[749] An R24A substitution rendered MCa ineffective to increase [^{3}H]ryanodine binding, to induce subconducting states on single RyR1, and to stimulate Ca^{2+} release in SR vesicles or intact myotubes.[749] Other single substitutions (K8A, K19A, K20A, K22A, R23A and T26A) were capable of reducing affinity of the parent peptide but appeared less critical components of MCa's binding site. Supposedly, the alanine substituting each of the above residues hampers, but does not disrupt, MCa's binding site.

Alanine scanning of $IpTx_a$ also revealed that the amino acid residues responsible for activation of RyR1 are localized in the C-terminal region and correspond (in order of importance) to R24, R31, R33, K22 and R23.[745] Furthermore, L7 appears to play an important role as point of hydrophobic interaction with RyR1. The 3-D structure of $IpTx_a$ shows that these six residues along with others make up a critical domain of this peptide with a surface area of ~1900 $Å^2$ (Fig. 19-1). This structural domain would form a functional surface with a putative binding site that interacts with a cytosolic region of the RyR1.[745]

The ability of peptide A to activate RyR1 has been correlated with both its capacity to adopt an α-helical structure[750-753] and with the orientation of its positive charges in a single surface of the molecule.[752,753] Peptide A displays a basic surface with five basic residues (R681-K685) clustered in the C-terminal region of an α-helix whereas $IpTx_a$ (and also MCa) aligns its basic residues (K22, R23, R24, R31 and R33) in a central region. In both $IpTx_a$ and peptide A, this basic surface is totally exposed to solvent and displays a characteristic shape that may be directly involved in the activation of RyR1. In the 3-D structure, the functional surface of $IpTx_a$ is large (~1900 $Å^2$), whereas the equivalent surface of peptide A is smaller (~800 $Å^2$) (Fig. 19-1). These differences could explain, at least in part, why $IpTx_a$ and peptide A compete for the same binding site with different affinities.[745]

$IpTx_a$ activates [^{3}H]ryanodine binding to RyR1 over a wide range of [Ca^{2+}], producing a generalized increment in the magnitude of the bell-shaped Ca^{2+}-dependence of [^{3}H]ryanodine binding curve (Fig. 19-3). On the other hand, $IpTx_a$ displays different effects on RyR2 (cardiac isoform), activating [^{3}H]ryanodine binding moderately at low [Ca^{2+}] and inhibiting it, also moderately, at high [Ca^{2+}]. These somewhat erratic effects of $IpTx_a$ on RyR2 transform the bell-shaped [^{3}H]ryanodine binding curve into a sigmoidal relationship,[736,754] suggesting that the Ca^{2+}-activation and Ca^{2+}-inhibition sites of RyR2 are differently affected by $IpTx_a$.

$IpTx_a$ and RyR isoforms

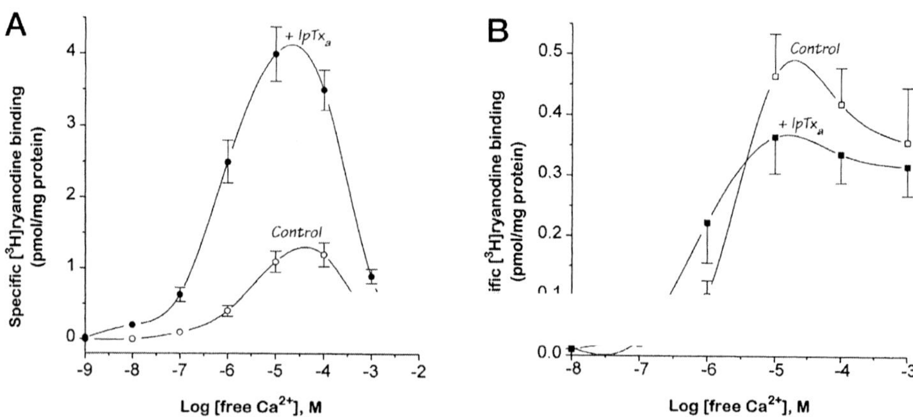

Figure 19-3. **Effect of $IpTx_a$ on the Ca^{2+}-dependence of [^{3}H]ryanodine binding curves** to (**A**) skeletal RyR (RyR1) and (**B**) cardiac RyR (RyR2). Taken, with permission, from El-Hayek *et al.*[736]

Tripathy *et al.*[754] showed that RyR2, although relatively insensitive to $IpTx_a$ in [^{3}H]ryanodine binding assays, is affected by $IpTx_a$ in a manner that is indistinguishable from RyR1. In single channel recordings, both RyR1 and RyR2 bind $IpTx_a$ and undergo conformational changes that induce the appearance of identical subconducting states (Fig. 19-4). $IpTx_a$, therefore, is a rare example of a RyR2 ligand that produces divergent effects on [^{3}H]ryanodine binding and single channel experiments.

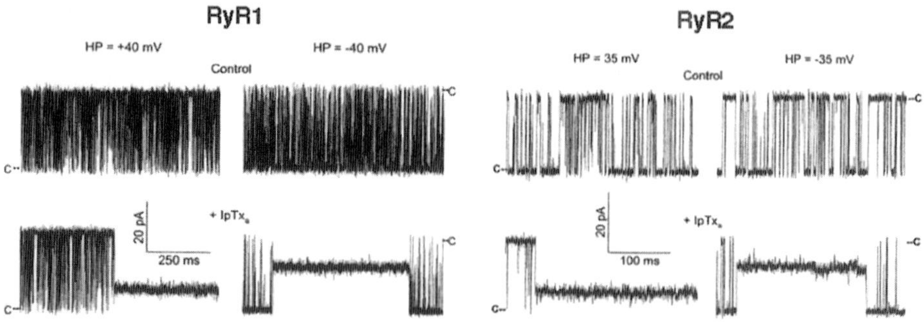

Figure 19-4. **Effect of $IpTx_a$ on single channel behavior of skeletal and cardiac RyRs.** Taken, with permission, from Tripathy *et al.*[754]

$IpTx_a$ stimulates [^{3}H]ryanodine binding to RyR3 (brain, smooth and skeletal muscle isoform), but at higher concentrations than required for effects on RyR1.[755] The effect of $IpTx_a$ on RyR3 is observed over a wide range of [Ca^{2+}] (0.1 μM to 10 mM), and single channel experiments show $IpTx_a$-induced subconducting states similar to those observed in RyR1 and RyR2. These results indicate that $IpTx_a$ is capable of inducing indistinguishable single channel effects on all three RyR isoforms, whereas its effect on [^{3}H]ryanodine binding is isoform-specific, with potencies ranking RyR1>RyR3>RyR2.[755]

The mechanism by which $IpTx_a$ exerts different effects on RyR isoforms when tested on [^{3}H]ryanodine binding and identical effects on single channel experiments is unknown, but an appealing hypothesis may be advanced by dividing the effect of the toxin into two distinct events. The first would be an event common to all RyR isoforms which induces a conformational change that leads to the subconducting state observed in single channel recordings; this event requires an open channel for $IpTx_a$ binding and is favored by conditions that promote high P_o.[754] The second event would be isoform-specific and affected by the RyR-ryanodine interaction, which is in turn dependent on the activity of the channel. As $IpTx_a$ and ryanodine bind to different sites on RyRs,[754] both sites may exert bi-modal cooperativity on each other. Thus, at low activity, [^{3}H]ryanodine binding is low and $IpTx_a$ exerts positive cooperativity, leading to additional increment on binding parameters. At high activity, [^{3}H]ryanodine binding is high and $IpTx_a$ may actually affect it adversely, by destabilizing the conformational state that favors binding of the alkaloid. This may explain why RyR1, which has intrinsically lower activity than RyR2, responds to $IpTx_a$ at all [Ca^{2+}], whereas [^{3}H]ryanodine binding to RyR2 is increased by $IpTx_a$ only at low [Ca^{2+}], where its activity is low.

RyR binding site(s) for $IpTx_a$ and stoichiometry of binding

The similarity in structure and function of $IpTx_a$ and MCa suggest that both peptides may share the same binding site in RyR1 and that this site may be overlapped with the activation site for peptide A of the DHPR,[748,750] although this scheme may not be that simple. Recently, it's been proposed that $IpTx_a$ displays three independent functional effects on RyR1 as well as on RyR2. Accordingly, $IpTx_a$ binds to three different sites on RyRs, one of high affinity, another of low affinity, and yet another of intermediate affinity that is responsible for inducing the subconducting states.[718]

Single channel experiments[754] and studies using frog skeletal fibers[756] concluded that one molecule of $IpTx_a$ interacts with one RyR tetramer during the induction of long Ca^{2+} releasing events. This 1:1 ($IpTx_a$-RyR) stoichiometry contrasts with results produced in [^{3}H]ryanodine binding[748] and electron microscopy[112] experiments, which suggest that up to 4 $IpTx_a$ molecules may bind to 1 RyR tetramer. The results may be reconciled if it is postulated that binding of a single molecule of $IpTx_a$ to any of its four potential binding sites is sufficient to activate the channel. In this scheme, both the long Ca^{2+} release events observed in permeabilized skeletal fibers[756] and the subconductance state observed in single channel recordings[754-756] represent long-dwelling events of a single $IpTx_a$ onto a single RyR channel.

The three-dimensional structure of RyR1 determined by cryo-electron microscopy revealed that the channel has a mushroom-like form with a squarely-shaped, bulky cytoplasmic domain containing four peripheral clamps.[57,106,107] The transmembrane (TM) region is composed of four subdomains (one for each subunit) that form the stem of the mushroom-like channel. Comparison of RyR1 in open and closed states show that there is a great range of conformational changes in the stem of the channel accompanied by opening of a central pore[106,112] The TM domain in the open state is rotated ~4° with respect to closed state in a movement similar to the movement of an iris and potentially involving the four TM subdomains.[106] A single $IpTx_a$ molecule binds to a single RyR1 subunit in a crevice between domain 3 and domain 7/8[112] (which is probably the site binding MCa as well). Domain 3 and domain 7/8 are connected to the central conducting vestibule through short "bridges". Based on this structural information, occupation of the toxin sites may transmit a great range of conformational changes through the region of the "bridges" that introduces a constriction of the conduction pathway. In this manner, binding of the toxin to any of the four RyR subunits may modify the conformational changes of the four subunits. Accordingly, $IpTx_a$ or MCa (and peptide A, if bound to the same site) may limit the counter-clockwise rotation predicted by cryo-electron microscopy to less than the ~4° required for a normal, fully-conducting opening, thus producing a partial rotation that leads to subconducting states (Fig. 19-5).[757]

Accessibility of $IpTx_a$ binding sites in intact cells

It has been long recognized that ionized peptide toxins are incapable of penetrating the plasmatic membrane unless aided by an active mechanism of transport. It is therefore logical that peptide toxins lack intracellular targets, although some peptide toxins are known to mimic external receptors and to unfold a series of intracellular events. $IpTx_a$ and MCa, however, are extremely basic peptides (net charge of +7 at physiological pH), a property that could confer them the capacity to permeate membranes.[758,759] Specifically, highly basic peptides translocate to cytosolic compartments after local perturbation of the lipid bilayer,[760] apparently by interaction of positively-charged basic amino acids with the negatively-charged polar heads of the phospholipids of the external membrane. Indeed, MCa has been recently shown to induce release of Ca^{2+} from intracellular stores of intact myotubes.[749] As the release of Ca^{2+} was evoked in the absence of external Ca^{2+}, it was inferred that MCa penetrated the external membrane and reached intracellular stores to open Ca^{2+} release channels.

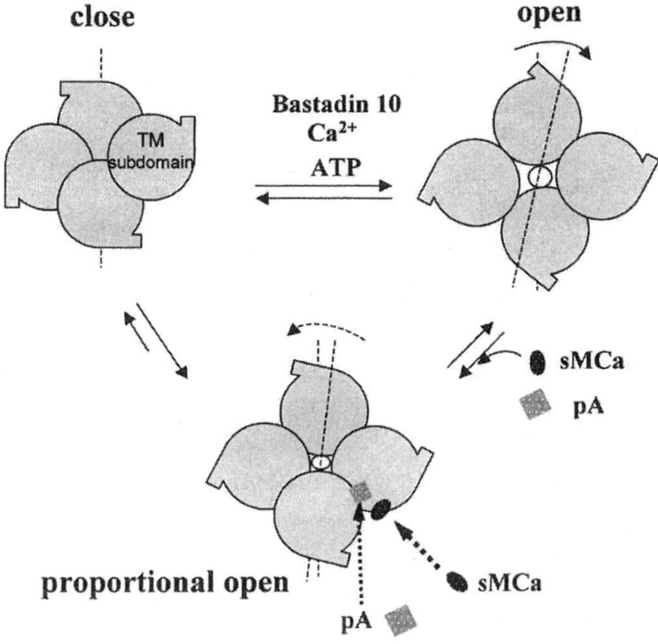

Figure 19-5. **Proposed mechanism of action of MCa and Peptide A on RyRs.** Taken, with permission, from Chen *et al.*[757]

Alternative hypotheses abound that could explain how these toxins reach their intended targets. RyRs have recently been found in unusual places, such as mitochondria[761] and possibly external membranes. It is possible that these oddly-localized RyRs are more frequent in insects and reptiles, scorpions' natural prey, than in mammals. Also, scorpion venoms contain a rich assortment of phospholipases[735] that may aid in the permeation of ionized molecules.

CONCLUDING REMARKS

$IpTx_a$ and MCa are representative of a group of high-affinity scorpion peptides that induce conformational changes in the RyR protein that ultimately evoke the release of Ca^{2+}. The specificity, high affinity, and reversibility of the peptide-RyR interaction make $IpTx_a$, MCa and the emerging group of new toxins useful tools for the study of the structural determinants of RyR gating and conduction. At the cellular level, this subclass of toxins may aid in the dissection of the chain of events that lead to the opening of RyRs during excitation-contraction coupling.

Chapter 20

REDOX SENSING BY THE RYANODINE RECEPTORS

Gerhard Meissner[1] and Jonathan S. Stamler[2]
[1]Depts. of Biochemistry and Biophysics, and Cell and Molecular Physiology, University of North Carolina, Chapel Hill, NC and [2]Depts. of Medicine and Biochemistry and Howard Hughes Medical Institute, Duke University Medical Center, Durham, NC

INTRODUCTION

The release of Ca^{2+} ions from intracellular membrane-bound stores is a key step in a wide variety of biological functions. In cardiac and skeletal muscle, the release of Ca^{2+} ions through Ca^{2+} release channels into the cytoplasm leads to muscle contraction. The Ca^{2+} release channels are also known as ryanodine receptors (RyRs) because the plant alkaloid ryanodine modifies their function by binding with high affinity and specificity.[109] The RyR ion channels are large protein complexes that are composed of four RyR 560 kDa polypeptides subunits, four small 12 kDa FK506 binding proteins (FKBP) and various associated proteins with a total molecular weight of greater than 2,500 kDa.[110,211] Numerous endogenous effectors ranging from divalent cations (Ca^{2+} and Mg^{2+}) to small molecules (e.g. ATP) and proteins (e.g. calmodulin, FKBP) regulate RyR function and thereby muscle function. The RyRs are also targets for redox active molecules. This chapter reviews the regulation of the skeletal muscle and cardiac muscle ryanodine receptors by glutathione, oxygen tension (pO_2), NADH, nitric oxide (NO) and related reactive oxygen and nitrogen species.

REGULATION OF RYRS BY OXYGEN TENSION AND GLUTATHIONE REDOX POTENTIAL

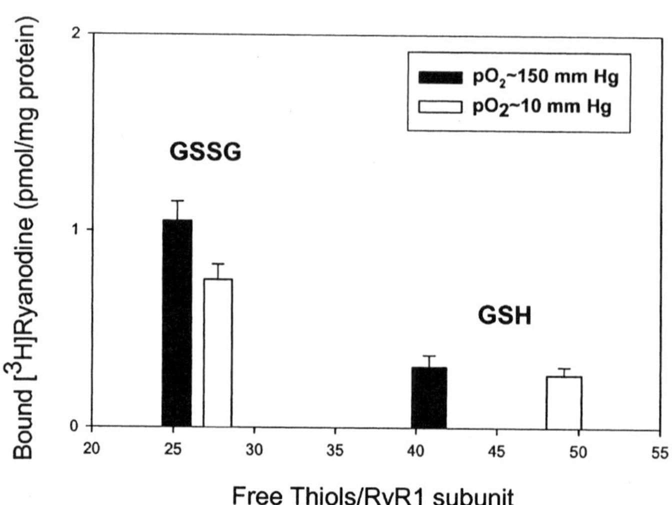

Figure 20-1. **RyR1 channel activity and redox state.** [^{3}H]-Ryanodine binding (as a measurement of RyR1 activity) and free thiol content were determined either at pO_2~10 mm Hg or 150 mm Hg in the presence of either 5 mM reduced (GSH) or oxidized (GSSG) glutathione. [^{3}H]-Ryanodine binding was determined by incubating skeletal muscle sarcoplasmic reticulum vesicles with [^{3}H]-ryanodine in the presence of 10 μM free Ca^{2+}. The free thiol content was determined by the monobromobimane method in the same condition From Xu *et al.*[611]

RyR ion channels contain reactive cysteines (i.e. thiols susceptible to redox-based modifications), which modulate RyR activity.[110] Heavy metals, alkylating agents such as N-ethylmaleimide (NEM) and oxidants such as diamide and H_2O_2 modulate the activity of the RyRs.[484,762,763] The experimental results in Fig. 20-1 show that RyR1 activity and the number of reduced cysteines (free thiols) depend on two principal determinants of cellular redox state - oxygen tension (pO_2) and reduced (GSH) or oxidized (GSSG) glutathione.[612] Studies using the lipophilic, thiol-specific probe monobromobimane have revealed that nearly half of the 404 cysteines within the tetrameric RyR1 channel complex are reduced in the presence of 5 mM GSH at pO_2 ~10 mm Hg, i.e. under conditions comparable to resting muscle.[764] In this situation, RyR1 activity was low, as measured by a ligand binding assay using the RyR-specific probe [^{3}H]-ryanodine. An increase in oxygen tension from ~10 mm Hg (simulating the tissue) to ambient air (pO_2

~150 mm Hg) in the presence of 5 mM GSH modifies the redox state of up to 8 thiols/RyR1 subunit without appreciably changing RyR1 activity. Exposure of RyR1 to oxidized glutathione (GSSG) at pO_2 ~10 mm Hg or at ambient conditions resulted in the oxidation of up to 24 thiols/RyR1 subunit and a large increase in activity. The results of Fig. 20-1 suggest that RyR1 has a large group of functionally 'silent' thiols that may protect the RyR1 from low oxidative stress (as might be seen in normal working muscle), and another group of reactive thiols that may control the channel's response to more hazardous levels of oxidants (e.g. produced during rigorous exercise).

Additional parameters determine the redox state of RyR1. Micromolar activating concentrations of Ca^{2+} lowered the redox potential of RyR1 and favored channel opening, whereas elevated inhibitory concentrations of Ca^{2+} and Mg^{2+} had opposite effects.[604] In mammalian cells, a cytosolic ratio of GSH/GSSG ≥ 30:1 creates a highly reducing redox potential.[765] However, a ratio of 3:1 to 1: 1 generates a more oxidizing environment in the ER lumen. In single channel measurements, RyR1 responded to redox potentials produced by both SR lumenal and cytoplasmic glutathione, indicating that the receptor is under the control of a transmembrane redox potential.[609] Studies with skeletal muscle membranes suggested that glutathione transport across the SR membrane may be facilitated by RyR1-dependent and -independent mechanisms.[609,766]

Fig. 20-2 examines the regulation of the skeletal muscle and cardiac muscle ryanodine receptors by glutathione at ambient oxygen tension in the presence of two endogenous channel effectors, MgATP and calmodulin. Reduced glutathione (5 mM GSH, i.e., concentrations similar to those found in cells) resulted in low RyR1 activity, whereas the addition of oxidized glutathione (5 mM GSSG) strongly activated [^{3}H]-ryanodine binding without appreciably affecting the Ca^{2+}-dependence of channel activity. In contrast, a change from oxidizing to reducing conditions shift the RyR2 Ca^{2+} activation curve to the right without appreciably altering the maximal levels of [^{3}H]-ryanodine binding at optimally activating Ca^{2+} concentrations. The results suggest that the effects of GSH/GSSG redox state on RyR1 and RyR2 activity are exerted by different mechanisms.

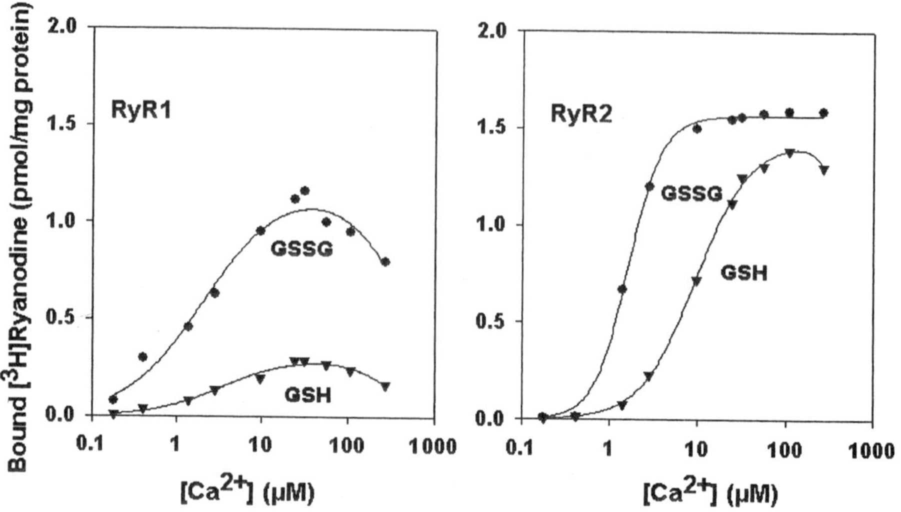

Figure 20-2. **Redox regulation of skeletal muscle and cardiac muscle ryanodine receptors by reduced and oxidized glutathione.** Specific [^{3}H]-ryanodine binding to rabbit skeletal and cardiac sarcoplasmic reticulum membranes was determined at ambient oxygen tension in the presence of two endogenous channel modulators, 5 mM Mg AMPPCP (an ATP analog) and 1 μM calmodulin, in assay media containing 0.25 M KCl, 20 mM imidazole, pH 7, 1 nM [^{3}H]-ryanodine and the indicated concentrations of free Ca^{2+}. From Balshaw *et al.*[331]

MODULATION OF RYRS BY REACTIVE OXYGEN SPECIES

Working muscle produces reactive oxygen species (ROS) at a low basal rate.[767] Enzymes that scavenge ROS such as superoxide anion (O_2^-) and hydrogen peroxide (H_2O_2) attenuate force development in muscle exposed to 95% O_2 (standard bioassay conditions), supporting a functional role. During strenuous muscle exercise or short episodes of ischemia followed by the resupply of oxygen, increased levels of ROS impose an oxidative stress by altering various cellular functions. Cells protect themselves against the excessive production of reactive oxygen species via the action of superoxide dismutase, which converts O_2^- to O_2 and H_2O_2 and catalase and glutathione peroxidase, which detoxify H_2O_2. Excessive levels of O_2^- decreased cardiac SR Ca^{2+} content by lowering SR pump activity[768] and displacing calmodulin from RyR2, resulting in increased release of Ca^{2+} from SR.[769]

Reactive oxygen species can be formed by several mechanisms, including the mitochondrial electron transport chain, xanthine oxidase and

NADH oxidase. In skeletal and cardiac muscle, SR-associated NADH oxidases are potential sources of $O_2^{\cdot-}$ production. NADH can stimulate RyR1 activity.[770] Activation of RyR1 was observed in the presence of mitochondrial electron transport inhibitors but was inhibited by superoxide dismutase, suggesting that a NADH oxidase activates RyR1 by producing $O_2^{\cdot}$. The skeletal muscle RyR1 has an N-terminal oxidoreductase-like domain and binds NAD^+ to sites other than the ATP binding site.[103] However, it remains to be established that the oxidoreductase-like domain is enzymatically active. Contrary to the results of Xia *et al.*[770], Baker *et al.*[103] observed that NADH had only minor effects on RyR1 activity.

In contrast to activation of RyR1, NADH decreased single RyR2 ion channel activity[771] and SR Ca^{2+} release.[772] Furthermore, NADH inhibition of RyR2 was not affected by superoxide dismutase and thus was independent on $O_2^{\cdot-}$ production.[768] Another remarkable difference was that mitochondrial electron transport inhibitors relieved the inhibition of RyR2 activity by NADH.[772] How then does NADH inhibit RyR2? RyR2 may sense changes in redox potential that may be influenced by either NADH/NAD^+ or cellular respiration or both. Alternatively, NADH may transfer reducing equivalents to RyR2 to reduce regulatory thiol groups. Such a mechanism would require a high local NADH concentration because the inhibition of RyR2 (as measured by Ca^{2+} sparks in permeabilized cells and in single channel measurements) was only seen at NADH/NAD^+ >1.[768,771] By comparison, the cytosolic NADH/NAD^+ in aerobically perfused working hearts is low (~0.1%).[773] Even during the extreme anaerobic condition of sustained ischemia, the cytosolic NADH/NAD^+ ratio[773] is below that required to inhibit SR Ca^{2+} release.[768,771] It may be of biological or experimental interest that thiols will add directly to nicotinamide at the 1:4 position of the nicotinamide ring of NAD^+.

MODULATION OF RYRS BY NO AND RELATED NITROGEN SPECIES

NO is formed by one of three major classes of nitric oxide synthases (NOSs): endothelial (eNOS), neuronal (nNOS) and inducible (iNOS). In skeletal muscle, the predominant isoform, nNOS, is targeted to neuronal postsynaptic densities by interacting with postsynaptic proteins, and to specialized invaginations of the sarcolemma, called caveolae, by binding to caveolin 3 and dystrophin-associated proteins.[774] In cardiac muscle, eNOS is the predominent NOS isoform. The enzyme is primarily expressed in the coronary and endocardial endothelia but has also been localized to caveolae and mitochondria of cardiomyocytes. Immunoelectron microscopy showed association of nNOS with cardiac but not skeletal muscle SR membranes.[775] A selective association of nNOS with RyR2 was described and the use of $eNOS^{-/-}$ and $nNOS^{-/-}$ mice demonstrated that nNOS has a specific role in regulating SR Ca^{2+} release.[776] RyR1[612] and RyR2[611] are endogenously S-nitrosylated, supporting a role of NO in skeletal and cardiac muscle EC coupling. The third isoform, iNOS, is transcribed in inflammatory cells and muscles in response to cytokines and bacterial endotoxins.

NO exerts its cellular effects via cGMP-dependent or -independent pathways.[777] In the cGMP-dependent pathway, the binding of NO to the heme group of guanylate cyclase results in enhanced production of intracellular cGMP and activation of cGMP-dependent kinase. The principal mechanism by which NO operates independently of cGMP is through S-nitrosylation, which occurs most often at a single cysteine residue within an acid-base or hydrophobic structural motif[778] (compounds such as glutathione which shuttles NO bioactivity in the form of GSNO may serve as intermediates). Pathological oxidation of RyR may involve other species, such as peroxynitrite ($OONO^-$), which extensively oxidizes the RyRs[611,779] and has been implicated in postischemic injury.[780]

NO or NO related species have been reported to activate[781] or inhibit[660] the skeletal RyR1. NO generated in situ from arginine by endogenous NOS and the NO donor S-nitroso-N-acetylpenicillamine reduced the rate of Ca^{2+} release from SR vesicles and the activity of single skeletal RyR1 channels incorporated in lipid bilayers.[660] In contrast, Stoyanovsky *et al.*[781] found that NO, delivered in the form of NO gas, and NO donors (NONOates, S-nitrosothiols) activated single RyR1 ion channels and Ca^{2+} release from SR vesicles. Aghdasi and colleagues[763] reported that NO donors had no detectable effects at low concentrations, but at higher concentrations were able to block intersubunit cross-links and prevented activation of the skeletal RyR channel by the disulfide inducing agent diamide. In two other studies, NO-generating agents both activated and inhibited RyR1 in lipid bilayers, depending on donor concentration, membrane potential, and the presence of channel agonists and other sufhydryl modifying reagents.[782,783]

In vitro, *S*-nitrosylation of the skeletal muscle RyR1 by NO depends on NO concentration and O_2 tension.[612] Physiological concentrations (<1 μM) of NO *S*-nitrosylated and activated RyR1 at pO_2~10 mm Hg but not in ambient air (pO_2~150 mm Hg). Changes in oxygen tension oxidized/reduced as many as 6-8 thiols in each RyR1 subunit, which may explain the responsiveness of RyR1 to NO at tissue pO_2 but not ambient air.[612] In contrast, other NO related molecules such as 3-morpholinosydnonimine (SIN-1), S-nitrosoglutathione or NOC12, which generate a variety of reactive nitrogen oxides can activate RyR1 independently of oxygen tension. NOC-12 activated by S-nitrosylation,[617] SIN-1 by oxidation of thiols,[617] and

S-nitrosoglutathione by *S*-nitrosylation/oxidation[617] and *S*-thionylation.[613] Site-directed mutagenesis studies demonstrated that at physiological O_2 concentrations, NO specifically S-nitrosylates Cys3635 among ~50 free cysteines per RyR1 subunit.[616] C3635 is located in the CaM binding domain of RyR1, which provides an explanation for the observation that NO transduces its functional effect only in the presence of calmodulin (Fig. 20-3).

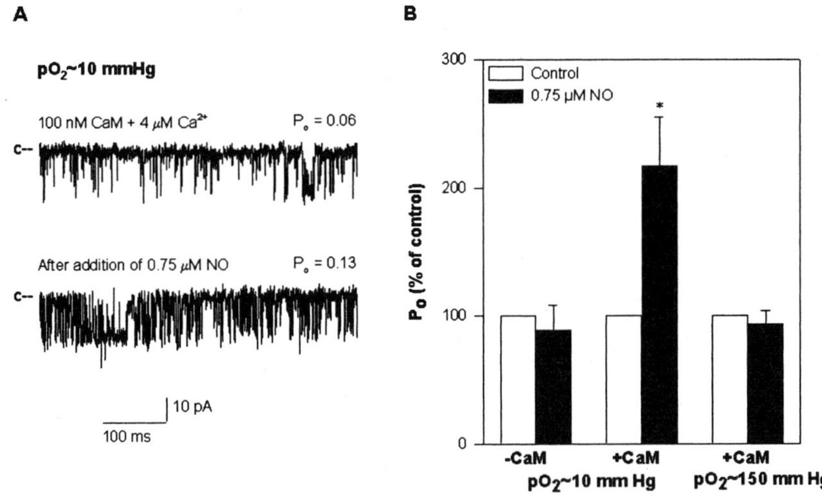

Figure 20-3. **NO modulates single RyR1 channel activity under physiological muscle O_2 tension in the presence of calmodulin. A**. Channel currents of two RyR1s, shown as downward deflections from closed (c--) levels, were recorded in a lipid bilayer chamber pre-equilibrated to pO_2 ~10 mm Hg with voltage held at -35 mV. Top trace: control with 100 nM CaM and 4 mM free Ca^{2+}, channel open probability (Po) = 0.06; second trace: 2 min after the addition of 0.75 mM NO to cytosolic side, Po=0.13. **B**. As compared to controls (open bars), 0.75 mM NO (filled bars) significantly increased Po of RyR1 (*, $p < 0.05$) at pO_2 ~10 mm Hg but not pO_2 ~150 mm Hg. NO did not significantly alter Po of RyR1 at pO_2 of ~10 mm Hg in the presence of 1 mM myosin light chain-derived calmodulin binding peptide that dissociates endogenously bound calmodulin (-CaM). From Eu *et al.*[612]

A recent study addressed the role of NO and O_2 tension in controlling SR Ca^{2+} release and contractile force generated by skeletal muscle. Eu *et al.*[764] compared the role of pO_2 on contractility of extensor digitorum longus muscle and on Ca^{2+} transients and cell shortening of flexor digitorium brevis myocytes, both prepared from normal and nNOS-deficient mice. Included were measurements at 95% O_2 (pO_2~700 mmHg) because studies with isolated skeletal muscle fibers are usually done at high O_2 concentrations. The measurements revealed an enhancement in muscle performance and the amplitude of the Ca^{2+} transients at low physiological O_2 tension, which depended on endogenous nNOS activity. At 95% O_2, which produced a high non-physiological core muscle pO_2 ~400 mmHg, force production was enhanced but response to NO was diminished. The findings show that contractility depends on O_2 tension and NO modulates O_2 dependence.

NO also fulfills many of the criteria of a physiological modulator of cardiac muscle EC coupling.[776,777,784,785] In *in vitro* studies, NO and NO-related molecules activated[611,781] or inactivated[661] RyR2, leading to reversible or irreversible alteration of RyR2 channel activity. The two NO-related species GSNO and CysNO S-nitrosylated and/or oxidized up to 12 sites per RyR2 subunit in ambient O_2 tension.[611] The level of S-nitrosylation appeared to be dependent on channel conformation because Mg^{2+}, a RyR inhibitor, reduced SNO content. 3-Morpholinosydnonimine (SIN-1), which produces effector peroxynitrite, activated and oxidized but did not S-nitrosylate RyR2.

CONCLUDING REMARKS

Current evidence suggests that the activity of the RyRs depends critically on redox state both at the whole cell level and at the level of the RyRs themselves: oxygen tension, GSH/GSSG, NADH/NAD^+ and NO can each modulate channel activity. Future work will need to address the isoform and tissue specificity of interaction of the RyRs with redox active molecules, the molecular basis of this specificity, and how "redox" regulation of the RyRs by NO/O_2 relates to the roles of NO and O_2 in overall muscle function.

ACKNOWLEDGMENTS

Support by National Institutes of Health grants AR18687 and HL27540 is gratefully acknowledged.

Chapter 21

RYANODINE RECEPTOR DYSFUNCTION IN THE DIABETIC HEART

Keshore R. Bidasee, Sarah Ingersoll, and Chun Hong Shao
Dept. of Pharmacology, University of Nebraska Medical Center, 985800 Nebraska Medical Center, Omaha, NE

INTRODUCTION

Diabetes mellitus (DM) is a major metabolic illness affecting populations worldwide. In America more than 17 million individuals are inflicted with this syndrome, which is clinically characterized as having fasting blood glucose levels of ≥126mg/dL (7mmol/L).[786] In addition to frank DM, a significant number of individuals also exhibit lesser degrees of impaired glucose regulation. DM is classified into three types, Type 1 (account for about 10% of all cases), Type 2 (≈ 85% of cases) and gestational diabetes (≈ 5% of cases). Type 1 DM arises when beta cells of the pancreas are unable to produce insulin. This defect can occur from chemical toxicity, lymphocytic infiltration following viral infection (autoimmune reaction) or from tumors.[787] Usually children and young adults are the ones inflicted with Type 1 DM. Type 2 DM results either from defects in beta cell signaling, insulin receptor signaling, glucose transport proteins, or combinations thereof. While genetics is an important predisposition, factors such as obesity and a sedentary lifestyle also increase risk for developing Type 2 diabetes. Although initially thought to occur only in adult life, recent data suggest that young obese children are also developing Type 2 diabetes. Gestational diabetes occurs in about 5% of all pregnancies. For the mother, gestational diabetes increases risk of preeclampsia, cesarean section and future risk of Type 2 diabetes. For the fetus or neonate, the disorder is associated with higher rates of perinatal mortality, macrosomia, birth trauma, hyperbilirubinemia and neonatal hypoglycemia.[788]

Persistent elevation in circulating glucose levels lead to the progressive loss of function of many components of the cardiovascular system, including the heart itself. This "diabetic cardiomyopathy" which occurs independent of coronary arteriosclerosis and/or hypertension, starts of as an asymptomatic slowing in relaxation kinetics.[789] As the syndrome progresses, systolic function also becomes compromised, increasing morbidity and mortality. To date, it is well accepted that the etiology underlying diabetic cardiomyopathy (DC) is multifactorial.[790] At the molecular level, DC reflects alterations in expression of several proteins. For example, increased myocardial stiffness has been attributed to increases in expression of extracellular fibronectin and collagen IV.[791] Changes in expression of β-adrenoreceptor complement and associated intracellular signal transduction proteins are also responsible in part for decrease in autonomic function.[792,793] Diabetes also decreases synthesis and release of thyroid hormones, T_3 and T_4.[794] This in turn decreases the ATPase activity of myosin heavy chain resulting in a decrease in the extent of myocyte shortening. Expression of several proteins intimately involved in excitation-contraction coupling is also altered in the heart during diabetes.

The UK Prospective Diabetes Study (UKPDS) and the Diabetes Control and Complications Trial (DCCT) clearly demonstrated that complications resulting from both Type 1 and Type 2 patients can be minimize with tight glycemic control (metformin/sulfonylureas/insulin).[795,796] Insulin pumps have made this goal more achievable for type 1 diabetic patients. Also, islet cell transplantation could become another widely use treatment strategy for regulating blood glucose levels in Type 1 diabetics if stem cell technology is able to reduce dependency on viable of pancreatic tissues. However, for the vast majority of patients, tight glycemic control is often difficult to achieve and can lead to more severe hypoglycemia. Persistent elevation in blood glucose levels lead to failure of several components of the cardiovascular system that requires treatment with therapeutics in order to manage the symptoms and improve quality of life. Among the drugs used are angiotensin-converting enzyme inhibitors (ramipril/perindopril), angiotensin receptor blockers (losartan, irbesartan), diuretics (thiazides) and lipid lowering drugs (chlorthalidone, atorvastatin).[797-801] While some of these drugs appear to exert secondary beneficial effects on the heart by reducing inflammation and triggering reverse remodeling, their primary mode of action is to reduce peripheral resistance and/or load. Carvedilol, a β_1-adrenoreceptor blocker widely used to treat DC also has α_1 blocking and antioxidant properties (10 x greater than that of vitamin E).[802] Multi-drug therapies in combination with diet and exercise are currently being explored to reduce cardiovascular complications.[803] However, economic cost and compliance may be inhibitory factors against this treatment strategy. Although, current pharmacotherapeutics improve cardiovascular hemodynamics, the beneficial effect on the diabetic heart *per se* remains modest. As such, heart failure continues to persist in the diabetic population. Two immediate challenges therefore are (i) to identify additional mechanisms that contribute to loss in left ventricular function, and (ii) identify/develop newer therapeutic strategies that can minimize these changes.

ROLE OF RYANODINE RECEPTORS (RYR2) IN THE ETIOLOGY OF DIABETIC CARDIOMYOPATHY

Decrease in the ability of the heart to effectively contract is one of the major causes for the increased incidence of morbidity and mortality in diabetic patients. Studies suggest that this defect is due in part to alterations in function of several proteins involved in excitation-contraction coupling. One of these proteins is RyR2, the channel through which calcium ions leaves the sarcoplasmic reticulum to effect contractions. Yu and McNeill[804] were the first to implicate RyR2 in the etiology of DC when they found that post-rest potentiation (Woodworth staircase: an enhancement in stimulated contraction following a long rest) was significantly reduced in hearts from diabetic rats. They also showed that membrane vesicles prepared from diabetic rat hearts bound significantly less [^{3}H]ryanodine when compared with age-matched, non-diabetic controls[805] and suggested that expression of RyR2 is being decreased during diabetes. We and others later showed that expression of RyR2 do indeed decrease in hearts of chronic diabetic patients[806,807] as well as in hearts of streptozotocin (STZ)-induced diabetic rats.[808-811] However, since critical calcium cycling proteins are usually expressed in amounts that exceed that required for minimal physiologic functioning, it seems unlikely that a decrease in expression of RyR2 *per se* could be solely responsible for the decrease in post-rest potentiation induced by diabetes. Eisner and co-workers also echoed this view when they suggested that a decrease in RyR2 protein density would be compensated for by an increase in the amount of releasable calcium inside the sarcoplasmic reticulum.[812] Moreover, using the streptozotocin-induced diabetic rat model we found that not all hearts with establish DC show a decrease in expression of RyR2 protein (Fig. 21-1, panels A, B and C). Zhong *et al.*[810] also found that loss of function precedes loss of protein expression. Thus, it seems likely that mechanisms other than changes in RyR2 expression are responsible for decrease in post-rest potentiation and loss in ventricular contractility associated with diabetes.

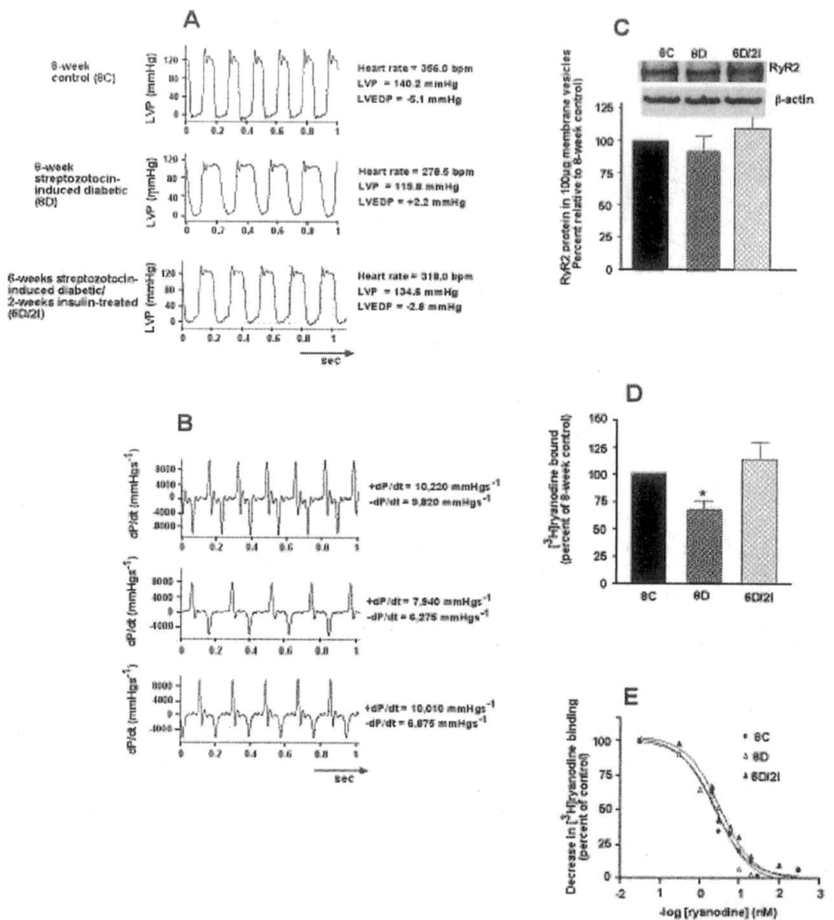

Figure 21-1. **Comparison of basal cardiac function in hearts from 8-week control (8C), 8-week diabetic (8D) and 6-week diabetic/2-week insulin-treated (6D/2I) animals and its correlation with expression and function of type 2 ryanodine receptors (RyR2). A-B.** comparision of *in vivo* cardiac function. For this, animals were lightly anesthetized with Inactin® (20mg/kg) and a pressure transducer attached to the end of a catheter was inserted into the left ventricle by way of a carotid artery. Basal heart rates, left ventricular pressures, and left ventricular end diastolic pressures were then directly obtained **A**. The first derivatives, ± dP/dt were also obtained to determine rates of changes **B**. **C**. Steady state level of RyR2 protein in hearts from 8C, 8D and 6D/2I. For this, Western blot analyses were carried out using standard procedures employing 50μg of membrane protein from 8C, 8D and 6D/2I. **D**. Comparison of the ability of 50 μg of membrane protein from 8C, 8D and 6D/2I to bind the specific ligand [^{3}H]ryanodine. **E**. Comparison of the relative affinities of RyR2 from these three groups of animals for ryanodine.[811,813,814]

RYR2 BECOMES DYSFUNCTIONAL DURING DIABETES

Using a lower dose of streptozotocin to induce experimental diabetes (50mg/kg instead of the typical 65mg/kg, IV), we recently discovered that equivalent amounts of RyR2 protein from diabetic rat hearts bind less of the specific ligand [^{3}H]ryanodine when compared with age-matched controls.[811] We also found that this defect preceded loss of expression of RyR2.[813] Interestingly, while the amount of accessible ryanodine binding sites decreased (lower B_{max}), the affinity of RyR2 for ryanodine (K_d) did not change. In other experiments, we also found that the electophoretic mobility of RyR2 from diabetic animals on SDS-PAGE gels was slowed, suggesting posttranslational modification.[814] Two salient questions that arises from these data are (i) can posttranslational modification decrease RyR2 function, and (ii) if so, what types of modifications are occurring on RyR2 as a result of diabetes. It should also be pointed out that since RyR2 appears to have multiple binding site for ryanodine/ryanoids, a decrease in B_{max} is possible without significant changes in K_d.[811] Studies have also shown that single point mutations on homologous RyR1 can significantly decrease its ability to bind [^{3}H]ryanodine.[815] Thus, it seems reasonable to conclude that posttranslational modifications on RyR2 can also decrease RyR2's ability to bind [^{3}H]ryanodine. Moreover, several point mutations on RyR2 are also known to trigger sudden cardiac death in children and young adults as is the case with catecholaminergic polymorphic ventricular tachycardia (CPVT) and arrhythmogenic right-ventricular dysplasia/cardiomyopathy (ARVD2).[294]

POSTTRANSLATIONAL MODIFICATION OF RYR2 DURING DIABETES

It has been known for a long time that the turnover rate of RyR2 is slow (half-life ≈ 8 days). It is therefore conceivable that alterations in intracellular milieu brought about by diabetes could trigger posttranslational modifications. Two types of modifications that can be readily be formed on RyR2 as a result of shifts in metabolism and biochemistry are oxidation of sulfhydryl groups on exposed cysteine residues and non-enzymatic glycation of lysine, arginine and histidine residues.

A: Oxidation reactions of sulfhydryl moieties on cysteine residues

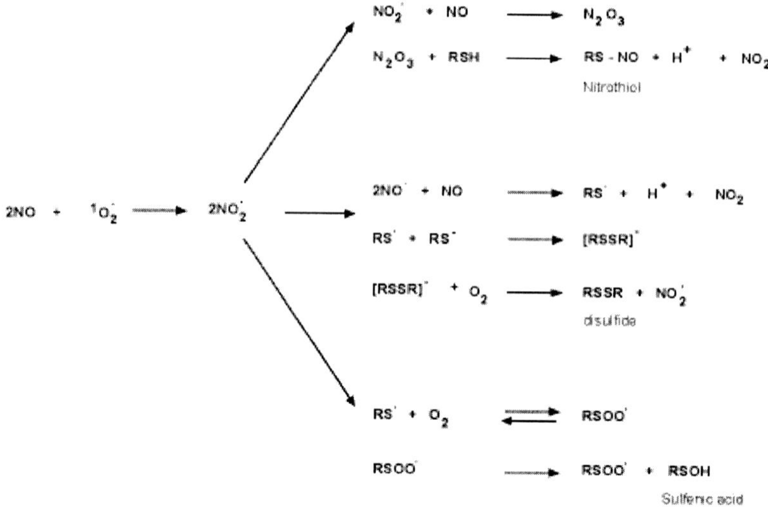

B: Formation of AGEs on arginine, histidine and lysine residues

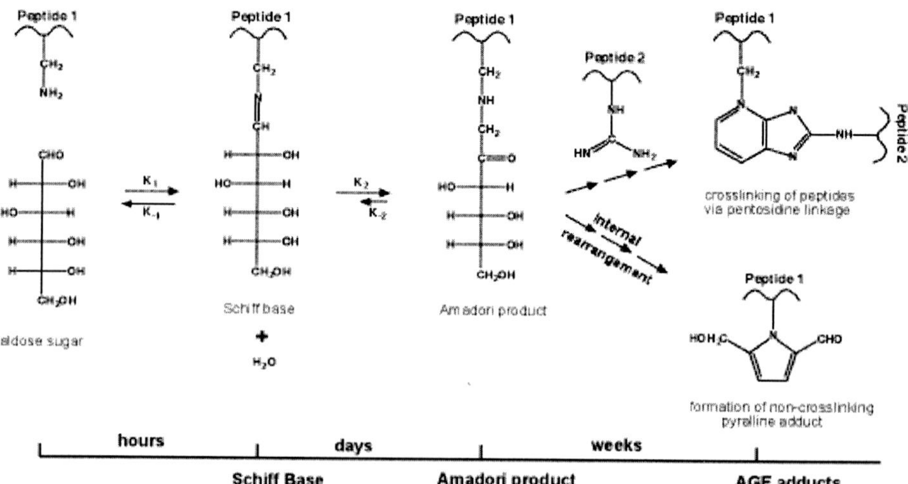

Figure 21-2. **Examples of posttranslational modification reactions that can occur on RyR2 during diabetes. A**. Select reactions that lead to the formation of nitrothiols, disulfide bonds and sulfenic acid adducts on sulfhydryl moieties of exposed cysteine residues, represented by "R". **B**. Reactions between aldose and arginine/lysine residues that lead to the formation of crosslinking (pentosidine) and non-crosslinking advanced glycation end products (AGEs) on RyR2.

Oxidation of cysteine residues on type 2 ryanodine receptors

Studies have shown that the activity of RyR2 is dependent on the oxidative state of several sulfhydryl groups (SH).[816] When the more reactive of these "exposed" sulfhydryl groups are oxidized, this usually trigger channel activation (increases P_o, increases [^{3}H]ryanodine binding). As the concentration of oxidants increases, other sulfhydryl groups also become oxidized, triggering a decrease in channel activity (decreases P_o/decreases[^{3}H]ryanodine binding). Studies have also shown that shifts in metabolism and biochemistry brought diabetes increases intracellular levels of reactive oxygen species (ROS) including superoxide anions [$O^{\cdot}$], hydroxy radicals [$OH^{\cdot}$], lipid peroxides [$ROO^{\cdot}$], singlet oxygen [$^1O_2^{\cdot}$], and hydrogen peroxide [H_2O_2]).[817] We recently found that expression of nitric oxide synthases (eNOS and iNOS) also increase in the heart during diabetes, suggesting an increase in production of nitric oxide (unpublished data). NO in turn can react with ROS increasing production of several reactive nitrogen species including nitrosonium cation [NO^+], nitroxyl anion [NO^-], and peroxynitrite [$ONOO^-$]) species. ROS and nitrogen species are also known to react rapidly reacts with the sulfhydryl moiety on cysteine residues forming nitrothiols, disulfide bonds and sulfenic acid derivatives (Fig. 21-2 A).

In a recent study, we found that when RyR2 from diabetic rat hearts were treated with 2mM dithiothreitol, its ability to bind [^{3}H]ryanodine was partially restored.[818] These data suggest that the reduced ability of RyR2 to bind [^{3}H]ryanodine stems in part from increased formation of disulfide bonds (S-S). Since there are several classes of reactive sulfhydryl groups on RyRs, further experiments were conducted to ascertain which class of sulfhydryl groups might be involved in disulfide bond formation. For this we synthesized the pyrrole sulfhydryl reagent, pyrocoll (5*H*,10*H*-Dipyrrolo[1,2-*a*:1',2'-*d*]pyrazine-5,10-dione). At nM concentrations, this drug interacts with one class of free sulfhydryl groups triggering channel deactivation (decreases RyR2 ability to bind [^{3}H]ryanodine). At higher μM concentrations, pyrocoll reacts with a second class of SH groups, triggering instead channel activation. Interesting, we found that pyrocoll at μM concentrations was unable increase [^{3}H]ryanodine binding to RyR2 from diabetic rat hearts, suggesting that a class of SH groups that trigger channel activation are not available. We have yet to determine the location of these specific SH groups (cysteine residues) on RyR2.

Non-enzymatic glycation of arginine, histidine and lysine residues on RyR2

Studies have also shown that glucose-6-phosphate levels increases in myocytes during chronic diabetes. High levels of this aldose sugar, as well as other reactive aldehydes formed as a result of diabetes will accelerate the formation of Schiff bases on lysine, arginine, and histidine residues (non-enzymatic glycation reactions). Over time, these Schiff bases undergo internal rearrangement to form more stable Amadori products. On long-lived proteins, Amadori products further undergo a series of oxidation, reduction, elimination and cyclization reactions to form advanced-glycation end products (AGEs, Fig. 21-2 B).[819] Once formed, these complexes remain attached to the protein throughout its lifetime. Studies have also shown that modification of proteins with AGEs ultimately lead to organ dysfunction. There are two major types of AGEs, those that are crosslinked (formed between adjacent amino acid residues), and those that are non-crosslinking. Also, some AGEs fluoresce while other do not.

In a recent study using matrix-assisted laser desorption ionization mass spectrometry in conjunction with an in-house PERL algorithm, we found that formation of non-crosslinking AGEs increases on RyR2 during diabetes and production of these complexes were attenuated with insulin-treatment[814] (also see Fig. 21-3 A). More recently, we also found that formation of pentosidine-type crosslinking AGEs also increases on RyR2 during diabetes (unpublished data). As an example, pentosidine AGEs were formed between arginine 870 and lysine 748 (see Fig. 21-3A, top left). Interestingly, this crosslinking AGE adduct was found in the highly conserved N-terminal, regions in which mutations trigger malignant hyperthermia (MH), central core disease (CCD), CPVT and ARDV2. Since RyR2 undergo conformation rearrangement when translocating calcium ions from the lumen of the SR to the cytosol, it seems likely crosslinking of the domains could significantly compromise function. Fig. 21-3 B show the approximate locations of select AGEs adducts identified thus far on RyR2.

A: AGE modifications on RyR2 peptides

${}_{869}$WKFMMK${}_{874}$

${}_{743}$KDGGVRK${}_{749}$

Pentosidine adduct

${}_{4677}$VAALDFSDAREK${}_{4687}$

Pyrraline adduct

${}_{3439}$MSKAAISDQER${}_{3449}$

Imidazolone B adduct

${}_{1606}$VDVSRISER${}_{1614}$

1-alkyl-2-formyl-3,4-glycosyl-pyrrole (AFGP) adduct

B: Approximate location of amino acid residues on RyR2 protein that are modified by advanced glycation end products (AGEs)

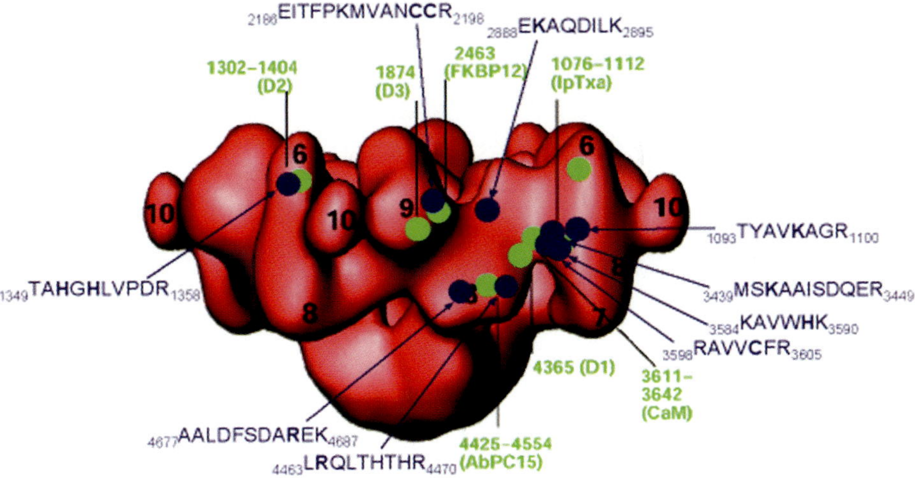

Figure 21-3. **Amino acid residues on RyR2 that are modified by advanced glycation end products and their relative locations on the 3D structure of RyR2. A**. Specific arginine, histidine or lysine residues on RyR2 that are modified by defined advanced glycation end products. Bold letters indicate the amino acid residue that is modified. The chemical structures of four structurally diverse AGEs are also shown. **B**. The approximate location of the amino acids that are modified by AGEs (blue filled circles). The green filled circles represent the locations of previously identified residues.

CONCLUDING REMARKS

In conclusion, we have shown that RyR2 becomes dysfunctional during diabetes. We have also identified two types of posttranslational modifications that occur on RyR2 during diabetes. Treatment with insulin reduced posttranslational modifications on RyR2 as well as partially attenuated loss of function induced by diabetes. Although suggestive, these data do not establish that posttranslational modifications are responsible for the loss of RyR2 activity and by extension, the decrease in ventricular contractility seen during diabetes. Experiments using site-directed mutagenesis studies, as well as treatment with drugs capable of preventing AGEs formation and oxidation of amino acid residues are ongoing.

ACKNOWLEDGMENTS

This work was supported in part by grants from the National Institutes of Health (RO1-HL66898). The authors thank Drs. Terrence Wagenknecht and Manjuli Sharma for providing the 3D structure of RyR2. The authors would also like to thank Drs. Kaushik Patel, Mu Wang and Henry R. Besch, Jr. for helpful discussions.

Chapter 22

MOLECULAR AND CLINICAL GENETICS OF RYR1 DISORDERS

Tommie V. McCarthy, James J.A. Heffron, and John Mackrill
Dept. of Biochemistry, University College Cork, Cork, Ireland

INTRODUCTION

Malignant hyperthermia (MH) is a potentially fatal pharmacogenetic disorder of skeletal muscle. It is triggered in susceptible people by exposure to commonly used volatile anaesthetics agents such as halothane, isoflurane, enfluorane and sevoflurane or depolarising muscle relaxants such as succinyl choline. A fulminant MH crisis is characterised by any combination of hyperthermia, skeletal muscle rigidity, tachycardia or arrhythmia, and respiratory and metabolic acidosis. Advances in patient monitoring during anaesthesia, intervention on the appearance of early MH indicators and the use of the drug dantrolene sodium (a skeletal muscle relaxant) has reduced the mortality rate in developed countries from 70% to below 10%. Individuals susceptible to MH are not clinically distinguishable from the general population and may present with none, some or all of the classical MH signs with variable intensity on any given exposure to trigger agents. As MH can be avoided by the use of non-triggering anaesthetic agents, knowledge of the susceptibility of individuals prior to anaesthesia is of vital importance for prevention of MH.[820]

The main accepted and validated test for diagnosing susceptibility to MH is an *in vitro* contracture test (IVCT) performed on skeletal muscle tissue obtained by biopsy from "at risk" cases such as individuals exhibiting unconfirmed MH during anaesthesia and relatives of such probands. The IVCT has been standardised independently by the European and North American Malignant Hyperthermia Groups.[821,822] In the test, individuals whose muscle exhibits hypersensitivity to caffeine and halothane induced contracture are diagnosed as MHS (MH susceptible). Individuals that are not hypersensitive to both agents are classified as MHN (MH normal) while hypersensitivity to either caffeine or halothane is diagnosed as MHE (MH equivocal). Clinically, MHE and MHS individuals are considered susceptible to MH. However, the MHE phenotype is somewhat enigmatic and its biochemical and genetic basis remains to be clarified. The European and North American IVCTs differ in several respects. The former has a sensitivity of 99% and a specificity of 93%[823] while the latter, referred to as the caffeine halothane contracture test (CHCT) has a sensitivity of 92-97% and a specificity of 78%.[824] The diagnostic thresholds are also somewhat different.

Clinical MH is considered autosomal dominant with low penetrance. By contrast, MHS in almost all families is an autosomal dominant pharmacogenetic trait with high penetrance. From a clinical perspective, MH is a relatively rare disorder with an incidence in the region of 1 in 10,000 to 1 in 50,000 administrations of triggering anaesthetic agents. By contrast, epidemiological evidence indicates that the frequency of MHS in the population is on the order of 1% while MHE frequencies are as high as 5%.[823] This suggests that genetic and/or environmental factors have a strong influence on expression of clinical MH.

A syndrome essentially identical to human MH was identified in pigs in the late 1960s. Porcine MH is associated with a high muscle to fat ratio in pigs and has proved to be an invaluable animal model for understanding the biochemical, physiological and genetic basis of human MH.[172] MH like syndromes have also been reported in a number of other species, most notably dogs, where several pedigrees have been described.

MHS has been associated with and/or observed in a variety of other conditions. The clinical congenital myopathy Central Core Disease (CCD) is consistently associated with MH. This disorder is characterised by hypotonia and proximal muscle weakness which presents in infancy and leads to delay of motor milestones.[825] CCD histology shows the presence of amorphous, mitochondria depleted central areas (cores) in type 1 muscle fibres and pathological SR changes.[826] Patients with CCD are at high risk for MH and in almost all cases are diagnosed as MHS by the IVCT. CCD exhibits great variability both clinically and histologically and can range from normal to severe within a single family.

THE GENETIC BASIS OF MHS

Biochemical and physiological studies on human MH and particularly on porcine MH, showed that calcium release from the sarcoplasmic reticulum in skeletal muscle was abnormal.[172] Genetics studies showed that the gene for the MH trait in pigs referred to as halothane sensitivity (HAL) gene was linked to the glucose phosphate isomerase (GPI) and the H blood group antigen locus. This prompted a genetic linkage analysis on Irish families, which showed that the human MHS locus was linked to the GPI gene on chromosome 19q12-13.2.[826] Independent linkage analysis showed that the skeletal muscle calcium release channel, the ryanodine receptor (RYR1) gene was the main candidate for MH by demonstrating that it mapped to chromosome 19q12-13.2 and was tightly linked to MHS in Canadian families.[827] A causative role for the RYR1 gene in MH was confirmed by sequence analysis of the porcine RYR1 gene on chromosome 6q12, which identified a single point mutation (Arg615Cys) in MH pigs.[21] Interestingly, the same mutation is present in all affected pigs indicating that the mutation arose through a founder effect and was disseminated through the domestic pig population through breeding and muscle quality selection practices. A causative role for the RYR1 gene in human MH was also confirmed by sequence analysis and demonstrated the presence of the analogous mutation (Arg614Cys) in humans.[828] Mutation screening of the RYR1 gene in CCD families confirmed that the gene was also mutated in CCD.[829,830] More recently, direct sequencing of the RYR1 gene in canine MH showed that MHS segregated precisely with a V547A mutation in MHS dogs.[831]

GENETIC HETEROGENEITY IN MALIGNANT HYPERTHERMIA

While there is considerable genetic, biochemical and electrophysiological evidence to support the role of RyR1 mutations in MH, a number of non-chromosome 19 linked families have also been reported. The first alternative MHS locus was assigned tentatively to chromosome 17q in North American families[832] but this finding has never been replicated despite considerable effort. The *CACNL2A* gene on chromosome 7q, encoding the α_2 and δ-subunits of the DHP receptor, has been tentatively linked to MHS in a single European family.[833] However, despite extensive efforts, sequencing of the *CACNL2A* gene has not led to the identification of a causative mutation. Genome wide analysis has also been performed using several large, apparently non-chromosome 19 linked European MH families. In one family, the MHS trait was found to co-segregate with a marker on chromosome 3q13.1 generating a lod score of 3.22.[834] However, extensive screening of candidate genes at this location has not confirmed any causative mutations. A very tentative locus on chromosome 5p and a new MHS loci on chromosome 1q and was also identified.[835] The *CACNL1A3* gene that encodes the α_1-subunit of the dihydropyridine (DHP) receptor maps to the chromosome 1q locus and sequence analysis identified an Arg1086His mutation in affected individuals in the MH family.[836] The DHP channel is known to directly interact with the RYR1 protein and the mutation is located in the loop between domains III and IV of the channel.

MUTATION SCREENING OF THE RYR1 GENE IN MHS

The RYR1 gene is one of the largest and most complex genes known with 106 exons and a transcript of over 15Kb. Mutation screening to date in MHS and CCD affected individuals has led to the identification of large number of mutations in the RYR1 gene. The mutations appear to cluster in three main regions of the RYR1 gene: an N-terminal region ranging from amino acid residues 35 to 614, a mid region from residues 2060 to 2458 and a C-terminal region from residues 4214 to 4940 with the latter region being predominantly associated with clinically expressed CCD.

The prevalence of RYR1 mutations in MHS patients varies across Europe and North America. The R614C mutation has been described in several families. The frequency of this mutation varies across Europe and North America with a prevalence of 1.3%, 1.4%, 4.5%, 8%, 11% and 11% in the UK, North America, Switzerland, Italy, France and Germany respectively.[837-840] The G341R mutation originally described as a relatively common mutation also varies across Europe and North America with a prevalence of 1.4%, 1.5%, 3%, 8.5% and 16% in Germany, Switzerland, the UK, France and Italy respectively.[837-840] The G2434R mutation also described as a relatively common mutation has a prevalence of 17.5%, 5.5%, 3.4%, 3%, 2.8% and 2.4% in the UK, North America, Germany, Switzerland, France and Italy respectively.[837-840] The prevalence of RYR1 mutations in other populations has not been extensively reported at this point. The variation of the relative prevalence of the mutations across populations infers different founder events. Investigation of the frequency of twenty-three RYR1 mutations in forty-eight unrelated Swiss MH families showed that 40% of families could be explained by the presence of RYR1 mutations. The mutation V2168M was found to have a particularly high incidence (27%). This mutation occurs at a much lower frequency in other populations suggesting a founder effect for this Swiss mutation.[839] Genotype-phenotype correlation of twenty one RYR1 mutations in one hundred and five MH families showed that three genotypes were discordant suggesting a sensitivity of 98.5% and a minimal specificity of 82% for the IVCT.[840] Analysis of seventy three unrelated North American MH families showed that ten mutations accounted for 22% of the susceptible individuals with the highest frequency observed for G2434R.[838] The frequencies reported for each of the mutations differed from the frequencies reported for European studies. A survey of fifteen RYR1 mutations in two hundred and ninety seven unrelated British families showed that eight mutations accounted for 29% of cases and that the mutation G2434R had the highest frequency at 17.5%.[837] In an assessment of the prevalence of fifteen RYR1 mutations in over five hundred unrelated European MHS individuals, RYR1 mutations were detected in 30% of families investigated. Phenotype genotype discordance in a single individual was observed in ten out of the one hundred and ninety six mutation-positive families. A mutation positive/IVCT normal individual was observed in five families and a mutation negative/IVCT positive was observed in the other five families.[837]

GENOTYPE-PHENOTYPE DISCORDANCE IN MHS

Linkage analysis in MHS families suggests that MHS has significant genetic heterogeneity with mutations in the RYR1 gene accounting for about 50% of families. However, reports suggest that the actual genetic heterogeneity in MHS may be much lower than originally estimated as the apparent heterogeneity may be explained in many cases by the less than 100% specificity of the IVCT and the unanticipated high incidence of the MHS phenotype in the population. Highly significant lod scores have only been reported for three of the six MHS loci.[832-836] Mutations in candidate genes have only been reported at two of the loci, namely RYR1 and CACNL1A3 with mutations in the latter accounting for less that 1% of MHS cases to date. Theoretically, one incorrect IVCT diagnosis in a family can exclude linkage to the *RYR1* gene and falsely suggest the presence of a second MHS locus. Given the specificity of the European and North American IVCT for MHS diagnosis, families excluded from linkage to RYR1 would be expected to appear relatively frequently. Linkage analysis to date has incorrectly assumed a very low frequency for the MHS trait in the population (typically 1 in 10,000). Epidemiological data indicate that the frequency of MHS is on the order of 1%.[823] This data is further supported by recent linkage, haplotype and/ or RYR1 mutation analysis of a panel of one hundred and four French MHS families, which showed that in six of the families both apparently unrelated parents of MHS probands were MHS. In three of the families, homozygous or compound heterozygous individuals for

RYR1 mutations were identified. In one family, a compound heterozygous patient harbouring a RYR1 mutation and a CACNA1S mutation was identified.[841] These data support the case for a high incidence of mutations causing a MHS phenotype in the population and could explain both the 3-5% discordance between RYR1 and MHS observed in families and provide an alternative explanation for the apparently high genetic heterogeneity in MHS.

GENETIC DIAGNOSIS

The major disadvantage of the IVCT for diagnosis of susceptibility to MH is the invasive nature of the test (fresh surgically removed skeletal muscle tissue is required). The advances in understanding the genetic basis of MHS have led to the possibility of genetic diagnosis of MHS. However, a main concern of introducing genetic diagnosis for the condition is the apparent discordance between the IVCT phenotype and the RYR1 genotype in certain MH susceptible families. Patients classified as MHS by IVCT but where the familial mutation or high risk haplotype is absent are problematic and they could be explained by a false positive IVCT or the presence of a different underlying MHS mutation. Such patients must be classified as at risk for MH unless they opt for a re-evaluation by IVCT. Patients classified as MHN by IVCT but where the familial mutation or a high risk haplotype is revealed on genetic analysis are also problematic and must be considered at risk of developing MH to avoid potentially fatal consequences. Current genetic testing strategies for MHS in Europe and North America take cognizance of these critical problems and mutation positive members of MH families are diagnosed as at risk for MH irrespective of their IVCT phenotype. To avoid the danger of false-negative diagnosis and formally exclude risk from MH, mutation negative people within a family with a known causative mutation are required to undergo diagnosis by the IVCT to confirm MH negative status.[842,843] On the basis of RYR1 mutation screening to date, fifteen and seventeen RYR1 mutations have been identified as priority mutations for MH genetic screening in Europe and North America.

Exercise-induced myopathy

MH, heat stroke and exercise-induced rhabdomyolysis (ER) have previously been considered related syndromes. Investigation of patients with ER using the IVCT diagnosed 10 out of 12 patients as MHS and 1 as MHE. Mutation analysis of limited sections of the RYR1 gene identified the RYR1 mutations R163C, G341R and G2434R (G7297A) in three unrelated patients.[844] In a separate study, three clinical investigations of MH associated with either non-specific myopathies or congenital disorders revealed a common R401C mutation. Two of the cases showed evidence of exercise-induced rhabdomyolysis[845] confirming that the genetic basis of ER can be explained by RYR1 mutations.

Genes influencing MHS

Although MHS is considered an autosomal dominant pharmacogenetic trait, a study aimed at identifying genes that influence susceptibility in individuals has indicated that several genes may contribute directly or indirectly to susceptibility. Using the extended transmission equilibrium test, the study indicated that loci on chromosomes 1q, 3q, 5p and 7q might influence MHS. Testing of these findings in an independent data set has confirmed a role for loci on 5p and 7q with the influence of the chromosome 1q and 3q being less clear.[846] These findings are somewhat inconsistent with MHS being an autosomal dominant trait. However, one possible explanation is that as families selected for IVCT invariably have at least one proband, such families may be enriched for loci that influence the clinical expression of MH rather that contribute to the MHS trait as defined by the IVCT.

Mutation screening of the RYR1 gene in CCD

Significant advances have been made in screening of the RYR1 gene for mutations in CCD and related myopathies. Mutations associated with clinically expressed CCD have been reported in all three MHS mutation hotspots in the RYR1 gene but are predominantly located in the C terminus. Screening of 3' region of RYR1 exons 93-105 in unrelated CCD cases showed that twenty mutations in these regions account for more than one third of CCD cases most of whom exhibit mild to severe expression of the disease.[845] CCD has been considered a congenital myopathy with an autosomal dominant inheritance. However, as linkage and mutation screening analysis progress, it is becoming evident that recessive forms of the disease are likely to exist. There are many clinical reports where CCD presents in a patient with an apparent complete absence of symptoms in both parents. Molecular genetic studies in one such family identified a V4849I homozygous mutation in the RYR1 gene consistent with a recessive form of inheritance.[847] *De novo* mutations would be expected to occur in a gene as large as RYR1. Analysis of the RYR1 gene in a panel of thirty four families expressing clinical and morphological aspects of CCD identified twelve different RYR1 C-terminal mutations in sixteen unrelated families. Three of the mutations were deletion mutations. In an additional four families, different neomutations were detected in exon 100, 101 and 102 of the RYR1 gene suggesting that neomutations may be a relatively frequent event in CCD.[848] Neomutations have not been reported in MHS. Nonetheless, the presence of neomutations in CCD at a significant frequency suggest that neomutations will also be found in MHS.

MULTI-MINICORE DISEASE

Multi-minicore disease is an autosomal recessive congenital myopathy characterised by the presence of multiple, short-length core lesions (minicores) in both muscle fibre types. In the disease, these lesions can be non-specific and the clinical phenotype heterogenous. A genome wide screen in a consanguineous family in which the children presented with moderate weakness in axial muscles, pelvic girdle and hands, joint hyperlaxity and multiple minicores mapped the recessive gene to chromosome 19q13 and subsequent mutation analysis revealed a homozygous mutation (P3527S) in the RYR1 gene in the family. This locus was excluded in 16 other multi-minicore disease families with a classical phenotype (axial weakness, scoliosis and respiratory insufficiency). New muscle biopsies from patients in the family demonstrated typical central core disease with rods. This indicates that this recessive variant of CCD can present transiently as multi minicore disease.[849] A futher mutation type has been reported in classical multi-minicore disease with ophthalmoplegia. This mutation led to the creation of a cryptic donor splice site and to the addition of an exon at the 101-102 exon junction in the RYR1 cDNA. A 90% decrease in the normal RYR1 transcript was observed in a patient homozygous for the mutation.[850]

FETAL AKINESIA

Fetal akinesia syndrome is an aetiologically heterogeneous group of development abnormalities resulting from lack of intra-uterine fetal movements and is well known in several congenital myopathies such as nemaline and myotubular myopathies. A study of seven patients from six unrelated CCD families presenting with CCD and fetal akinesia syndrome led to the identification of RYR1 gene mutations in three families. Two of the cases were consistent with autosomal recessive inheritance and the third was consistent with autosomal dominant inheritance. In the latter case, the proband's mother had clinical symptoms of CCD. The mutations identified were R614C/G215E, L4650P/K4724Q and G4899E respectively.[851]

CONCLUDING REMARKS

Linkage analysis and mutation screening of the RYR1 gene has substantially advanced our knowledge of this large and complex calcium channel in human and animal disease. Unexpectedly, mutations in the gene underlie and link a variety of different conditions ranging from hypertrophy in the pig to MH, CCD, ER, multi-minicore disease and fetal akinesia in human. It is likely that analysis of this gene in other conditions will add to this list. Furthermore, genetic insights gained from genetic analysis of RYR1 in animal and human disease is already providing a background for identifying diseases linked to the RYR2 gene and may in the future assist in identifying RYR3 linked disease.

Chapter 23

PATHOPHYSIOLOGY OF MUSCLE DISORDERS LINKED TO MUTATIONS IN THE SKELETAL MUSCLE RYANODINE RECEPTOR

Robert T. Dirksen[1] and Guillermo Avila[2]
[1] *Dept. of Pharmacology and Physiology, University of Rochester Medical Center, Rochester, USA;* [2] *Dept. of Biochemistry, Cinvestav-IPN, Mexico City, Mexico*

INTRODUCTION

Skeletal muscle excitation contraction (EC) coupling involves a unique, bi-directional mechanical interaction between two different types of calcium channels: a sarcolemmal voltage-gated L-type calcium channel (dihydropyridine receptor, DHPR) and the ryanodine receptor (RyR1), a ligand-gated intracellular Ca^{2+} release channel located in the sarcoplasmic reticulum (SR) (see Dirksen[852] for review). In response to sarcolemma depolarization, the DHPR undergoes a conformational change that results in activation of nearby RyR1 release channels and subsequent massive release of SR Ca^{2+} into the myoplasm (see Melzer *et al.*[169] for review). Thus, the DHPR and RyR1 proteins are essential components of the EC coupling machinery in skeletal muscle, and thus, play a central role in muscle Ca^{2+} homeostasis. Not surprisingly, mutations and/or deletions in the genes that encode the skeletal muscle DHPR and RyR1 proteins are linked to at least five different human diseases: Malignant hyperthermia (MH), hypokalemic periodic paralysis, central core disease (CCD), multiminicore disease (MmD) and nemaline rod myopathy (NM). Mutations in RyR1 result in MH, CCD, MmD and NM, whereas DHPR mutations are linked only to MH and hypokalemic periodic paralysis. The genetic bases of these diseases, as well as the cellular mechanisms involved, have been thoroughly reviewed elsewhere.[853,854] This chapter will focus on the clinical manifestations and functional defects associated with human RyR1 disease mutations and how these defects might contribute to the pathophysiology of the skeletal muscle ryanodinopathies.

CLINICAL FEATURES

MH is a clinical syndrome in which genetically susceptible individuals respond to inhalation anesthetics (e.g. halothane) and muscle relaxants (e.g. succinylcholine) with attacks of high fever, skeletal muscle rigidity, hypermetabolism, lactic acidosis, hypoxia and tachycardia.[172,174] MH episodes may be life threatening if not corrected immediately by suspension of administration of the triggering agent, treatment with dantrolene sodium, and hyperventilation with 100% O_2. The incidence of MH has been estimated to be ~1 in 15,000 anesthetized children and ~1 in 50,000-100,000 anesthetized adults. In nearly 50-80% of families with MH the disorder has be linked to mutations in the RyR1 gene (Table 23-1). An *in vitro* contracture test (IVCT) is used to detect MH susceptibility. This test determines the sensitivity of muscle biopsies to contractures induced by caffeine and halothane. If certain contracture thresholds are reached in the presence of low concentrations of caffeine and/or halothane, then a diagnosis of MH susceptibility is made. Patients with CCD are at risk for MH and are often diagnosed as MH susceptible by the IVCT.[825]

Table 23-1. **Human mutations in RyR1**

Region	Number	Mutation	Phenotype	Dominant/Recessive
Region 1	1	C35R	MH	Dominant
	2	R163C	MH, CCD	Dominant
	3	G248R	MH	Dominant
	4	R328W	MH	Dominant
	5	G341R	MH	Dominant
	6	R401C	MH	Dominant
	7	I403M	CCD	Dominant
	8	Y522S	MH, CCD	Dominant
	9	R552W	MH	Dominant
	10	R614C	MH	Dominant
	11	R614L	MH	Dominant
Region 2	12	D2129E	MH	Dominant
	13	R2163C	MH	Dominant
	14	R2163H	MH, CCD	Dominant
	15	V2168M	MH, CCD	Dominant
	16	T2206M	MH	Dominant
	17	T2206R	MH	Dominant

Region	Number	Mutation	Phenotype	Dominant/Recessive
	18	V2214I	MH	Dominant
	19	V2280I	MH	Dominant
	20	Δ(E2347)	MH	Dominant
	21	A2350T	MH	Dominant
	22	A2367T	MH	Dominant
	23	D2431N	MH	Dominant
	24	G2434R	MH	Dominant
	25	R2435H	MH, CCD	Dominant
	26	R2435L	MH, CCD	Dominant
	27	I2453T	MH, CCD	Dominant
	28	R2454C	MH	Dominant
	29	R2454H	MH	Dominant
	30	R2458C	MH	Dominant
	31	R2458H	MH	Dominant
------	32	P3527S	MmD, CCD	Recessive
Region 3	33	I3916M	MH	Dominant
	34	R4136S	MH	Dominant
	35	Δ(4214-4216)	CCD	Dominant
	36	V4234L	MH	Dominant
	37	T4637A	MH,CCD,NM	Dominant
	38	T4637I	MH,CCD,NM	Dominant
	39	G4638D	CCD	Dominant
	40	Δ(4647-4648)	CCD	Dominant
	41	H4651P	CCD	Dominant
	42	R4737W	MH	Dominant
	43	L4793P	CCD	Dominant
	44	Y4796C	MH,CCD,NM	Dominant
	45	F4808N	CCD	Dominant
	46	R4825C	CCD	Dominant
	47	T4826I	MH	Dominant
	48	L4838V	MH	Dominant
	49	V4849I	MmD, CCD	Recessive
	50	DF4860	CCD	Dominant
	51	R4861C	MH, CCD	Dominant
	52	R4861H	CCD	Dominant
	53	Δ(4863-4869)	CCD	Dominant
	54	T4864C	CCD	Dominant
	55	14646+2.99 kb	MmD, CCD	Recessive
	56	G4891R	CCD	Dominant
	57	R4893W	MH, CCD	Dominant
	58	R4893Q	CCD	Dominant

Region	Number	Mutation	Phenotype	Dominant/Recessive
	59	I4898T	CCD	Dominant
	60	G4899R	CCD	Dominant
	61	G4899E	CCD	Dominant
	62	A4906V	CCD	Dominant
	63	R4914T	CCD	Dominant
	64	Δ4927-4928	CCD	Dominant
	65	A4940T	CCD	Dominant
	66	G4942V	MH	Dominant
	67	P4973L	MH	Dominant

Residues are numbered according to the human ryanodine receptor (RyR1) sequence (accession number J05200). MH susceptibility has not yet been explicitly ruled out for many of the C-terminal mutations that result in clinically expressed CCD.

CCD, MmD and NM are congenital myopathies, a heterogeneous group of early-onset neuromuscular disorders that exhibit a number of shared characteristics. The most common symptoms observed for each of these myopathies are fetal hypotonia and proximal muscle weakness during infancy. Although the clinical severity for these disorders varies considerably (both within and between disorders), symptoms can at times be fatal during the first few months of life. A significant predominance and atrophy of type 1 skeletal muscle fibers is typically observed and diagnosis is made on the basis of identification of characteristic histochemical or structural abnormalities linked to each myopathy.[855]

CCD is the most frequently observed congenital myopathy and is associated to mutations in the RyR1 gene.[171,856] Although CCD is primarily inherited in an autosomal dominant manner, recessive forms have also been confirmed.[847,849,850,857] Diagnosis of CCD is based on histochemical identification of amorphous areas (cores), which lack mitochondria and oxidative enzyme activity in type 1 muscle fibers.[848] Cores exhibit clearly circumscribed boundaries and can be located in central (Fig. 23-1 A), eccentric (Fig. 23-1 C), or multiple peripheral regions (Fig. 23-1 B) of individual type I muscle fibers. In addition, cores in CCD are often large and can run throughout the length of the muscle fiber (Fig. 23-2 A and B). CCD patients are often, but not always, found to be MH susceptible and may also exhibit foot/thoracic deformities and/or other skeletal defects.[825]

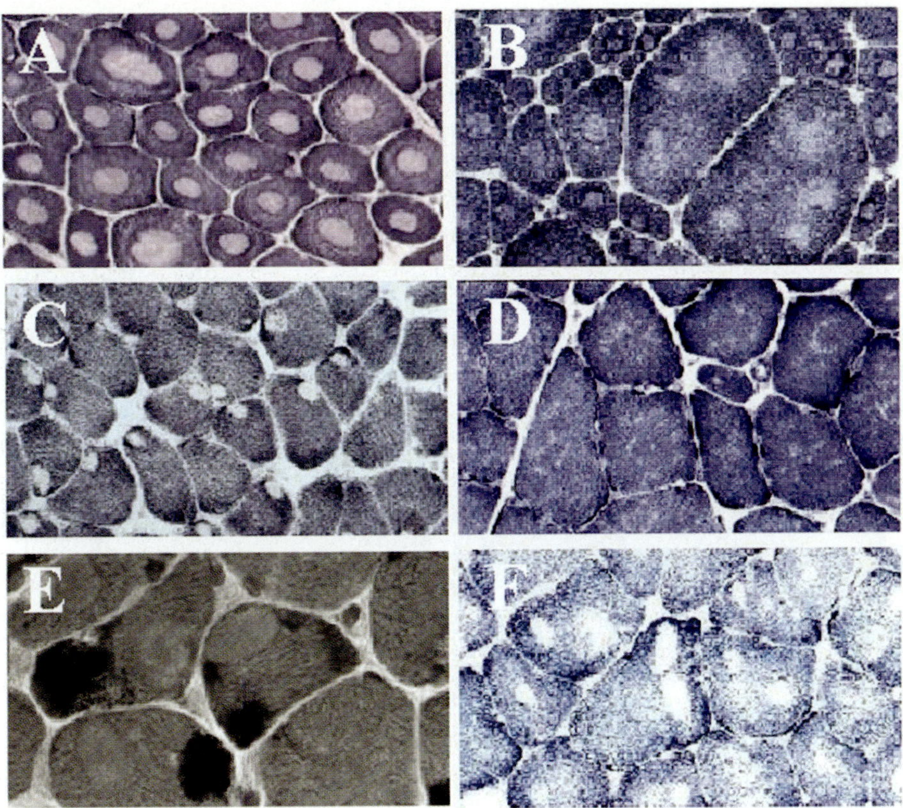

Figure 23-1. **Spectrum of histological phenotypes observed in serial transverse sections of skeletal muscle biopsies obtained from individuals possessing disease mutations in RyR1. A**. Classic unique central cores shown using NADH tetrazolium staining of a skeletal muscle section obtained from a patient with autosomal dominant CCD (L4793P). **B-D**. Succinate dehydrogenase staining of skeletal muscle obtained from patients with autosomal dominant CCD showing unique cores in small fibers and multiple cores in large fibers (**B**, D4214-4216), autosomal dominant CCD with unique eccentric cores near the sarcolemma (**C**, R4893W), and autosomal recessive multiple minicores (**D**, P3527S). **E- F**. Gomori staining (**E**) and succinate dehydrogenase staining (**F**) of muscle samples obtained from a patient exhibiting coincidence of autosomal dominant CCD with rods (Y4796C). Figures **A-D** are adapted from Monnier *et al.*[848]; figures **E-F** from Monnier *et al.*[858]

Multiminicore disease (MmD), or minicore myopathy, is morphologically characterized by the presence of multiple small core-like areas (minicores), which lack mitochondria and oxidative activity (Fig. 23-1 D and 23-2 C). In contrast to conventional cores observed in CCD patients, minicores are poorly circumscribed, multi-focal, and found in both type 1 and type 2 muscle fibers. The longitudinal length of minicores represents another major difference between minicores (Fig. 23-2 D) and classic cores

(Fig. 23-2 B). Clinical features of MmD are widely variable and include at least three distinct subgroups. The most common or classical phenotype (including an ophthalmoplegic subgroup associated with a severe facial weakness) exhibits axial muscle weakness, neonatal hypotonia, scoliosis and respiratory failure. The second group represents an early onset form and arthogryposis (persistent joint contracture). The third group is a slowly progressive form with hand involvement. MmD clinically overlaps with other neuromuscular disorders including CCD.[855,856,859] Interestingly, MmD is genetically heterogeneous and, in contrast to CCD, typically exhibits an autosomal-recessive mode of inheritance. The recent identification of recessively inherited mutations in RyR1 linked to MmD provides a genetic explanation for the clinical overlap between CCD and a subset of MmD patients.[847,849,850,857]

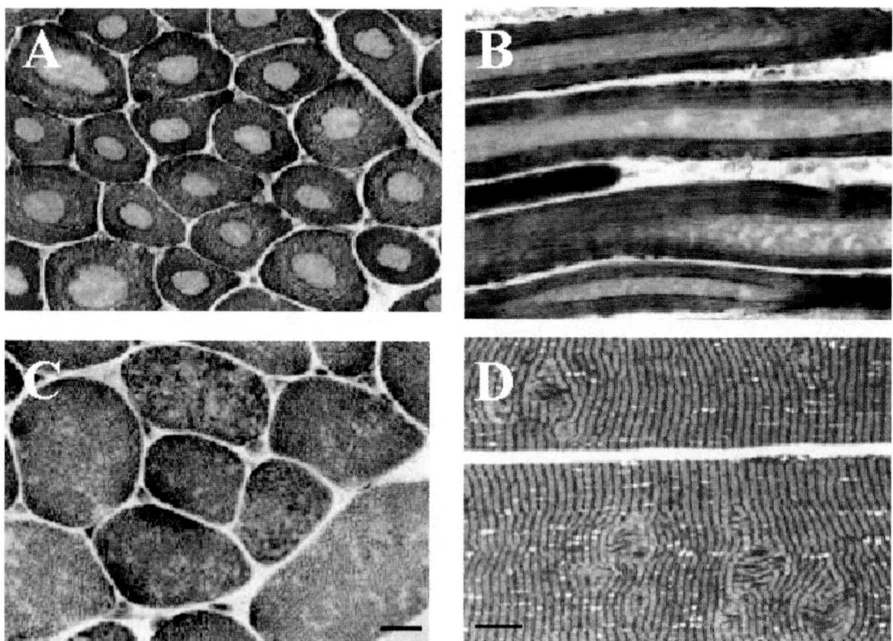

Figure 23-2. **Histological comparison of classic central cores and multiple minicores. A-B**. Transverse (**A**) and longitudinal (**B**) sections showing classic central cores following staining with NADH tetrazolium. Note that central cores are large, exhibit clearly circumscribed boundaries, and run throughout the length of the fiber. **C**. NADH tetrazolium staining of a transverse muscle section exhibiting multiple minicores. **D**. Minicores observed in two adjacent fibers in a longitudinal semithin section stained with toluidine blue. Minicores are characterized by multiple short regions of diffuse negative staining and are coincident with a disruption of the normal sarcomeric pattern. Panel **A** is adapted from Monnier *et al.*[848]; and panels **C-D** are adapted from Monnier *et al.*[858] Panel **B** was kindly provided by Dr. Joël Lunardi.

NM is a congenital neuromuscular disorder affecting 1 in every 50,000 live births. The clinical spectrum of NM is wide and ranges from a severe fatal neonatal form to only mildly affected adults. The most common symptoms of NM are congenital hypotonia and generalized skeletal muscle weakness, predominantly affecting facial and axial muscles. NM is also characterized by the presence of nemaline bodies (or rods), visualized using Gomori's trichrome stain,[858,860] composed primarily of α-actinin and other Z-disc proteins arranged in irregular clusters in the periphery and/or at the Z-line (Fig. 23-1 E). Nemaline myopathy typically arises from mutations in genes encoding thin filament proteins including α-tropomyosin-3 (*TPM3*,), α-actin (*ACTA1*), nebulin (*NEB*), β-tropomyosin (*TPM2*) and troponin T (*TNNT1*).[855,856,859] However, studies have also reported the simultaneous occurrence of both central cores and nemaline rods in the same muscle biopsy, suggesting a "core-rod myopathy" that represents a clinical overlap between CCD and NM. In some cases, core-rod myopathy has been linked to mutations in the RyR1 gene.[845,858,860] In these families, both central cores and nemaline rods can be found within the same muscle biopsy (Fig. 23-1 E and F).

FUNCTIONAL DEFECTS OF RYR1 DISEASE MUTANTS

Most disease-linked mutations in RyR1 are distributed among three distinct regions of the RyR1 protein, known as MH/CCD region 1 (amino acids 35-614), MH/CCD region 2 (amino acids 2129-2458), and MH/CCD region 3 (C-terminal domain) (Table 23-1). MH/CCD region 3 contains all of the putative transmembrane (TM) segments including the selectivity filter/pore-lining region,[8] whereas MH/CCD regions 1 and 2 are located in the large cytosolic aspect of RyR1. For certain RyR1 mutations, individuals exhibit both MH and CCD (MH+CCD mutants), whereas others appear to result in either a pure MH phenotype (MH-only) or CCD in the apparent absence of enhanced MH-susceptibility (CCD-only). Because MH and CCD are inherited primarily in an autosomal dominant manner (except for instances of MmD and CCD coincidence), it is widely believed that the majority of these mutations produce "gain-of-function" or "change-in-function" effects on the activity of the SR Ca^{2+} release channel. In fact, as outlined below, functional studies have provided compelling evidence in support of this prediction for at least some of the disease mutations in RyR1.

Initial pioneering studies designed to characterize the functional effects of MH-linked mutations were conducted using muscle samples from pigs carrying the R615C RyR1 mutation (equivalent to the human R614C mutation). These studies found that MH-susceptible muscle exhibited higher specific ryanodine binding, an increased sensitivity to activation by micromolar Ca^{2+}, and a higher resistance to Ca^{2+}-dependent inactivation. In addition, MH-susceptible muscle exhibits increased sensitivity to activation by caffeine and 4-chloro-m-cresol (4-cmc) (see for reviews[172,174]). These abnormalities may be potentiated by inhalation anesthetics and depolarizing skeletal muscle relaxants, and thus, result in supersensitive or overactive SR Ca^{2+} release channels.

The increased sensitivity of RyR1 release channels to activation by exogenous agents (including caffeine, halothane, and 4-cmc) also extends to the physiologic trigger. In skeletal muscle bundles and myotubes obtained from MH pigs, contractions exhibit enhanced sensitivity to activation via sarcolemmal depolarization.[861,862] The increased contractile sensitivity to depolarization arises from a hyperpolarizing shift in the voltage dependence of SR Ca^{2+} release that occurs in the absence of an effect on the magnitude of voltage-gated SR Ca^{2+} release or the magnitude/voltage-dependence of DHPR L-type Ca^{2+} currents.[863] Thus, the porcine MH mutation (R615C) results in an enhanced release channel sensitivity to activation by the voltage sensor (i.e. a leftward shift in the release versus voltage relationship).

Many RyR1 mutations, particularly those in MH/CCD regions 1 and 2, result in the co-occurrence of both MH and CCD (Table 23-1). Several studies have provided evidence that the MH+CCD mutations in regions 1 and 2 result in the formation of "overactive" or "leaky" SR Ca^{2+} release channels. In line with this view, heterologous expression in HEK 293 cells of RyR1 mutations in regions 1 and 2 that result in co-occurrence of both MH and CCD lead to varying degrees of both a reduction in luminal endoplasmic reticulum (ER) Ca^{2+} content and an increase in resting Ca^{2+} levels.[864] Similarly, homologous expression of the same mutant RyR1 proteins in RyR1-deficient (dyspedic) skeletal myotubes also results in SR Ca^{2+} depletion and elevations in resting Ca^{2+} levels that follow a similar rank order as that observed in HEK 293 cells.[177,865] In contrast, SR Ca^{2+} depletion does not appear to occur following expression of RyR1 mutants that only result in MH and not CCD in either HEK 293 cells[864] or dyspedic myotubes.[176] Apparently, significant ER/SR Ca^{2+} leak only occurs for RyR1 disease mutants that result in coincidence of MH and CCD.

Interestingly, similar to that observed for the porcine MH mutation, the MH+CCD mutations in MH/CCD regions 1 and 2 also reduce the threshold for voltage activation of SR Ca^{2+} release in the absence of a change in L-type Ca^{2+} channel activity.[865] In addition, voltage sensitivity of SR Ca^{2+} release is also increased for a number of MH-only mutations in RyR1.[176] However, in contrast to MH-only mutations, maximal amplitude of voltage-gated SR Ca^{2+} release is reduced following expression of MH+CCD mutations, suggesting that store depletion results in a reduction in Ca^{2+} available for release during EC coupling. Moreover, the degree of enhanced sensitivity to activation by voltage observed for the MH+CCD mutations in RyR1 tested strongly correlated with the degree of SR Ca^{2+} store depletion, elevation in resting Ca^{2+}, and reduction in maximal voltage-gated Ca^{2+} release.[865] Together, these results suggest that reduced Ca^{2+} release during EC coupling that results from enhanced SR Ca^{2+} leak and store depletion, contributes to generalized muscle weakness experienced in CCD.

Lynch *et al.*[151] were the first to identify a mutation in the extreme C-terminus of RyR1 (I4898T) that results in an unusually severe and highly penetrant form of CCD, but did not appear to result in clinical MH. More recent genetic studies (reviewed in Lueck *et al.*[856] and Dirksen and Avila[171]) have identified an additional 26 CCD mutations in the C-terminal region of RyR1 (MH/CCD region 3), demonstrating that MH/CCD region 3 represents a primary molecular hot-spot for CCD. In addition, several MH-selective mutations have now been identified in this region (Table 23-1). Functional measurements of the I4897T mutation (the human I4898T mutation engineered into the analogous position of the rabbit RyR1) expressed in HEK 293 cells suggested that this mutation also promotes Ca^{2+} leak and subsequent store depletion.[151] A similar conclusion was reached in experiments utilizing human B-lymphocytes (which express functional RyR1 Ca^{2+} release channels) obtained from patients possessing the I4898T CCD mutation.[866] However, neither HEK 293 cells nor B-lymphocytes contain all of the many triadic proteins (e.g. DHPR, calsequestrin, triadin junctin, FKBP12) known to regulate RyR1 channel activity in skeletal muscle. In particular, these systems lack RyR1 regulatory control imparted by the skeletal muscle DHPR, which acts as an activator at depolarized membrane potentials and a key negative modulator at resting membrane potentials.[487]

For these reasons, the impact of the I4897T CCD mutation on Ca^{2+} release channel function was also characterized following homologous expression in dyspedic skeletal myotubes.[177,867] In contrast to that observed in non-muscle cells, expression of I4897T-containing release channels within a skeletal muscle environment did not promote SR Ca^{2+} leak and store depletion (no change in resting Ca^{2+} or releasable SR Ca^{2+} content). Nevertheless, voltage-gated Ca^{2+} release was either absent or reduced by 50% following expression in dyspedic myotubes of I4897T alone or in combination with wild-type RyR1, respectively. Thus, the I4897T mutation exerts a dominant-negative reduction in voltage-gated SR Ca^{2+} release, consistent with the autosomal-dominant nature of this disorder. Based on these results, it was concluded that the I4897T mutation reduces Ca^{2+} release during skeletal muscle EC coupling via a mechanism distinct from that of

SR Ca^{2+} leak. Rather, the mutation appears to produce a functional uncoupling of excitation from the efficient release of SR Ca^{2+} (termed EC uncoupling, Fig. 23-3).

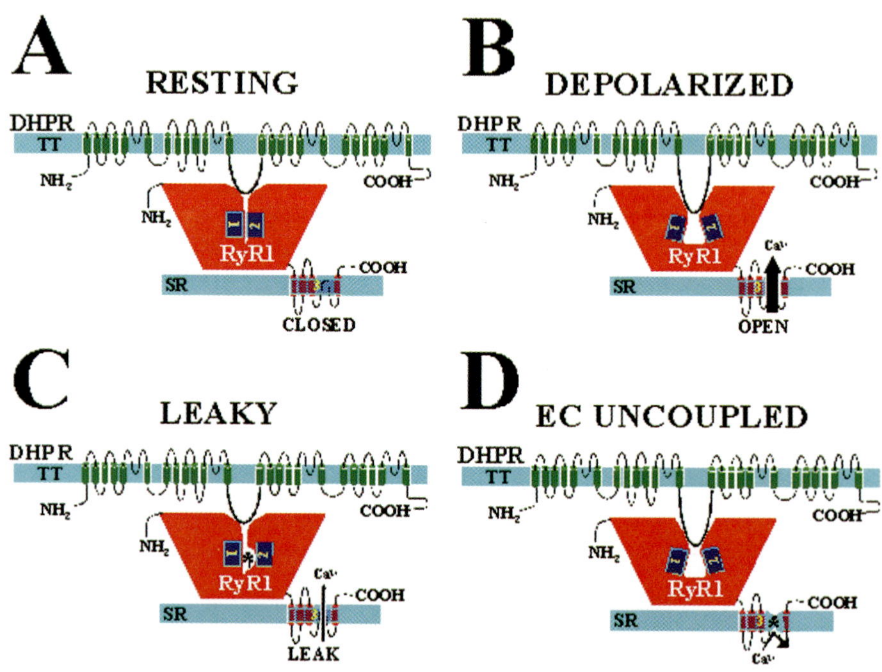

Figure 23-3. **A conceptual model to account for two distinct mechanisms by which CCD mutations in RyR1 alter SR Ca^{2+} release channel function. A**. In the domain-switch model (see Ikemoto *et al.*[180] and Chapter 6 for details), the II-III loop of the skeletal muscle DHPR interacts with a binding site in RyR1 that is functionally coupled to two domains (MH/CCD regions 1 and 2) that interact and regulate the opening of the release channel pore. Under resting conditions, the DHPR promotes interactions between domains 1 and 2 ("zipped" state), which stabilize the resting closed state of the release channel. **B**. During skeletal muscle EC coupling, membrane depolarization causes a voltage-driven conformational change in the DHPR that disrupts the interaction between domains 1 and 2 ("unzipped" state), and subsequently leads to rapid opening of the release channel. **C**. Mutations in MH/CCD regions 1 and 2 alter this interdomain interaction, and thus, cause a partial unzipping of the domains such that release channel sensitivity to activation by endogenous (i.e. voltage sensor) and exogenous (e.g. caffeine, halothane, 4-cmc) triggers is increased. CCD mutations in regions 1 and 2 are shown to cause a degree of unzipping that is sufficient to cause Ca^{2+} leak through the channel at resting membrane potentials. **D**. CCD mutations in the selectivity filter/pore-lining region of the channel disrupt Ca^{2+} permeation through the channel without affecting voltage sensor unzipping of domains 1 and 2.

Interestingly, single channel measurements of mutations in I4897 and neighboring amino acids have provided strong evidence that this region of the protein comprises the pore-lining region of the channel.[37,38] Thus, mutations to residues strategically located in this highly conserved pore-lining/selectivity filter region would be expected to dramatically reduce Ca^{2+} permeation/gating of the activated channel. The validity of this conclusion is reinforced by experiments demonstrating that elevations in resting Ca^{2+} levels and store depletion produced by leaky CCD mutant release channels (e.g. Y523S) are completely corrected by the additional incorporation of the I4897T mutation (Y523S/I4897T).[177] This observation can best be explained by the I4897T mutation interfering with enhanced Ca^{2+} leak promoted by the Y523S mutation. If reduced Ca^{2+} permeation and EC uncoupling represent an important cellular mechanism for muscle weakness in CCD, then other mutations in the pore-lining/selectivity filter of the channel would also be expected to result in EC uncoupling. Consistent with this notion, all of the CCD mutations tested so far that are located in the pore-lining region of the channel (including G4890R, R4892W, I4897T, G4898E, G4898R, A4905V, and R4913G) lead to varying degrees of EC uncoupling. Specifically, mutations to the key "GIGD" selectivity filter residues (e.g. I4897T, G4898E, and G4898R) result in complete EC uncoupling (under homozygous conditions), while mutations to more peripheral pore-lining residues (e.g. R4892W and A4905V) can result in lesser degrees of EC uncoupling.[177]

TWO DISTINCT CELLULAR MECHANISMS FOR MUSCLE WEAKNESS IN CCD

Experiments investigating the effects of CCD mutations on RyR1 function[151,177,864,865,867] have lead to the proposal of two distinct cellular mechanisms by which mutations in RyR1 contribute to muscle weakness in CCD (see Fig. 23-3). The conceptual model presented in Fig. 23-3 combines information gleaned from the functional measurements described above as applied to the "domain-switch" hypothesis proposed by Ikemoto and colleagues (see Ikemoto *et al.*[180] and Chapter 6 for further details). The domain-switch hypothesis predicts that under resting conditions the closed state of the release channel is stabilized by strong interactions between MH/CCD regions 1 and 2 (the "zipped" state). Moreover, agents that promote unzipping of regions 1 and 2 cause a conformational change in the complex that results in rapid activation and opening of the release channel pore ("unzipped" state). According to this model, both release channel triggers (e.g. DHPR, caffeine, halothane, 4-cmc) and mutations that promote unzipping result in a destabilization of the channel closed state that lowers the energy required to open the channel.

The domain-switch model provides a simple conceptual framework for interpreting the functional effects of RyR1 MH and CCD mutations on EC coupling and Ca^{2+} homeostasis discussed above. At resting membrane potentials, the II-III loop of the skeletal muscle DHPR is shown to interact with a specific DHPR binding core formed by disparate regions of the cytoplasmic aspect of the release channel (Fig. 23-3 A). This interaction between the DHPR and RyR1 stabilizes the closed state of the release channel at hyperpolarized membrane potentials.[487] During EC coupling, voltage-driven conformational changes in the skeletal muscle DHPR promote the unzipping of MH/CCD domains 1 and 2, and resulting in rapid release channel activation, opening, and a massive release of Ca^{2+} into the myoplasm (Fig. 23-3 B). According to this model, CCD mutations in regions 1 and 2 promote SR Ca^{2+} leak (and subsequent store depletion) by destabilizing the critical interactions between MH/CCD regions 1 and 2 in a manner sufficient to cause a partial unzipping and increased channel opening even under resting conditions (Fig. 23-3 C). MH-selective mutations in regions 1 and 2 may disrupt this regulatory domain-domain interaction to a lesser degree, and thus cause increased sensitivity to activation by all RyR1 triggers (e.g. voltage sensor, caffeine, halothane, 4-cmc) without enhanced SR Ca^{2+} leak. In contrast, mutations in the selectivity filter/pore-lining region of the channel act downstream of the interdomain regulatory mechanism. Although voltage-driven unzipping may be unaffected by the pore mutations, Ca^{2+} permeation through the pore of the activated channel is nevertheless disrupted (Fig. 23-3 D). Thus, both leaky and EC uncoupled release channels would lead to reduced Ca^{2+} release during EC coupling and muscle weakness, although via distinct cellular mechanisms (SR Ca^{2+} leak/store depletion vs. reduced Ca^{2+} permeation). The ability of the I4897T pore mutation to abolish severe Ca^{2+} leak and store depletion caused by the Y523S mutation in MH/CCD region 1 is entirely consistent with this model.[177]

CONCLUDING REMARKS

It will be important for future work to characterize the effects of CCD mutations in MH/CCD region 3 that lie outside the putative selectivity filter/pore-lining region of the channel. Interestingly, a mutation in MH/CCD region 3 (Y4796C) was recently shown to exhibit all the hallmarks of a leaky channel following expression in dyspedic myotubes (including elevated resting Ca^{2+}, store depletion, increased sensitivity to activation by voltage, and reduced maximal voltage-gated Ca^{2+} release).[177] Thus, this portion of the C-terminal region of RyR1 may function as hinge that integrates/transmits regulatory signals coming from cytoplasmic regions of the channel. Mutations in residues that contribute to such a hinge region could promote leak via alterations in this relay function. In addition, a number of CCD mutations identified in MH/CCD region 3 (T4637A/I, D4647-4648, L4650P, and H4651P) are clustered in one of the highly conserved RyR1 TM segments (M2 in the model of Takeshima *et al.*[3] or M6 in the model of MacLennan *et al.*[8]). However, effects on channel gating/permeation of mutations located in this transmembrane segment are unknown.

Mutations that alter Ca^{2+} permeation of the pore might not be the only mechanism of EC uncoupling. In fact, it is conceivable that EC uncoupling (reduced Ca^{2+} release during EC coupling in the absence of store depletion) could also result from mutations that dramatically reduce DHPR or RyR1 expression, perturb RyR1 or DHPR junctional targeting, alter the proper formation of DHPR tetrads or RyR1 arrays, or disrupt functional coupling between properly targeted DHPR and RyR1 proteins.[171] In fact, a recently discovered, cryptic splice-site mutation in the RyR1 gene (14646+2.99 kb, see Table 23-1) results in recessive MmD/CCD and an ~90% reduction in skeletal muscle RyR1 transcript/protein levels. Thus, this splicing mutation would be expected to result in EC uncoupling via a mechanism involving markedly reduced RyR1 expression.[850]

Finally, because of the very recent association of MmD and NM to alterations in the RyR1 gene, almost nothing is known regarding how MmD- or NM-linked RyR1 mutations modify SR Ca^{2+} release channel activity and/or trigger MmD- and NM-specific phenotypes. In addition, as RyR1 Ca^{2+} release channels are also expressed in B-lymphocytes and certain neuronal cells (including cerebellar Purkinje cells, dentate gyrus of the hippocampus, CA1 and CA3 cells of the Ammons' horn and the olfactory bulb),[868] it seems likely that future work may identify specific clinical manifestations of the RyR1 ryanodinopathies that extend to certain non-muscle related phenotypes/disorders. In any event, these unanswered questions provide substantial fertile ground for future mechanistic studies regarding the molecular mechanisms and pathophysiology that underlie the skeletal muscle ryanodinopathies.

ACKNOWLEDGEMENTS

The authors thank Dr. J. Lunardi for providing micrographs of the cores and nemaline rods depicted in Figs. 23-1 and 23-2 and to Dr. N. Ikemoto for helpful discussions regarding intramolecular RyR1 domain-domain interactions. This work is supported by research grants from the National Institutes of Health (AR44657) and the Muscular Dystrophy Association.

Chapter 24

THE DANTROLENE BINDING SITE ON RYR1

Implications for clinical therapy

Jerome Parness

Depts. of Anesthesia, Pharmacology, Physiology and Biophysics, and Pediatrics, UMDNJ-Robert Wood Johnson Medical School, New Brunswick, NJ

INTRODUCTION

Dantrolene sodium, a hydantoin derivative with a unique ability to suppress the release of intracellular calcium in skeletal muscle cells, has primarily been used clinically in the treatment of malignant hyperthermia, a potentially deadly pharmacogenetic sensitivity to volatile anesthetics and depolarizing skeletal muscle relaxants (see Chapters 22-23). The pharmacology of dantrolene has been excellently reviewed if somewhat sporadically over the years, and the reader is referred to these for their for their historical value and for their views on the potential mechanism.[869,870] The purpose of this review is to give fresh insight into the potential mechanism of action of this fascinating compound, and how this may reflect on mechanisms that may regulate RyR-dependent Ca^{2+} release. Furthermore, I will speculate on potential therapeutic uses of dantrolene and/or its derivatives in the future.

HISTORY

Dantrolene and its congeners were originally synthesized by Snyder and colleagues in 1967 and reported to have intracellular muscle relaxant activity.[871,872] For a number of years after its introduction, dantrolene sodium began to be used clinically in oral formulation to treat the spasms and discomfort of contractures resulting from a variety of upper motor neuron diseases, though the evidence supporting its efficacy has remained limited.[873,874] Though, as a clinical entity MH was described in the mid-1960s, not until the early 1970s was it suspected that the contractures and high temperatures in this syndrome were associated with abnormalities in the SR and intracellular Ca^{2+}. The studies from the laboratories of Kim and Nelson a decade later first demonstrated that MH might be associated with a defect in sarcoplasmic reticulum and an exaggerated rise in intramyoplasmic Ca^{2+}.[875,876] Yet, given the fact that MH was associated with hypercontracture of skeletal muscle and that dantrolene was an intracellular skeletal muscle relaxant, a remarkably astute South African clinician, G.G. Harrison, who had discovered the porcine model for MH, in 1975 hypothesized that dantrolene might be effective in the treatment of MH. In a fascinating story of discovery, Harrison laboriously dissolved hydrophobic dantrolene from tablets in aqueous solution containing NaOH and mannitol, and experimentally demonstrated the efficacy of this compound inhibiting porcine MH (see Introduction, in Britt *et al.*[877]). With the rapid introduction of dantrolene into clinical use, death rates from MH plummeted over the next decade from ~80% to ~7%, a value not improved upon to this day.[869,870]

MOLECULAR PHYSIOLOGY AND PHARMACOLOGY

Dantrolene (Fig. 24-1) is a planar, lipophilic, hydantoin derivative (hydrated 1-(((5-(4-nitrophenyl)-2-furanyl)-methylene)-amino)-2,4-imidazolidinedione sodium) whose phenolic ring is rotated approximately 30° out of the plane of the furane ring.[878] It is poorly soluble in aqueous solutions, with a solubility maximum in buffered solution of about 50 μM at room temperature, and best solubilized for stock solutions in DMSO, DMF or ethanol. Ellis and colleagues established early that dantrolene and some of its derivatives were directly acting intracellular skeletal muscle relaxants.[878-881] With the work of Nelson and Kim described above, it became clear that dantrolene somehow interfered with the release of skeletal muscle Ca^{2+} from its intracellular storage site, and this somehow was related to its ability to truncate an episode of MH.

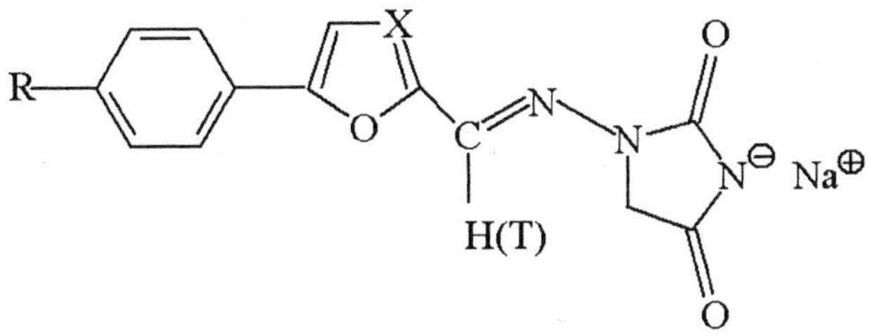

Dantrolene	X = CH, R = NO_2
Azidodantrolene	X = CH, R = N_3
Azumolene	X = N, R = Br

Figure 24-1. **The structure of dantrolene, its equipotent congener azumolene, and the photoaffinity label, azidodantrolene.** The non-exchangeable site used for tritiation in [^{3}H]dantrolene and [^{3}H]azidodantrolene is denoted by (T).

MH (see Chapters 22-23) is a pharmacogenetic sensitivity to volatile anesthetics and depolarizing skeletal muscle relaxants such as succinylcholine that results in an exaggerated release of intracellular Ca^{2+} from SR stores, the aberrant signal involved in the hypercontracture and hypermetabolism so characteristic of this clinical entity.[172,882,883] Understanding the detailed pathophysiology of MH and the molecular mechanism of action of dantrolene in the suppression of intracellular Ca^{2+} release should shed light on the mechanisms of normal and aberrant skeletal muscle excitation contraction coupling. A brief description of skeletal muscle excitation-contraction coupling is therefore in order.

Sarcolemmal excitation and the resultant voltage change of depolarization is sensed by a specific, membrane-bound voltage sensor, the skeletal muscle isoform of the L-type, voltage dependent Ca^{2+} channel, also known as the dihydropyridine receptor (DHPR), residing in the membrane of the interdigitating transverse tubules. Depolarization induces intramembranous charge movement in the DHPR that results in movement of the cytoplasmic loop between transmembrane segments II and III of the α-1 subunit of this voltage sensor. The II-III loop then directly contacts the primary Ca^{2+} release channel of sarcoplasmic reticulum, the type 1 ryanodine receptor (RyR1), with which it is has an intimate organizational and physiological relationship, and induces the RyR1 to open and release Ca^{2+} into the myoplasm, thereby disinhibiting troponin C and allowing for the ATP-dependent actin-myosin interactions that result in contraction. Relaxation of muscle is accomplished by the uptake of Ca^{2+} against its concentration gradient into SR via SERCA1, the skeletal muscle isoform of sarcoplasmic/endoplasmic reticulum Ca^{2+}-ATPase (for reviews, see MacLennan[884] and Protasi[885]).

The precise mechanisms underlying the triggering of MH are unclear, but the following broad outline seems well founded in experimental and clinical evidence. Upon exposure to volatile anesthetics, the RyR1 opens in a poorly regulated manner releasing exaggerated amounts of Ca^{2+} into the myoplasm. Contraction and mitochondrial respiration are inappropriately and continually activated, resulting in hypercontracture and hypermetabolism. The connection of MH to genetic and physiologically relevant changes in RyR1 seem clear: the genetic change in the porcine model of MH has been identified as the Arg615Cys mutation,[827] approximately 50% of human families that are MH sensitive have genetic changes in RyR1,[174,886] SR from MH sensitive individuals bind [^{3}H]ryanodine with higher affinity and a left-shifted Ca^{2+} activation curve,[887] when RyR1 cDNA with MH mutations is expressed in heterologous cells the resultant channels are more leaky to Ca^{2+},[175,864] and RyR1 channels with MH mutations have a longer open time and are more sensitive to triggers of channel opening.[888,889] The evidence that mutations in RyR1 are largely responsible for MH sensitivity is formidable, but not absolute. There are still ~50% of human families whose susceptibility to MH does not map to RyR1.

Dantrolene, however, seems to be therapeutic in MH no matter what the genetic mutation, and effects its therapeusis in temporal association with a dramatic decrease in intracellular Ca^{2+}. Indeed, in a beautiful study using Ca^{2+}-selective electrodes impaled in MH susceptible swine, Allen and Lopez and colleagues demonstrated that azumolene (Fig. 24-1), an equipotent congener of dantrolene, was able to suppress the Ca^{2+} release and truncate the clinical phenomena of a triggered MH episode.[890] The question remained as to where in the pathway of excitation-contraction coupling does dantrolene work. Van Winkle first suggested that dantrolene might act at the level of the SR by demonstrating that dantrolene inhibited Ca^{2+} release from these vesicles *in vitro*.[891] In 1983 Ohnishi demonstrated that dantrolene was capable of inhibiting Ca^{2+} release from SR isolated from MH sensitive pigs despite that fact that three earlier studies were unable to demonstrate any effect.[892-895] These findings suggested that the abnormality in MH and the site of action of dantrolene were to be found in SR and led to other work to better define the specific site of action of dantrolene.

Early attempts to find the binding site of dantrolene in SR were inconclusive, and were hampered by techniques, which could not distinguish between specific and nonspecific binding.[896,897] Using [^{3}H]dantrolene, we first demonstrated specific binding to porcine skeletal muscle SR, despite a signal to noise ratio of 0.25 for this hydrophobic drug.[898] Binding of [^{3}H]dantrolene to subcellular membrane fractions of skeletal muscle paralleled that of [^{3}H]ryanodine, i.e., its specific binding was confined to SR. In contradistinction to the solution requirements for [^{3}H]ryanodine binding, [^{3}H]dantrolene binding to SR required low ionic strength buffer and was Ca^{2+} and Mg^{2+} insensitive. In our hands, dantrolene did not inhibit [^{3}H]ryanodine binding and ryanodine did not inhibit [^{3}H]dantrolene binding to SR.[899] Indeed, optimizing solution conditions that allowed for both dantrolene and ryanodine binding still did not produce reciprocal inhibition of drug binding (K. Paul-Pletzer and J. Parness, *unpublished results*). Furthermore, measuring [^{3}H]dantrolene and [^{3}H]ryanodine binding to SR fractionated on linear sucrose gradients revealed separable but overlapping peaks of binding.[899] These results led us to postulate that dantrolene and ryanodine might bind to separate molecular entities.

On the other hand, Fruen and colleagues demonstrated that dantrolene was able to inhibit Ca^{2+} release from to porcine skeletal muscle SR, and [^{3}H]ryanodine binding to both SR and purified RyR1 incorporated into artificial liposomes. Furthermore, dantrolene inhibited Ca^{2+} release in heterologous cells transfected with either RyR1 or RyR3 cDNA, but not in those transfected with RyR2.[900,901] These results taken together indicated that dantrolene acted either directly on RyR1 or on a ubiquitous protein that regulates RyR1.

In order to directly define the molecular target of dantrolene in skeletal SR, we synthesized a radiolabeled photoaffinity analog of dantrolene, [^{3}H]azidodantrolene (Fig. 24-1), to use in photoaffinity labeling experiments to identify the dantrolene binding site.[902] Specific dantrolene binding was further enhanced three-to-four fold by the addition of AMP-PCP, a non-hydrolyzable analog of ATP, and allowed for a better signal. [^{3}H]Azidodantrolene was shown to inhibit dantrolene binding to SR in the dark and specifically photolabel the 565 kDa RyR1 and a ~172 kDa band that was shown to be the amino terminal fragment of RyR1 cleaved at position 1400 (of 5037 amino acids) by an endogenous, SR-membrane bound, n-calpain - a thiol- and nanomolar Ca^{2+}-activated protease.[903] Using photoaffinity labeling, synthetic domain peptides from RyR1, and an anti-RyR1 monoclonal antibody, we identified a dantrolene binding sequence of amino acids 590-609.[187] This sequence corresponds to the synthetic domain peptide 1 (DP1) shown by Ikemoto and colleagues to activate RyR1.[181,904] The DP1 region of RyR1 seems to be involved in channel activation, as anti-DP1 antibodies enhance Ca^{2+} release from and [^{3}H]ryanodine binding to skeletal muscle SR, and induce a conformational change detectable in fluorescence quenching experiments.[905] The dantrolene binding site is therefore on a conformationally active region of RyR1. We hypothesize that in order to inhibit Ca^{2+} release, dantrolene must stabilize interdomain interactions of conformationally active regions of RyR1, thereby suppressing the ability of the channel to open.

Despite the evidence described above, the physiological data regarding the mechanism of action of dantrolene are complex. Data from the Nelson laboratory show that dantrolene has a biphasic effect on RyR1 channel open time in lipid bilayers: first inducing a rapid opening and then shutting the channel down.[906] These authors also demonstrate that dantrolene first enhances the basal contractile state of MH sensitive skeletal muscle before it causes relaxation. Interestingly, no other laboratory has reported an effect of dantrolene on RyR1 in lipid bilayers. Indeed, results from Csernoch's laboratory demonstrate that not only does dantrolene have no effect on RyR1 Ca^{2+} channel function in lipid bilayers, it does not activate SR Ca^{2+} release, and even at 25 μM dantrolene never completely inhibits Ca^{2+} release in muscle fibers.[907] If dantrolene eventually causes the channel to completely close, as Nelson *et al.* propose, skeletal muscle should not just relax in the presence of dantrolene, but also become completely flaccid. Animals and humans treated with dantrolene never become completely flaccid. How are these contradictory findings to be approached?

Nelson's findings might be explained by the presence of two compounds in their experiment, i.e., breakdown products of dantrolene, one rapidly activating, the other of slower onset and inhibiting. In preliminary experiments, we examined dantrolene that had been allowed to sit in solution at 4°C for a month and compared the effect of this solution with that of freshly prepared dantrolene on [^{3}H]ryanodine binding to rabbit SR, as a measure of the open state of the channel. Freshly prepared dantrolene had no effect on [^{3}H]ryanodine binding, while "aged" dantrolene enhanced [^{3}H]ryanodine approximately two-fold (K. Paul-Pletzer, J. Parness, unpublished results). While we have yet no time frame for the rapidity of this process or whether it might occur in crystalline dantrolene exposed to humidity, it is possible that in the experiments of Nelson *et al.*, dantrolene might have degraded to compounds that are both activating and inhibiting. The inability of dantrolene to inhibit RyR1 channel activity in lipid bilayers may be the result of the purification procedure and loss of quaternary structure necessary for dantrolene interaction, though Fruen and colleagues were able to see a dantrolene effect on purified RyR1 reconstituted into liposomes.[900] Therefore, trivial but functionally significant differences between experimental systems might explain the contradictory results. Differences in lipid composition of the bilayers or liposome might play a role in engendering a dantrolene-sensitive conformation in RyR1. Experimental temperature may also play a role since single channel recordings in lipid bilayers are presently performed at room temperature.

Ohta has shown that dantrolene inhibits Ca^{2+}-induced Ca^{2+} release in skinned guinea pig muscle at 38°C, but not at 20°C.[908]

In summary, the direct evidence of photoaffinity labeling experiments demonstrates that a dantrolene binding site is present on RyR1 and comprises amino acids 590-609. While ~50% of human MH families map to RyR1 mutations, only 7% of affected individuals do not respond to dantrolene. Whatever dantrolene does to RyR1 in inhibiting skeletal muscle Ca^{2+} release, it does so in some final common pathway. Unraveling a more intimate picture of the mechanism of action of this compound should shed light on how RyR1 functions in regulating Ca^{2+} release.

DANTROLENE ACTION ON OTHER RYR ISOFORMS

The data cited above suggest that the dantrolene binding site on RyR1 is the DP1 sequence. Surprisingly, this sequence is nearly identical except for a few highly conserved changes in both RyR2 (amino acids 601-620, NCBI Accession #: P30957) and RyR3 (amino acids 556-675, NCBI Accession #: NP_808320). This suggests that all three isoforms should be sensitive to the pharmacological effects of dantrolene. Yet, there is much contradictory data regarding the interaction of dantrolene with RyR2, the cardiac ryanodine receptor. Some data seems to suggest that dantrolene has no effect on this isoform. For example, in direct photoaffinity labeling experiments of isolated cardiac SR with [^{3}H]azidodantrolene, we were unable to demonstrate specific photolabeling of RyR2 even in the presence of AMP-PCP.[903] Fruen and colleagues did not find any dantrolene inhibition of Ca^{2+} release by expressed RyR2 in CHO cells.[900] Yet, the physiological literature suggests that dantrolene might affect cardiac function, presumably through an effect on RyR2, particularly during experimental pre-treatment for physiological stresses associated with enhanced intracellular Ca^{2+} release: hyperthyroid cardiomyopathy,[909] heart failure,[910] myocardial stunning and ischemia,[911-913] post-infarction contractility and responsiveness to isoproterenol,[914] and endotoxin- or thermal injury related suppression of myocardial function.[915,916] Indeed, recent evidence, in contradistinction to those of Fruen *et al.* above, suggests that dantrolene *can* inhibit Ca^{2+} release via RyR2 expressed in CHO cells.[917] Taken together, the evidence suggests that under certain pathophysiological conditions, RyR2 may be capable of interacting with dantrolene, i.e., accessibility to the putative dantrolene-binding site on RyR2 may conformationally regulated. This suggestion may have profound consequences for clinical cardiac pharmacotherapy.

Aberrant myocardial regulation of intracellular Ca^{2+} in common pathophysiological states such as myocardial ischemia/stunning and heart failure, as well as some rare syndromes such as Long QT Syndrome, have been been linked to the development of cardiac arrhythmias.[294,918-920] In recent years, two genetic syndromes of SCD, arrhythmogenic right ventricular dysplasia type II (ARVD II) and catecholaminergic (familial) polymorphic ventricular tachycardia (C(F)PVT), have been traced to mutations in three regions of RyR2 that are homologous to the three mutationally "hot" regions of RyR1 associated with MH and central core disease, a rare myopathy, and associated with leaky myocardial SR (Fig. 24-2).[294,921-923] These results strongly suggest that Ca^{2+} leakage from myocardial SR via dysfunctional RyR2 is associated with the development of ventricular arrhythmias. Drugs such as dantrolene that have the potential to suppress this aberrant Ca^{2+} release might be efficacious in stemming the development of these potentially fatal arrhythmias. The dantrolene-binding site on RyR1 lies within the first of the mutationally "hot" regions associated with dysregulated Ca^{2+} release (Fig. 24-2), and we have presented evidence that a putative dantrolene binding site may exist in the homologous region of RyR2. The development of RyR2-specific dantrolene derivatives as an entirely new class of antiarrhythmics would present us with potential new agents for a novel target in the treatment of lethal ventricular arrhythmias.

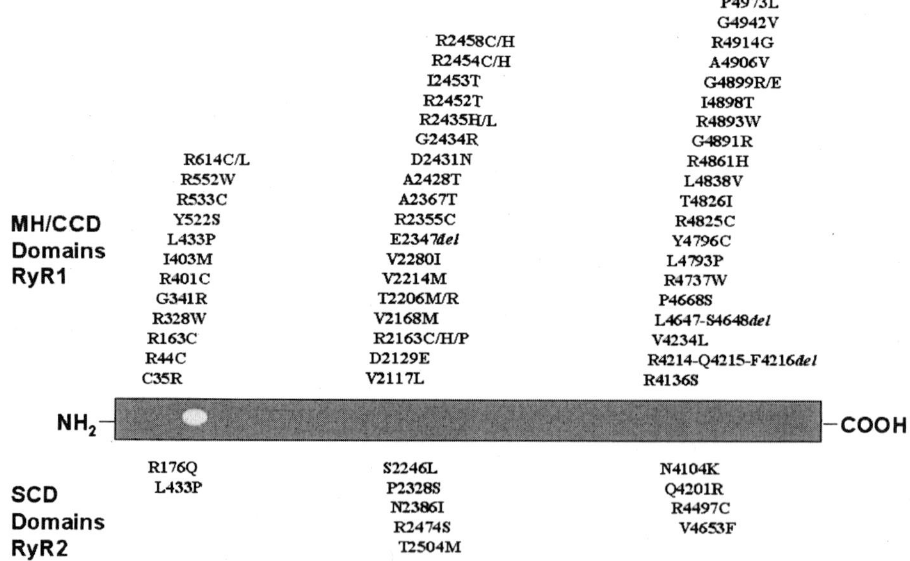

Figure 24-2. **Schematic denoting the mutationally active domains of RyR1 in MH and CCD, and RyR2 in ARVD2 and C(F)PVT** (after Marks[924]). The ellipse denotes the approximate location of the dantrolene binding site.

While there are not yet any pathophysiological processes or genetic diseases known to be associated with RyR3, one can speculate these are yet to be discovered as diseases of various forms of smooth muscle, at the very least. If they involve leaky channels, dantrolene or derivatives thereof, may be efficacious in managing those, as well. The future brings promise both in the delineation of the roles of these channel isoforms and their attendant regulatory proteins in the generation of normal physiology, pathophysiology and disease, as well as the definition of the pharmacological mechanisms by which these may be therapeutically modulated with dantrolene as a model drug.

CONCLUDING REMARKS

Dantrolene sodium is an intracellular skeletal muscle relaxant, and is the only therapeutic agent in use for the treatment of malignant hyperthermia, a pharmacogenetic sensitivity to volatile anesthetics and the depolarizing muscle relaxant, succinylcholine. Once triggered, MH results in exaggerated intracellular calcium release, hypercontracture of skeletal muscle and hypermetabolism, and, unless treated with dantrolene, >90% of patients succumb. Physiological and pharmacological studies have demonstrated that dantrolene suppresses the release of RyR1-dependent calcium from sarcoplasmic reticulum (SR) in skeletal muscle of normal and MH susceptible tissue. The mechanism of action of this compound is still somewhat mysterious. Recent advances using photoaffinity labeling, RyR1-peptide domain mimics and monoclonal antibodies have pinpointed the drug-binding site to amino acids 590-609 of the amino terminal domain of this RyR isoform. An identical sequence exists in RyR2 and RyR3, but the available evidence is that dantrolene interacts well with only RyR1 and RyR3. The physiological evidence, however, suggests that a dantrolene binding site on RyR2 may become available under periods of cardiac stress that renders this tissue sensitive to the development of lethal arrhythmias. Hence, this site may be available for therapeutic manipulation by dantrolene or one of its congeners under these conditions. Pathophysiological states of RyR3 function have not yet been defined, but these too should be favorable treated by dantrolene or its congeners when they are identified.

Chapter 25

RYANODINE RECEPTOR DYSFUNCTION IN HEART FAILURE AND ARRHYTHMIAS

Stephan E. Lehnart, Xander H.T. Wehrens, and Andrew R. Marks
Dept. of Physiology and Cellular Biophysics, Center for Molecular Cardiology, College of Physicians and Surgeons, Columbia University, New York, NY

INTRODUCTION

Ventricular tachycardias and sudden cardiac death (SCD) are associated with underlying cardiac disease including ischemic heart disease and heart failure. Although arrhythmias are a relatively common cause of sudden cardiac death, the mechanisms that trigger and sustain electrical instability of the heart are not well understood. Abnormalities in intracellular Ca^{2+} cycling have been associated with heart failure (HF), cardiac hypertrophy, and in several genetic forms of arrhythmias. Aberrant diastolic sarcoplasmic reticulum (SR) Ca^{2+} release provides a mechanism for the initiation of arrhythmias. Abnormal SR Ca^{2+} release during the relaxation phase of the heart (diastole), when intracellular Ca^{2+} concentrations are low, causes delayed afterdepolarizations (DADs). Afterdepolarizations caused by abnormal diastolic SR Ca^{2+} release cause electrical instability of the membrane potential which may degenerate into arrhythmias. In both the failing heart and in genetic forms of arrhythmias, defective cardiac ryanodine receptor (RyR2) Ca^{2+} release channels have been associated with abnormal SR Ca^{2+} release. Patients with missense mutations in the *RyR2* gene exhibit exercise-induced arrhythmias in the structurally normal hearts, which implies a dominant role for aberrant diastolic SR Ca^{2+} release as a trigger for cardiac arrhythmias. We will review recent findings that indicate RyR2-dependent diastolic SR Ca^{2+} leak as an arrhythmogenic trigger mechanism and as a new therapeutic target.

HEART FAILURE RESULTS IN DEFECTIVE Ca^{2+} HANDLING

About 50% of patients with HF die suddenly and a majority of these deaths are related to ventricular tachycardias. Heart failure is characterized by neurohumoral activation as a futile compensatory mechanism to counteract reduced cardiac output, resulting in increased catecholamine concentrations in the plasma and heart.[925,926] Chronically increased stimulation of the β-adrenergic signaling cascade has been shown to result in maladaptive changes that sustain and worsen HF.[927] Regardless of the etiology, HF results in defective Ca^{2+} homeostasis in cardiomyocytes.[928,929] Relative to the normal heart, the whole cell Ca^{2+} transient is reduced in amplitude and the decay of the Ca^{2+} transients slowed in cardiomyocytes and heart muscles from HF patients and in animal models of HF.[930,931] The reduced amplitude of the intracellular Ca^{2+} transient underlies the reduced force production of failing heart muscle[932] and is associated with decreased SR Ca^{2+} concentrations.[933-935]

SR Ca^{2+} depletion has been linked to decreased SR Ca^{2+} uptake in HF. Reduced SR Ca^{2+} uptake is related to decreased SR Ca^{2+} ATPase (SERCA2a) pump function and decreased SR Ca^{2+} uptake rate due to relative upregulation of, and hypo-phosphorylation of phospholamban (PLB),[936] which inhibits SERCA2a.[937] The net result of increased SR Ca^{2+} leak via RyR2 (see below) and decreased SERCA2a function is reduced SR Ca^{2+} concentrations and prolonged decay of the SR Ca^{2+} release transient, which impairs contractility.[306,931,933]

Chronic stimulation of the sympathetic nervous system in HF causes hyperactivity of protein kinase A (PKA) in the terminal or junctional SR (see Chapter 4). PKA hyperphosphorylation of RyR2 Ca^{2+} release channels results in depletion of the channel-stabilizing subunit calstabin2 (FKBP12.6) from the RyR2 channel complex (see Chapter 15), resulting in increased RyR2 channel activity due to enhanced Ca^{2+}-dependent activation.[5] A chronic defect in diastolic RyR2 closure may contribute to SR Ca^{2+} store depletion.[5,938] Our group and others have recently shown that RyR2 is a macromolecular signaling complex in which mAKAP (AKAP6) targets PKA specifically to the RyR2 Ca^{2+} release channel, thereby establishing compartmentalized PKA phosphorylation-dependent modulation of SR Ca^{2+} release which is distinct from other Ca^{2+} handling proteins.[6,525,939] In hearts of HF patients, decreased levels of protein phosphatases PP1 and PP2A were observed in the RyR2 channel complex, contributing to chronic RyR2 PKA hyperphosphorylation.[5,940] Thus, PKA hyperphosphorylation of RyR2-Ser[2809] and calstabin2 depletion result in "leaky" RyR2 channels[5,940,941] and increased diastolic SR Ca^{2+} leak[189,938], which have been demonstrated in HF patients and multiple animal models of HF (Fig. 25-1 A).

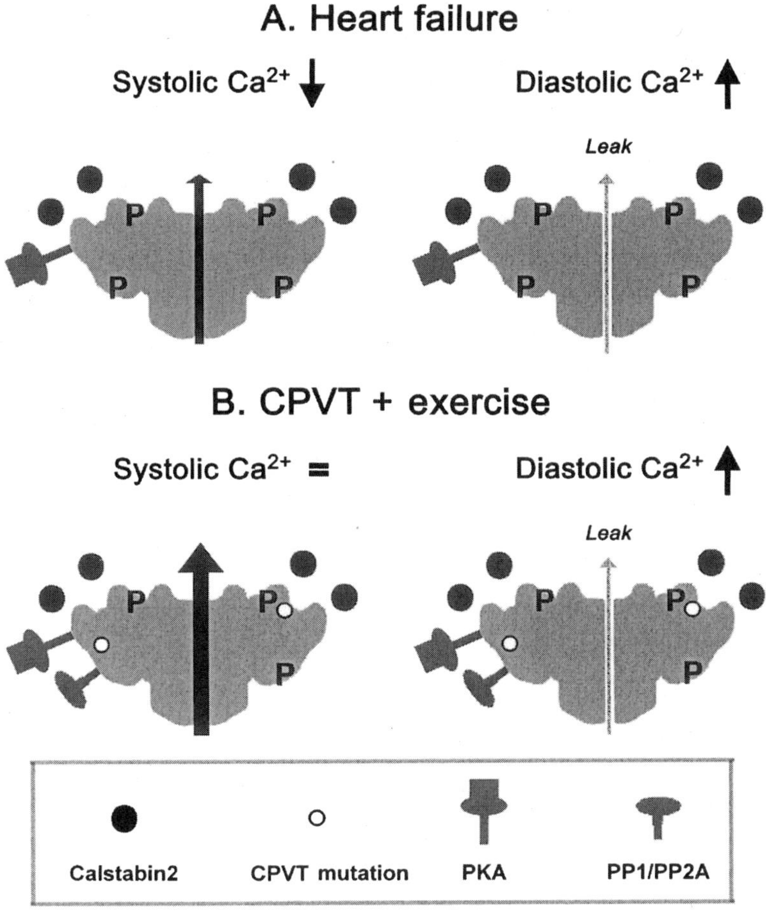

Figure 25-1. **Model of the RyR2 Ca^{2+} release channel in heart failure and CPVT. A.** In failing hearts, PKA hyperphosphorylation of Ser^{2809} in RyR2 due to chronic activation of the sympathetic nervous system and reduced amounts of protein phosphatases 1 and 2A (PP1, PP2A) in the RyR2 macromolecular complex, depletes calstabin2 (FKBP12.6) from the RyR2 complex. Increased diastolic RyR2 open probability results in depletion of SR Ca^{2+} stores, contributing to reduced systolic RyR2 Ca^{2+} release. In addition, Ca^{2+} leak during diastole can initiate arrhythmias. **B.** In CPVT, inherited RyR2 missense mutations reduce the calstabin2 binding affinity for RyR2. During exercise, PKA phosphorylation of RyR2 further depletes calstabin2 from the channel complex leading to increased Ca^{2+}-dependent activation and aberrant diastolic SR Ca^{2+} release that can activate DADs and trigger fatal ventricular arrhythmias.

The diastolic SR Ca^{2+} leak via PKA hyperphosphorylated RyR2 in cardiomyocytes from failing hearts, combined with decreased SR Ca^{2+} uptake due to decreased SERCA2a activity, results in partial SR Ca^{2+} depletion such that action potentials leading to activation of Ca^{2+} induced Ca^{2+} release (CICR) release less Ca^{2+} resulting in decreased contractility.[5,305] Chronic sympathetic stimulation that characterizes heart failure causes PKA-hyperphosphorylation of RyR2, thereby further increasing SR Ca^{2+} leak in HF.[296,298,562,942,943] Additional changes occurring in HF contribute to defective intracellular Ca^{2+} homeostasis. Increased Na^+/Ca^{2+} exchanger (NCX) expression and function have been demonstrated in HF.[302,944] Since NCX and SERCA2a compete for Ca^{2+} extrusion, more Ca^{2+} is extruded from the cytosol to the extracellular space, contributing to SR Ca^{2+} store depletion in HF.[919] In the context of a prolonged intracellular Ca^{2+} transient, Na^+-dependent Ca^{2+} extrusion via NCX compensates for decreased SR Ca^{2+} uptake at the cost of increased membrane depolarization.[302,945,946] On the other hand, reverse mode NCX Ca^{2+} influx during the late phase of the action potential has been demonstrated to contribute to increased intracellular Ca^{2+} in HF cardiomyocytes.[947] To summarize, HF results in altered function of several key Ca^{2+} handling proteins involved in excitation-contraction coupling resulting in partial SR Ca^{2+} store depletion that is associated with RyR2-dependent diastolic SR Ca^{2+} leak.

ARRHYTHMIC MECHANISMS IN HEART FAILURE

Alterations of intracellular Ca^{2+} cycling have been described consistently in failing hearts, and represent a candidate mechanism for the initiation of DADs and triggered arrhythmias. Alterations in transmembrane ion transport exacerbate the electrical instability of the cardiomyocyte membrane. Among several alterations in HF, expression and function of the Na^+/K^+-ATPase is decreased, resulting in a reduction of outward repolarizing current, increased intracellular Na^+ concentrations, increased reverse-mode NCX current and intracellular Ca^{2+} concentrations.[948,949] Functional downregulation of K^+ currents delays repolarization and shifts the resting membrane potential to more positive levels.[950,951] Abnormalities in membrane repolarization and action potential prolongation contribute to arrhythmogenesis and sudden death in HF patients.[952]

Diastolic SR Ca^{2+} leak can activate a transient inward current (I_{ti}), which causes membrane depolarizations resulting in DADs and triggered arrhythmias.[943,953,954] It is thought that I_{ti} results from forward mode NCX net Na^+ influx[955] or from a Ca^{2+}-activated Cl^- current ($I_{Ca/Cl}$).[956] In the failing heart, a prominent increase in NCX function contributes significantly more depolarizing current, and increases the propensity for arrhythmias triggered by DADs[957,958] and early afterdepolarizations (EADs).[959] Acutely, the propensity for triggered arrhythmias may be further increased by activation of β-adrenergic signaling due to upregulation of SR Ca^{2+} uptake and Ca^{2+} leak in the context of reduced repolarizing K^+ currents in HF.[301] Indeed, mapping studies in animal models and in patients with heart failure have identified repetitive focal activity as a mechanism underlying ventricular tachycardia consistent with DADs due to SR Ca^{2+} leak in cardiomyocytes.[960]

INHERITED CARDIAC ARRHYTHMIA SYNDROMES DISTURBING INTRACELLULAR Ca^{2+} CYCLING

Inherited mutations in genes that are involved in intracellular Ca^{2+} handling increase the propensity for SCD and ventricular tachycardias (VT). Autosomal-dominant inherited missense mutations in the *RyR2* gene have been linked to exercise-induced arrhythmias,[961] known as catecholaminergic polymorphic ventricular tachycardia (CPVT).[53,54] Mutation carriers characteristically develop arrhythmias during exercise or emotional stress but not during rest (Fig. 25-2 A). Overall mortality rates are 30-50% at age 35 (Fig. 25-2 B),[53,54,573,962,963] and only partial protection from syncope and SCD can be achieved by treatment with β-blocker treatment.[962,963] RyR2 missense mutations have also been linked to arrhythmogenic right ventricular dysplasia/cardiomyopathy type 2 (ARVD/C2).[178] Importantly, arrhythmias in CPVT mutation carriers occur in the structurally normal heart, whereas ARDV/C2 is associated with dysplasia of the right ventricle.

Studies of single RyR2 channels containing missense mutations found in CPVT patients demonstrated a gain-of-function defect following PKA phosphorylation, consistent with 'leaky' RyR2 channels (diastolic SR Ca^{2+} leak) during stress/exercise.[294,573] Consistent with these findings, intracellular Ca^{2+} leak was observed after β-adrenergic stimulation in atrial tumor cells expressing the same CPVT mutant RyR2 channels.[922] The observation that RyR2 missense mutations only result in leaky Ca^{2+} release channels under conditions that mimic activation of the β-adrenergic signaling cascade[294,573] is in agreement with the finding in affected mutation carriers that arrhythmias only occur during stress or exercise.[962,963] An important finding in CPVT mutant RyR2 channels is a decreased binding affinity of the channel-stabilizing subunit calstabin2, contributing to enhanced dissociation of calstabin2 from the RyR2 channel complex during PKA phosphorylation, which enhances diastolic SR Ca^{2+} leak.[5,189,294,941,964] However, it is important to understand that calstabin2 is bound to CPVT mutant RyR2 channels under resting conditions, in contrast to calstabin2-depletion due to PKA hyperphosphorylation of RyR2 in failing hearts, which sustains diastolic SR Ca^{2+} leak even at rest (Fig. 25-1).

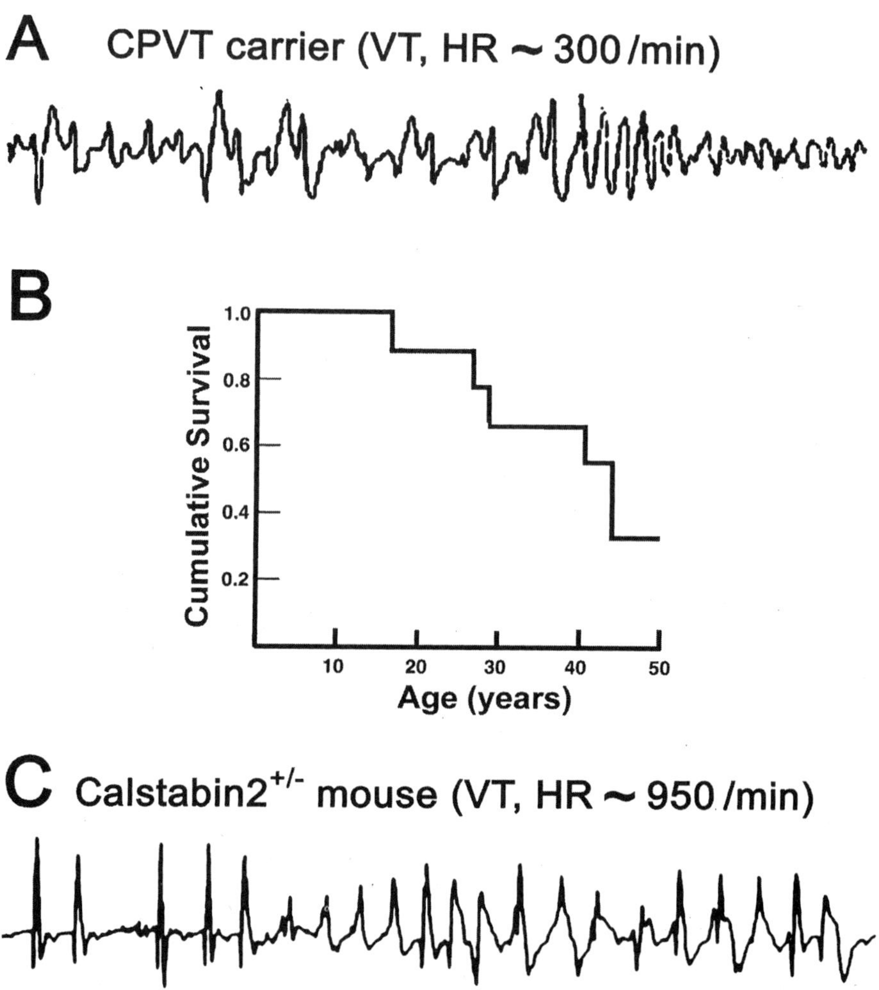

Figure 25-2. **Ryanodine receptor dysfunction causes ventricular arrhythmias in CPVT patients and calstabin2-deficient mice. A.** Example of a ventricular tachycardia degenerating into ventricular fibrillation in a CPVT patient carrying a RyR2 missense mutation. Reproduced with permission from Priori *et al.*[963] **B.** Kaplan-Meyer curve showing high mortality rates in carriers of the RyR2-Q4201R missense mutation linked to CPVT. Reproduced with permission from Lehnart *et al.*[573] **C.** Electrocardiogram of a *calstabin2*$^{+/-}$ haploinsufficient mouse, showing polymorphic ventricular tachycardia recorded by telemetry during exercise testing. Reproduced with permission from Wehrens *et al.*[299]

Missense or nonsense mutations in the calsequestrin 2 gene (*CSQ2*) have been liked to an autosomal-recessive form of CPVT.[203,204] Calsequestrin 2 is the most abundant Ca^{2+} binding protein within the SR Ca^{2+} store of cardiomyocytes, and functions as a high capacity low affinity Ca^{2+} buffer presumably regulating RyR2 function. It was proposed that *CSQ2* missense mutations decrease intra-SR Ca^{2+} binding, which would increase the concentration of free SR Ca^{2+} consistent with SR Ca^{2+} overload and diastolic SR Ca^{2+} leak as a mechanism causing DADs and arrhythmias.[206,957] For details about RyR2 regulation by luminal SR Ca^{2+} and calsequestrin, please refer to Chapter 7. An autosomal-dominant form of the long-QT syndrome (LQT4), associated with cardiac arrhythmias and sudden cardiac death, was linked to inactivating point mutations in the ankyrin-B gene (*AnkB*).[965] Interestingly, arrhythmias and SCD typically occurred in *AnkB* mutation carriers after physical exertion and emotional stress.[966] It is thought that *AnkB* mutations cause defective membrane targeting of Ca^{2+} handling proteins, including the inositol 1,4,5-trisphosphate receptor (IP_3R), NCX and the Na^+/K^+-ATPase, resulting in SR Ca^{2+} overload and diastolic SR Ca^{2+} leak as a trigger of DADs and arrhythmias.[965] To summarize, a variety of mutations that affect intracellular Ca^{2+} handling directly or indirectly cause arrhythmias by alterations in intracellular Ca^{2+} cycling all of which are consistent with diastolic SR Ca^{2+} serving as the trigger for fatal cardiac arrhythmias. Functional defects in intracellular Ca^{2+} handling become exaggerated during β-adrenergic stimulation, activating inward depolarizing currents and DADs that are the likely trigger mechanism for cardiac arrhythmias.

MOUSE MODELS OF TRIGGERED ARRHYTHMIAS

Genetic mouse models have been employed to explore defective intracellular Ca^{2+} cycling as a trigger mechanism of arrhythmias. Since CPVT mutant RyR2 channels display decreased calstabin2 binding affinities,[294,573] we hypothesized that depletion of calstabin2 from the RyR2 channel complex facilitates RyR2 Ca^{2+} leak which may cause DADs and initiate arrhythmias.[299] Indeed, *calstabin2*$^{-/-}$ knockout mice consistently develop DADs, ventricular tachycardias, and SCD following exercise and β-adrenergic stimulation (Fig. 25-2 C).[294,299] These observations are supported by our findings that missense mutations in RyR2 linked to CPVT reduce the affinity of calstabin2 for RyR2 and increase single-channel activity under conditions that simulate exercise during diastole.[294,573]

Previous studies have found that interventions that reduce calstabin2 binding to RyR2 increase the channel open probability causing SR Ca^{2+} leak and altered EC coupling.[5,522,559,941,967] Consistent with these findings, RyR2 channels from *calstabin*$^{-/-}$ knockout mice show increased open probabilities under exercised conditions during diastole.[294] Whereas diastolic SR Ca^{2+} leak may become effectively buffered under resting conditions,[968] the pronounced gain-of-function defect seen during exercise and sympathetic activation causes pronounced diastolic SR Ca^{2+} leak, which triggers DADs and arrhythmias.[294]

PHARMACOLOGIC TARGETING OF DEFECTIVE INTRACELLULAR Ca^{2+} RELEASE

There are only a few antiarrhythmic drugs that reduce the incidence of SCD, however, with a low efficacy providing only partial protection. The beneficial effects of β-blockers in heart failure are, at least in part, related to the reduction of RyR2 PKA hyperphosphorylation and normalization of RyR2 open probability.[940,969,970] It has become clear that drugs that block Na^+ or K^+ channel function may increase mortality from arrhythmias.[971,972] Therefore, an alternative rationale would be to develop drugs that stabilize, rather than block channel function. Since calstabin2 stabilizes the RyR2 closed state, we hypothesized that rebinding of calstabin2 to the channel complex may reduce SR Ca^{2+} leak and prevent cardiac arrhythmias.

We showed that a calstabin2 (FKBP12.6)-D37S mutant subunit binds to PKA hyperphosphorylated RyR2 with a higher affinity compared to wild-type calstabin2, which has markedly reduced affinity for PKA phosphorylated RyR2 as compared to unphosphorylated RyR2.[294] Calstabin2-D37S reduced the open probability of the PKA hyperphosphorylated RyR2 channel and rescued the gain-of-function defect that causes diastolic SR Ca^{2+} leak.[294] Adenoviral overexpression of wild-type calstabin2 in cardiomyocytes may also reduce SR Ca^{2+} leak, implying that supra-physiologic intracellular calstabin2 levels may promote calstabin2 binding to PKA phosphorylated RyR2.[973] Recently, we demonstrated that the 1,4-benzothiazepine derivative JTV519 can prevent arrhythmias and sudden cardiac death in *calstabin2*$^{+/-}$ haploinsufficient but not *calstabin2*$^{-/-}$ deficient mice, by increasing the binding of calstabin2 to the RyR2 channel complex.[299] Moreover, JTV519 normalizes the gain-of-function defect in CPVT-mutant RyR2 channels.[573] These results strongly support the concept that JTV519 inhibits diastolic SR Ca^{2+} leak and cardiac arrhythmias by increasing the binding of calstabin2 to RyR2 (see also Chapter 26).

CONCLUDING REMARKS

Altered RyR2 function plays an important role in heart failure and in genetic forms of arrhythmias. RyR2 dysfunction causes diastolic SR Ca^{2+} leak, which can deplete SR Ca^{2+} stores in failing hearts, and induce delayed afterdepolarizations that trigger arrhythmias. New pharmacological interventions that increase calstabin2 binding to PKA-phosphorylated RyR2 have been shown to increase contractility in a dog model of heart failure. and prevent cardiac arrhythmias in a mouse model of arrhythmias and sudden cardiac death. These studies have identified prevention of diastolic SR Ca^{2+} leak as a new therapeutic strategy for heart failure and certain forms of sudden cardiac death.

ACKNOWLEDGMENTS

Supported by grants to A.R.M. from the NIH and a postdoctoral grant from the Deutsche Forschungsgemeinschaft (DFG) to S.E.L. A.R.M. is the Doris Duke Charitable Foundation Distinguished Clinical Scientist; X.H.T.W. is a recipient of the Glorney-Raisbeck fellowship of the New York Academy of Medicine.

Chapter 26

STABILIZATION OF RYANODINE RECEPTOR AS A NOVEL THERAPEUTIC STRATEGY AGAINST HEART FAILURE

Masafumi Yano, Takeshi Yamamoto, and Masunori Matsuzaki
Dept. of Medical Bioregulation, Div. of Cardiovascular Medicine, Yamaguchi University School of Medicine, Ube, Yamaguchi, Japan

INTRODUCTION

Heart failure is a progressively disabling and ultimately fatal disease, which is characterized by a decline in the heart's ability to pump the blood efficiently enough to meet the body's metabolic demands. Recent studies have shown that the abnormal regulation of intracellular Ca^{2+} by sarcoplasmic reticulum (SR) is involved in the mechanism of contractile and relaxation dysfunction in heart failure. The Ca^{2+} uptake by SR was found to decrease in association with the decreased density of Ca^{2+}-ATPase in cardiac hypertrophy and/or failure.[974-976] The alteration of SR Ca^{2+} release is considered also as a cause of the slowed Ca^{2+} transient frequently observed in dilated cardiomyopathy[930] or failing heart.[977] However, little information is available concerning the functions of SR Ca^{2+} release channel in heart failure. In this chapter, we will review the recent advances in the treatment of heart failure from a viewpoint of stabilization of SR Ca^{2+} release channel, often referred to as ryanodine receptor (RyR).

REGULATION OF SR Ca^{2+} RELEASE IN HEART FAILURE

We have demonstrated that the rate of Ca^{2+} release induced by polylysine, RyR-specific Ca^{2+} release trigger, decreased in failing SR vesicles and that the polylysine concentration dependence of the initial rate of Ca^{2+} release and that of [^{3}H]-ryanodine binding were shifted toward a lower concentration of polylysine in failing SR vesicles.[978] This suggests that the channel gating function of the RyR is altered in heart failure.

Regarding the regulation of channel gating in RyR, a satellite protein, FKBP12 has been found to associate with RyR during sucrose density gradient centrifugation.[531] The physiological function of FKBP12 is modulation of RyR1, the skeletal muscle isoform of the Ca^{2+} release channel, possibly by enhancing the coordination among its four subunits.[522,531,979] FKBP with a different electrophoretic mobility (FKBP12.6) was found to associate specially with RyR2, the cardiac muscle isoform of the Ca^{2+} release channel.[533,980] FKBP12.6 has 85 % homology with FKBP12.[981] The stoichiometry of binding is approximately four moles of FKBP per one RyR tetramer (or one FKBP to one RyR monomer) in both skeletal muscle and cardiac muscle.

In previous studies,[941,964] we have shown several important features suggesting the involvement of FKBP12.6 in the pathogenesis of cardiac failure. For instance, (i) dissociation of FKBP12.6 from RyR2 induced by immunosuppressant agent FK506 causes Ca^{2+} leak in normal SR vesicles. (ii) The Ca^{2+} leak showed a close parallelism with the conformational change in RyR2. (iii) the stoichiometry of FKBP12.6 with respect to RyR2 was significantly decreased in failing SR vesicles, leading to an abnormal Ca^{2+} leak in heart failure. (iv) The dramatic reduction in FKBP12.6 by means of FK506 did not cause any further reduction in the rate of Ca^{2+} release from failing SR. This suggests that in heart failure the regulation of FKBP12.6 on RYR2 is absent, resulting in abnormal and maximal Ca^{2+} leak. Thus, the aforementioned modification of the polylysine-induced SR Ca^{2+} release in heart failure may be at least partly due to the reduced amount of FKBP12.6. Namely, when a sufficiently high concentration of FK506 (or rapamycin) is applied to normal cardiac myocytes, cooperation among the four RyR2 subunits is disrupted, thus destabilizing the channel. This in turn induces abnormalities in the channel-gating function of RyR2. Thus, failing channels behave as normal channels that are treated with FKBP-dissociating agents.

PROTEIN KINASE A (PKA)-MEDIATED HYPERPHOSPHORYLATION OF RYR

Marx *et al.*[5] have proposed the concept that a macromolecular complex in cardiac muscle is formed by RyR2, FKBP12.6, PKA, protein phospatases PP1 and PP2A and mAKAP (anchoring structure). They demonstrated that hyperphosphorylation of RyR2 by PKA in failing hearts causes a dissociation of FKBP12.6 from RyR2, resulting in the following abnormal single-channel properties: (i) increased Ca^{2+} sensitivity for activation and (ii) elevated channel activity associated with destabilization of the tetrameric channel complex. They proposed a model where, in normal hearts, a discrete phosphorylation of the complex due to β-stimulation could increase the Po of the channel and so increase the gain of E-C coupling (i.e. more Ca^{2+} release for the same cytoplasmic Ca^{2+} trigger). The hyperphosphorylated state of RyR2 of the failing myocardium would offset this regulation to its maximum, so that β-stimulation would not produce any further increase in Po (blunt β-stimulation response). The maximum RyR2-FKBP12.6 dissociation would also increase the Ca^{2+} leak from the SR to produce a reduction in the SR Ca^{2+} content and increased diastolic $[Ca^{2+}]$.

Not all previous results agree with the view that RyR2 is hyperphosphorylated in heart failure. Li *et al.*[297] showed that PKA-phosphorylation of RyR does not affect calcium sparks in permeabilized myocytes although experiments were done at subphysiological intracellular Ca^{2+} concentrations. There are also conflicting results as to the role of phophorylation at Serine2808 or 2809 on FKBP12.6 binding to RyR2, although Marks and colleagues[5,294] showed that in failing hearts RyR2 were hyperphosphorylated at serine-2808 (corresponding to serine- 2809 in rabbit RyR2), and this resulted in a dissociation of FKBP12.6 from RyR2. Recently, it has been reported that the constitutive phosphorylation of serine2808 or 2809 by mutations (S2808D or S2809D) failed to disrupt FKBP12.6-RyR2 interaction.[325,326] Differences in the experimental conditions may account for the difference in FKBP12.6 binding among those studies. Nevertheless, there is considerable evidence that SR leak as well as reduced SR Ca^{2+} uptake may be important for disturbed SR function in heart failure, and that FKBP is an important regulator for SR Ca^{2+} handling. For further details of the concept of PKA mediated hyperphosphorylation in failing heart, see Chapters 15 and 25.

STABILIZATION OF RYR: A NOVEL THERAPEUTIC TARGET

β-receptor blocker

A common finding in the patients with heart failure is that a hyperadrenergic state and elevated levels of circulating catecholamines are markers for increased risk of mortality.[982] Recent clinical trials have shown that the treatment with β-receptor blockers restores cardiac function and reduces the rate of mortality in the patients with heart failure.[983] The mechanisms for the benefits of β-blocker therapy include a reduction in sympathetic nervous activity, restoration of the β-receptor density with improved contractile and relaxation functions, and an improved cardiac efficiency with an associated reduction in heart rate. However, the basis of the adrenergic cascade-related myocyte abnormalities remains unclear.

Reiken *et al.*[940] reported that the β1-selective blocker metoprolol reversed PKA-mediated hyperphosphorylation of RyR2, restored the stoichiometry of RyR2 macromolecular complex, and restored normal single-channel function in a canine model of heart failure. We have also shown that in tachycardia-induced canine heart failure, low-dose propranolol, which had only a negative chronotropic but not a negative inotropic effect in normal dogs, restored channel regulation in RyR2 and thereby improved cardiac function.[970] In our study, treatment with propranolol had no effect on the protein expression of SR Ca^{2+}-ATPase or on Ca^{2+} uptake function. Treatment with propranolol reversed the phosphorylation of RyR2 in conjunction with a reassociation of FKBP12.6 back to RyR2. Taken together with the recent finding that in heart failure PKA-mediated hyperphosphorylation of RyR2 leads to a defective FKBP12.6-mediated channel regulation of RyR2, our results make it very likely that the mechanism by which propranolol improves cardiac function and prevents LV remodeling, without a change in Ca^{2+} uptake function, is an inhibition of Ca^{2+} leak through RyR2. As shown in Fig. 26-1, addition of the Ca^{2+}-ATPase blocker, thapsigargin to normal SR vesicles produced little Ca^{2+} leak, whereas addition of FK506 together with thapsigargin produced a much more pronounced leak. In contrast, in failing (propranolol-untreated) SR vesicles, addition of thapsigargin alone produced a prominent Ca^{2+} leak, but addition of FK506 produced no additional increase. In SR vesicles from paced, propranolol-treated dogs, a spontaneous Ca^{2+} leak was not observed, and FK506 had the same effect as in normal SR (that is, it greatly increased the Ca^{2+} leak).

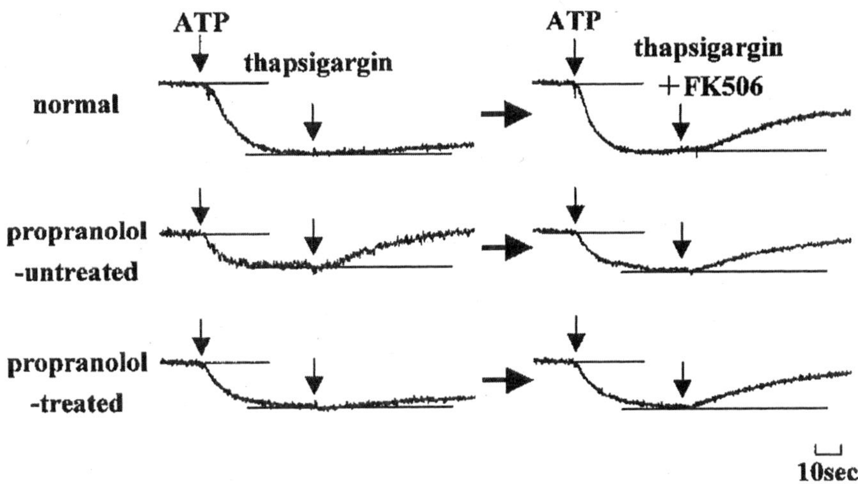

Figure 26-1. **Representative time courses of Ca^{2+} uptake and the ensuing Ca^{2+} leak from SR vesicles obtained from normal and failing hearts.** Note that after propranolol treatment for 4 weeks immediately after RV rapid pacing, the spontaneous Ca^{2+} leak seen in failing SR vesicles disappeared. Note also that FK506 (30 μmol/L) enhanced the Ca^{2+} leak in the paced, propranolol-treated dog and in the normal dog but not in the paced, propranolol-untreated dog. From Doi *et al.*[970] with permission.

These results may provide a molecular basis for the common clinical observation that the use of β-receptor blockers improves prognosis among patients with heart failure.

We have reported that a new compound, the 1,4-benzothiazepine derivative JTV519, prevents heart failure by stabilizing RyR2.[189] JTV519 shares an analogous chemical structure with the dihydropyridine-binding Ca^{2+}-channel blocker diltiazem and is known to have a protective effect against Ca^{2+} overload–induced myocardial injury.[984] In JTV519-treated dogs, no signs of heart failure were observed after 4 weeks of chronic RV rapid pacing, LV systolic and diastolic functions were preserved, and LV remodeling was prevented. JTV519 acutely inhibited both the FK506-induced Ca^{2+} leak from RyR2 in normal SR and the spontaneous Ca^{2+} leak in failing SR. There was no abnormal Ca^{2+} leak in the SR vesicles isolated from JTV519-treated hearts. As shown in Fig. 26-2, in JTV519-treated hearts the amount of RyR2-bound FKBP12.6 were restored in a normal level. In JTV519-untreated hearts, RyR2 was PKA-hyperphosphorylated, whereas it was reversed in JTV519-treated hearts, returning the channel phosphorylation toward the levels seen in normal hearts.

A novel RyR stabilizer: JTV519

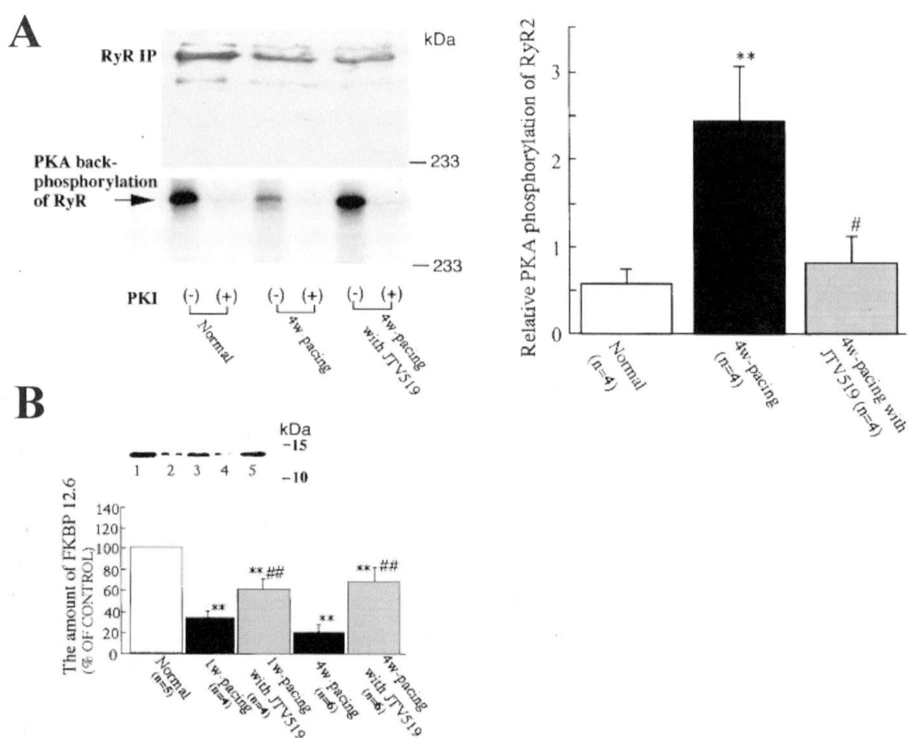

Figure 26-2. **Chronic effect of JTV519 on PKA-phosphorylation of RyR2 and on the amount of FKBP12.6 A**. PKA-mediated phosphorylation of RyR2 confirmed by back-phosphorylation. Nonspecific phosphorylation (not inhibited by PKA inhibitor) was subtracted, and the resulting value was divided by the amount of RyR2 protein (determined by immunoblotting and densitometry) and expressed as the inverse of the specific PKA-dependent [^{32}P]-ATP signal. **P<0.01 vs normal, #P<0.05 vs 4 week-pacing. IP indicates immunoprecipitation. PKI: PKA inhibitor. **B**. Amount of FKBP12.6 associated with RyR in SR vesicles: lane 1, normal; lane 2, 1w of pacing; lane 3, 1w of pacing with JTV519; lane 4, 4w of pacing; lane 5, 4w of pacing with JTV519. **P<0.01 vs normal, ##P<0.01 vs 1w- or 4w-pacing. From Yano *et al.*[189] with permission.

The improvement in LV relaxation induced by JTV519 may also be mediated through an enhancement of SR Ca^{2+}-ATPase activity because both Ca^{2+} uptake and the amount of Ca^{2+}-ATPase were increased at 4 weeks of RV pacing, concurrently with the increase in the basal level of Ser16 phosphorylated PLB. In both normal and failing SR vesicles, JTV519 had no direct effect of PLB-phosphorylation induced by cAMP *in vitro* (*unpublished data*). Therefore, these benefits of JTV519 on Ca^{2+} uptake property may be due to a secondary effect after an improvement of cardiac function. As mentioned by Marks *et al.*[550], PKA phosphorylation of specific targets within cardiomyocytes appears to be compartmentalized such that some proteins (e.g. RyR2) are PKA-hyperphosphorylated in failing hearts, whereas other Ca^{2+} handling proteins (eg, PLB) are hypophosphorylated in the same hearts.

These results indicate that this cardioprotective effect is produced by restoring the normal FKBP12.6-mediated stabilization of the RyR2, defectiveness of which is the major cause of a variety of abnormal channel functions in the failing heart.

Angiotensin II receptor antagonist

Angiotensin II antagonism has been found to attenuate the downregulation of Ca^{2+}-ATPase (SERCA) and improve intracellular Ca^{2+} handling.[985,986] The corrections in SR function due to angiotensin II antagonism may be partly responsible for the favorable effects of angiotensin II antagonism on contractile and relaxation functions. In a canine model of heart failure, we recently demonstrated that during the development of pacing-induced heart failure, valsartan preserved the density of β-receptors and concurrently restored SR function (increased Ca^{2+} uptake and prevention of Ca^{2+} leak) without improving resting cardiac function.[987] By acting on the presynaptic angiotensin II receptor, valsartan may inhibit norepinephrine release and stimulate norepinephrine uptake back into the synaptic pool, and thus less adrenergic signal being transmitted into the cell, associated with a decrease in the level of RyR2-phosphorylation and thereby with an inhibition of Ca^{2+} leak through RyR2. Although valsartan did not improve resting cardiac function, valsartan treatment increased the contractility reserve as suggested by an enhanced dobutamine response. This improved hemodynamic response may be caused by normalization of the Ca^{2+} regulatory process and thereby, improved exercise tolerance. Also, inhibition of an aberrant SR Ca^{2+} leak, which can trigger arrhythmias by initiating delayed after-depolarizations,[550] may lead to a better prognosis in patients with heart failure.

DOMAIN-DOMAIN INTERACTION: A KEY MECHANISM TO STABILIZE RYR

Recently, several disease-linked mutations in the RyR2 have been reported in human patients. These mutation sites are distributed in three limited regions of the RyR2. Interestingly, the first and second regions are similar to those of malignant hyperthermia (MH) linked mutation sites in RyR (see Chapters 22-23). This fact suggests that these two regions represent the domains that are critical for the regulation of both RyR1 and RyR2, and that these domains are involved also in the pathogenesis of the RyR-linked skeletal and cardiac muscle diseases. Using domain peptide probe studies with the peptides corresponding to the portions of the N-terminal and central domains of the RyR1, Ikemoto and colleagues proposed the hypothesis that the mode of interaction between the two domains controls the functional state of the channel (see Chapter 6). According to their hypothesis, a tight zipping of the interacting domain stabilizes the channel. A mutation in either domain weakens the inter-domain interaction increasing the tendency of being unzipped, causing activation and leakage of the Ca^{2+} channel. They demonstrated a cardiac domain peptide corresponding to the Gly2459-Pro2494 region of RyR2 (DPc10) produced significant activation of the RyR2 Ca^{2+} channel.[188] The activation effect of the peptide has a quite significant impact on the cardiac channel regulation, especially in the low Ca^{2+} concentration range, where the muscle is supposed to relax (Fig. 26-3). DPc10 produced an appreciable decrease in the AC50 for the activation of the RyR2 by polylysine. The Arg-to-Ser mutation made in the peptide mimicking the Arg2474-to-Ser2474 human polymorphic VT mutation completely abolished both of these hyperactivation and hyper-sensitization effects seen with the DPc10. According to the hypothesis, these findings suggest that the *in vivo* domain of the RyR2 corresponding to DPc10 (i.e., the Gly2460-Pro2495 region of the RyR2) plays an important role in the cardiac channel regulation, and that the mutation occurring in this domain will produce hyper-activation and hyper-sensitization effects on the channel, particularly at relaxing concentrations of Ca^{2+}. Based upon these data, Ikemoto and colleagues anticipated that the mutation occurred in the Gly2460-Pro2495 domain of the RyR2 not only makes the Ca^{2+} channel leaky but also increases its sensitivity to various pharmacological agonists, which lead to the diastolic Ca^{2+} overload as widely seen in cardiac diseases.

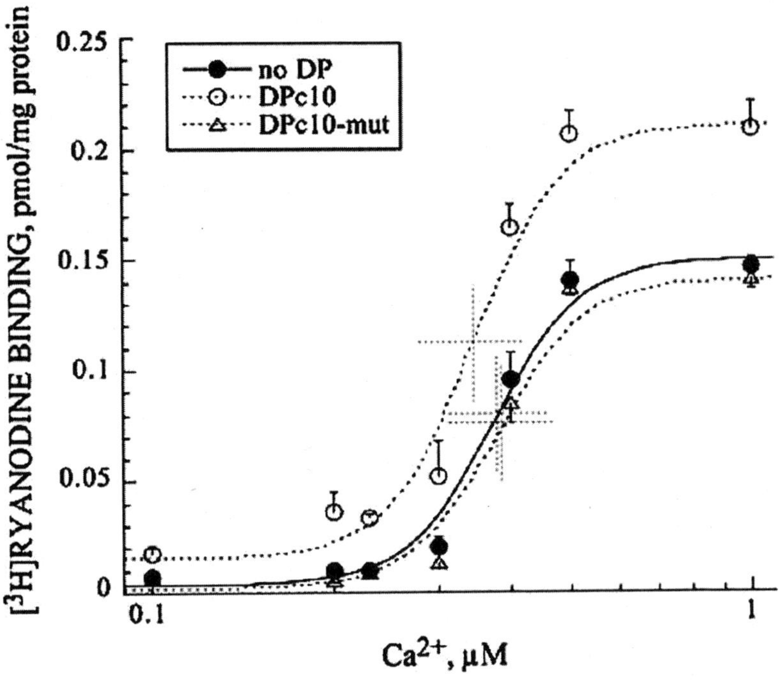

Figure 26-3. **Effect of Dpc10 on [Ca^{2+}]-dependence of ryanodine binding to RyR2.** The [Ca^{2+}]-dependence of the ryanodine binding activityof RyR2 in the absence of added domain peptide (solid circle), and in the presence of DPc10 (100 µM :open circle) or DPc10-mutant (100 µM: triangle). In the presence of DPc10, the ryanodine binding activity was much higher than the control at all Ca^{2+}concentrations examined. However, the magnitude of peptide activation was much higher in the lower concentration range of Ca^{2+}. From Yamamoto *et al.*[188] with permission.

More recently, we have found that DPc10 induces SR Ca^{2+} leak via a partial dissociation of FKBP12.6 from RyR, indicating that inter-domain interaction mechanism is likely to be involved in the FKBP12.6-mediated stabilization of RyR2 (*unpublished data*). Importantly, DPc10 produced the essentially identical abnormalities in both SR vesicles and cardiac myocytes as those seen in the SR and myocytes isolated from the failing heart, such as dissociation of FKBP12.6 and an increased Ca^{2+} leak. Furthermore, JTV519 prevented DPc10-induced domain unzipping and prevented both FKBP dissociation and Ca^{2+} leakage. These findings suggest that destabilization of the zipped state of the interacting domains is a key mechanism for the development of various problems seen in the RyR2 of failing heart.

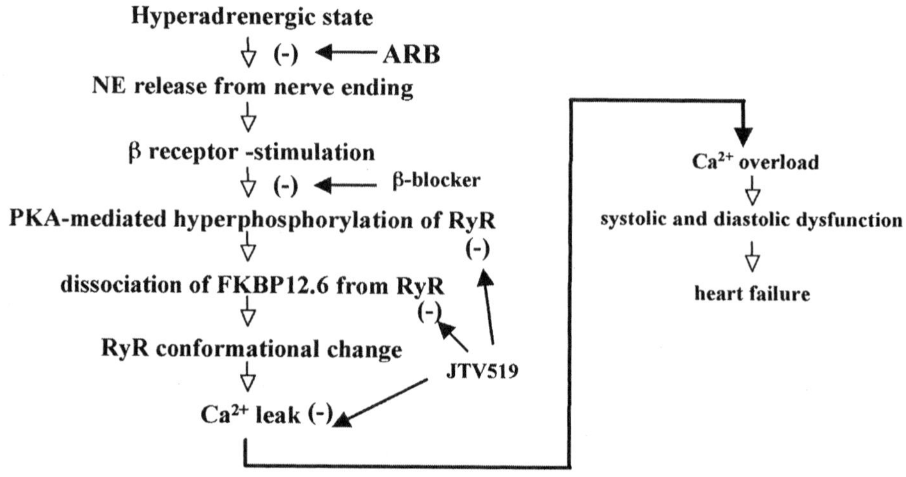

Figure 26-4. **FKBP12.6 mediated stabilization of RyR can be elicited at various levels of β-adrenergic signal transduction.** Excess β-stimulation induces PKA-mediated hyperphosphorylation, which leads to the dissociation of FKBP12.6 from RyR2, conformational change of RyR2, and then Ca^{2+} leak. This series of abnormal events within RyR2 might cause intracellular Ca^{2+} overload, and in turn cardiac dysfunction toward heart failure. FKBP12.6-mediated stabilization by β-receptor blocker, JTV519 or angiotensinII receptor antagonist (valsartan) might play an important role for prevention of the development of heart failure. ARB, angiotensinII-receptor antagonist.

CONCLUDING REMARKS

In heart failure, delicate interactions between SR Ca^{2+} release complex molecules could transform a highly specialized regulatory mechanism into a structure "out of control". The disrupted relationship between FKBP12.6 and RyR2 has been found to be involved in the pathogenesis of heart failure. We summarized how various drugs prevent the development of heart failure through stabilization of RyR in Fig. 26-4. This new concept may advance the understanding of the mechanism for contractile and relaxation dysfunctions in heart failure, and also may provide a valuable clue for the development of new methods of the treatment to prevent and cure heart failure.

Chapter 27

RYANODINE RECEPTOR ANTIBODIES AND MYASTHENIA GRAVIS

Frederik Romi
Dept. of Neurology, Haukeland University Hospital, Bergen, Norway

MYASTHENIA GRAVIS

Myasthenia gravis (MG) is an autoimmune disease characterized by a fluctuating pathological fatigue involving one or several skeletal muscle groups, mainly caused by antibodies to the acetylcholine receptor (AChR) at the post-synaptic site of the neuromuscular junction.[988,989] MG has a prevalence of 85-125 per million, and an annual incidence of 2-4 per million.[988,990] The disease has two peaks: one between 20 and 40 years dominated by women; and the other between 60 and 80 years equally shared by men and women.[991] Ocular symptoms with diplopia and ptosis occur early in the majority of patients, and can be the only manifestation of the disease. In 85% of the patients, however, MG becomes generalized, usually within three years, affecting limbs – especially the proximal parts, axial muscular groups such as the neck muscles, and facial and bulbar musculature causing loss of facial expression, speech difficulties, and chewing and swallowing disorders. The muscular weakness increases typically after exercise. When the respiratory muscles are affected, MG becomes life threatening and the patient may enter a MG crisis, requiring intensive care including mechanical ventilation.[992] Death due to respiratory failure or cardio-pulmonary complications can be the end result of such a crisis.[988,990]

The diagnosis of MG is based on the history and typical clinical findings. It can be confirmed pharmacologically by edrophonium test, where this acetylcholine esterase inhibiting drug gives an immediate and reproducible improvement of the MG signs after intravenous administration.[990] Failure of neuromuscular transmission in MG leads to a decremental response to repetitive nerve stimulation by electromyographical (EMG) examination. Increased jitter on single fiber EMG (SFEMG) is even more sensitive than repetitive nerve stimulation. The diagnosis is confirmed by the detection of AChR antibodies, which are present in about 85% of the patients' sera.[989] The prognosis of MG is generally good. MG related crisis occurs with an annual incidence of 2.5% among MG patients, but death during a MG crisis occurs very rarely in developed countries today.[993]

The etiology of MG is still enigmatic. There is a genetic predisposition, however, not completely understood. This may involve the MHC class I and II regions, the AChR-α-subunit, IgG heavy and light chain, FcγRII, and TCR genes. Although infection is postulated in the initiation of most autoimmune diseases through tissue damage, exposure of self-antigen, and activation of self-reactive T cells that recognize homologous sequences of a microorganism through molecular mimicry, there is so far no clear evidence that microbial infections can cause autoimmune disease. It is, however, generally believed that the initial triggering of an autoimmune reaction in MG takes place inside the thymus.[994] In MG patients who are younger than 40-50 years, the thymus is hyperplastic with germinal centers, indicating high immunological activity. Older patients usually have atrophic thymuses but germinal centers are present in some of them.[995,996] In 10-15% of the patients the disease is paraneoplastic and caused by a thymic tumour.

Auto-antibodies in MG

In 1960, John Simpson suggested that MG is an autoimmune disease caused by an autoimmune attack on the motor endplate. Patrick and Lindstrøm in 1973, demonstrated that this autoimmune attack was caused by antibodies to the AChR at the post-synaptic site of the motor endplate. AChR antibodies are present in the sera of more than 85% of MG patients with generalized MG.[989]

Also in 1960, Strauss *et al.* detected the presence of non-AChR antibodies in MG. These antibodies were found to bind to muscle antigens in a cross-striational pattern when muscle tissue was incubated with sera from MG patients. Later, several non-AChR antigens and antibodies were recognized, such as titin, myosin, actomyosin, rapsyn, muscle-specific kinase (MuSK), and ryanodine receptor (RyR).[989]

Titin is a giant protein molecule extending from the Z-disc to the M-line, providing the sarcomere with elasticity and controlling it's layout. Titin antibodies are present in sera from 80-90% of thymoma MG patients and about half of the late-onset MG patients, but occur only very infrequently in early-onset MG.[997]

Thymoma MG patients have higher titers of anti-myosin and anti-actomyosin antibodies than MG patients without thymoma. Cultured, dissociated thymic lymphocytes from MG patients secrete monoclonal striational antibodies that bind to myosin, α-actinin, or actin of skeletal muscles, suggesting that these antibodies may be involved in the pathogenesis of MG.

Antibodies against rapsyn have also been identified in MG, but they are found in patients with lupus and chronic procainamide associated myopathy as well. Any pathogenic role of these antibodies is not proven.

During formation of the neuromuscular junction, the basal membrane protein agrin initiates the aggregation of AChR on the surface of myotubes, where MuSK becomes phosphorylated upon incubation with agrin. MuSK is also expressed at the mature neuromuscular junction. 30% of AChR antibody negative MG patients, but no AChR antibody positive MG patients, have serum autoantibodies against MuSK, indicating the involvement of MuSK antibodies in the pathogenesis of AChR antibody negative MG. The pathogenetic mechanism for the MuSK antibodies is not known.

RyR antibodies

RyR antibodies belong to the non-AChR antibody group. The MG patient's RyR antibodies bind both to the skeletal (RyR1) and the cardiac (RyR2) form of the RyR.[998] RyR antibodies, especially RyR1, are implemented in the pathophysiology of MG. Antibody-binding sites on the so-called handle domains of the RyR's cytoplasmic assembly, near its junction with the transmembrane assembly have been identified to be RyR antigen epitopes.[999] A main immunogenic region (MIR) for MG patient RyR antibodies is located near the N terminus (residues 799-1172) of the RyR.[1000] Some sera also react with a shorter and more centrally located region (residues 2595-2935). These two parts of the molecule are probably located close to each other in the three dimensional naive conformation.[606] MG patient RyR antibodies recognize the MIR on the RyR, which seems to be of importance for RyR regulation. These RyR antibodies cause allosteric inhibition of RyR function in vitro, inhibiting Ca^{2+} release from sarcoplasmic reticulum. This inhibition is antibody-concentration dependent. Binding of ryanodine to the receptor is inhibited even at very high ryanodine concentrations, indicating a high antibody affinity for the receptor.[1001] The inhibition of ryanodine binding by RyR antibodies from MG patients indicates that the antibodies affect Ca^{2+}-release from sarcoplasmic reticulum by causing conformational changes that close the RyR ion-channel. RyR antibodies in MG patient's sera are usually detected by Western blot technique or by ELISA.[1002]

RYR ANTIBODIES IN MG

RyR antibodies and the pathogenesis of MG

It is generally accepted that the initial steps in the triggering of humoral immunity in MG take place inside the thymus.[994] Thymomas, especially those of cortical-type, are associated with MG in about 50% of the cases. The presence of muscle-like epitopes in thymomas has been demonstrated.[1003] MG-associated thymomas are enriched in AChR-like epitopes[1004] and AChR-specific T-cells.[994] Also RyR-like epitopes have been identified in the thymoma.[1005] In MG associated thymoma, the mechanisms involved in the initial autosensitization against RyR are probably similar to those implicated in the autosensitization against AChR. In all cases there is an over-expression of muscle-like epitopes and co-stimulatory molecules indicating that the T-cell autoimmunization is actively promoted by the pathogenic microenvironment inside the thymoma. In one study, RyR epitopes were also co-expressed along with LFA3 and B7 (BB1) co-stimulatory molecules on thymoma antigen presenting cells in cortical thymoma, indicating a role in the autosensitization process.[1006]

The events triggering the immune response against RyR in MG are not known. It is possible that the in vivo antibody response is confined to the MIR region in the initial phase of the immune response against RyR. The reactivity also against the centrally located region may be caused by epitope spreading which is typical for T cell driven autoimmune reactions such as in MG.[1007] The immunization is not only secondary to muscle destruction caused by AChR antibodies as RyR antibodies do not occur in early-onset MG which has the same anti-AChR autoimmune reactivity pattern. Moreover, RyR antibodies are not found after myocardial infarction, in muscle dystrophy or in other diseases involving muscle destruction.[998] There is some sequence homology between the transmembrane regions of the AChR-subunit and the RyR COOH terminal transmembrane regions.[3] Epitopes shared by RyR and AChR could play a part in the initial sensitization of autoreactive T cells. However, in a few thymoma patients RyR antibodies occur without detectable AChR antibodies, proving that RyR antibodies are not always coexistent with or secondary to AChR antibodies. A separate immunization against the different striated muscle antigens is therefore more likely.

The pathogenicity of RyR antibodies in MG

All four IgG isotypes are represented in RyR antibodies but with IgG 1 predominance.[1002,1008] The IgG 1 antibodies fix complement through the classical complement activation pathway, which is fast and efficient. RyR antibodies in one study were found to activate complement in vitro[1002], and could therefore be involved in the pathophysiology of MG through classical pathway complement activation.

Unlike AChR which is a cell-membrane antigen obviously exposed to circulating antibodies, RyR is a cytoplasmic sarcoplasmic reticulum membrane protein. Antibodies against RyR might have to penetrate the cell membrane to participate in any immune damage, either passively through a by-standing immune-mediated cell membrane damage or by active transport. This issue of cell membrane antibody penetration is not unique for RyR antibodies. Anti-DNA antibodies have been shown to penetrate the intact cell membrane by a receptor-mediated mechanism.[1009] Intracellular antibodies have also been used in therapeutic approaches for cancer and infectious disease.[1010] Further investigations are required to clarify cell membrane-penetrating capability of RyR antibodies and complement in MG patients.

There is circumstantial evidence for an in vivo effect of RyR antibodies. In one study, a rat strain with spontaneous thymomas, muscular weakness, and fatiguability resembling MG had electrophysiological signs of a defect excitation-contraction coupling. These rats had RyR antibodies but no detectable AChR antibodies.[1011] The presence of the muscle titin autoantibodies, was found to correlate with electromyography (EMG) evidence of myopathy in MG patients.[1012] Myopathy could be a plausible mechanism for muscle weakness caused by non-AChR muscle autoantibodies such as RyR antibodies.

The presence of RyR antibodies in MG patients correlates with a higher frequency of cardiac disease with sudden death.[1013,1014] The AChR antibodies cannot explain the cardiac involvement seen in some MG patients as nicotinic AChR is not found in the heart. The MG patient RyR antibodies bind both to the skeletal (RyR1) and the cardiac (RyR2) form of the RyR,[998] and this may explain a cardiopathogenic effect of RyR antibodies in MG patients.

RyR antibodies in subgroups of MG

Several MG subgroups have been identified: early-onset (type I MG) with MG start before the age of 50 years; late-onset (type II MG) with MG start at 50 years or later; AChR antibody negative MG (type III MG); and thymoma MG.[1015] RyR antibodies occur in 14% of the late-onset MG patients, and in 70% of the thymoma MG patients, and do not occur in other subgroups of MG.[997] The presence of RyR antibodies in a young MG patient strongly suggests the presence of a thymoma. The late-onset MG patients with RyR antibodies share immunological similarities with thymoma MG patients.[1016] It has been postulated that a pre-neoplastic (a process with potential malignant transformation) condition can lead to a paraneoplastic disease (autoimmune response induced by a tumour).[1017]

RyR antibodies have a 70% sensitivity and positive predictive value, 95% specificity and negative predictive value, and a test accuracy of 85% for the presence of a thymoma in a MG patient.[1018] The positive predictive value for thymoma is significantly higher for RyR antibodies than for the other known muscle antibodies in MG.[1019] This makes RyR antibodies useful in the serological diagnosis of thymoma in MG.

The RyR antibodies are found more often in patients where the thymoma is invasive and malignant.[1014] A surgical approach that ensures a complete removal of the thymoma should therefore be chosen in a thymoma patient with RyR antibodies.

RyR antibodies and the severity of MG

MG is often a more severe disease in patients with thymoma than in patients with early-onset MG.[1019] The presence of non-AChR muscle autoantibodies is associated with a more severe disease in all MG subgroups, and RyR antibodies occur significantly more often among patients with severe MG than among patients with less severe disease.[1013,1014,1019] RyR antibodies are therefore useful when assessing MG prognosis.

In one study, complement-activating RyR antibodies occurred with higher frequency in sera from thymoma MG patients than in sera from late-onset MG patients, and RyR IgG 1 antibodies occurred more often in severe MG than in mild and moderate disease groups. In the same study, mean total IgG and IgG 1 RyR antibody titers fell during long-time patient observation together with an improvement of the MG symptoms.[1002] Complement activation is therefore a possible mechanism for the correlation between RyR antibodies and a more severe MG. In another study, MG patients with RyR antibodies inhibiting ryanodine binding had a more severe disease than patients with RyR antibodies that did not inhibit ryanodine binding,[1001] suggesting a correlation between MG severity and the antibody effect on the RyR *in vitro*.

RyR antibodies and thymectomy in MG

Early-onset MG patients benefit from thymectomy.[1020,1021] However, the AChR antibody concentration does not influence the outcome of thymectomy in these patients, and non-AChR antibodies do not occur in this subgroup of MG.[1021]

Late-onset MG patients benefit far less from thymectomy,[1022,1023] and any limited improvement is even less likely in cases with RyR antibodies.[1023] MG severity and outcome over the course of years seem to be the same in thymoma and non-thymoma MG,[1021,1024] but the presence of RyR antibodies indicates a less favorable prognosis in both thymoma and non-thymoma MG.[1021]

CONCLUDING REMARKS

MG is an autoimmune disease caused by AChR antibodies. Some MG patients, especially those with a thymoma and those with late-onset MG, have other non-AChR antibodies, such as RyR antibodies. The events triggering the immune response against RyR in MG are not known, but RyR antibodies in a young MG patient strongly suggest the presence of a thymoma. RyR antibodies occur significantly more often among patients with severe MG. Many MG patients benefit from thymectomy, but the presence of RyR antibodies indicates a less favorable thymectomy outcome.

References

1. Bers DM. *Nature*. 2002;415:198-205.
2. Carafoli E. *Proc Natl Acad Sci U S A*. 2002;99:1115-22.
3. Takeshima H, Nishimura S, Matsumoto T, Ishida H, Kangawa K, Minamino N, Matsuo H, Ueda M, Hanaoka M, Hirose T, Numa S. *Nature*. 1989;339:439-445.
4. Otsu K, Willard HF, Khanna VK, Zorzato F, Green NM, MacLennan DH. *J Biol Chem*. 1990;265:13472-13483.
5. Marx SO, Reiken S, Hisamatsu Y, Jayaraman T, Burkhoff D, Rosemblit N, Marks AR. *Cell*. 2000;101:365-376.
6. Marx SO, Reiken S, Hisamatsu Y, Gaburjakova M, Gaburjakova J, Yang YM, Rosemblit N, Marks AR. *J Cell Biol*. 2001;153:699-708.
7. Zorzato F, Fujii J, Otso K, Phillips M, Green NM, Lai FA, Meissner G, MacLennan DH. *J Biol Chem*. 1990;265:2244-56.
8. Du GG, Sandhu B, Khanna VK, Guo XH, MacLennan DH. *Proc Natl Acad Sci U S A*. 2002;99:16725-30.
9. Doyle DA, Morais Cabral J, Pfuetzner RA, Kuo A, Gulbis JM, Cohen SL, Chait BT, MacKinnon R. *Science*. 1998;280:69-77.
10. Marks AR, Tempst P, Hwang KS, Taubman MB, Inui M, Chadwick C, Fleischer S, Nadal-Ginard B. *Proc Natl Acad Sci U S A*. 1989;86:8683-87.
11. Giannini G, Clementi E, Ceci R, Marziali G, Sorrentino V. *Science*. 1992;257:91-93.
12. Hakamata Y, Nakai J, Takeshima H, Imoto K. *FEBS*. 1992;312:229-235.
13. Ottini L, Marziali G, Conti A, Charlesworth A, Sorrentino V. *Biochem. J.* 1996;315:207-216.
14. Franck JPC, Morrissette J, Keen JE, Londraville RL, Beamsley M, Block BA. *Am J Physiol*. 1998;275:C401-15.
15. Oyamada H, Murayama T, Takagi T, Iino M, Iwabe N, Miyata T, Ogawa Y, Endo M. *J Biol Chem*. 1994;269:17206-14.
16. Maryon EB, Coronado R, Anderson P. *J Cell Biol*. 1996;134:885-93.

17. Takeshima H, Nishi M, Iwabe N, Miyata T, Hosoya T, Masai I, Hotta Y. *FEBS Lett.* 1994;337:81-87.
18. Tunwell RE, Wickenden C, Bertrand BM, Shevchenko VI, Walsh MB, Allen PD, Lai FA. *Biochem J.* 1996;318:477-87.
19. Leeb T, Brenig B. *FEBS Lett.* 1998;423:367-70.
20. Marziali G, Rossi D, Giannini G, Charlesworth A, Sorrentino V. *FEBS Lett.* 1996;394:76-82.
21. Fujii J, Otsu K, Zorzato F, de Leon S, Khanna VK, Weiler JE, O'Brien PJ, MacLennan DH. *Science.* 1991;253:448-51.
22. http://www.ensembl.org/Anopheles_gambiae/
23. Takeshima H, Iino M, Takekura H, Nishi M, Kuno J, Minowa O, Takano H, Noda T. *Nature.* 1994;369:556-9.
24. Shiwa M, Murayama T, Ogawa Y. *Am J Physiol Regul Integr Comp Physiol.* 2002;282:R727-37.
25. Mattei MG, Giannini G, Moscatelli F, Sorrentino V. *Genomics.* 1994;22:202-4.
26. Hughes AL. *Proc R Soc Lond B Biol Sci.* 1994;256:119-24.
27. Nakai J, Imagawa T, Hakamata Y, Shigekawa M, Takeshima H, Numa S. *FEBS.* 1990;271:169-177.
28. Futatsugi A, Kuwajima G, Mikoshiba K. *Biochem J.* 1995;305:373-78.
29. Xu X, Bhat MB, Nishi M, Takeshima H, Ma J. *Biophys J.* 2000;78:1270-81.
30. Jiang D, Xiao B, Li X, Chen SR. *J Biol Chem.* 2003;278:4763-69.
31. Puente E, Suner M, Evans AD, McCaffery AR, Windass JD. *Insect Biochem Mol Biol.* 2000;30:335-47.
32. Vazquez-Martinez O, Canedo-Merino R, Diaz-Munoz M, Riesgo-Escovar JR. *J Cell Sci.* 2003;116:2483-94.
33. Michikawa T, Hamanaka H, Otsu H, Yamamoto A, Miyawaki A, Furuichi T, Tashiro Y, Mikoshiba K. *J Biol Chem.* 1994;269:9184-9.
34. Wu Y, Kuzma J, Marechal E, Graeff R, Lee HC, Foster R, Chua NH. *Science.* 1997;278:2126-30.
35. Sorrentino V, Barone V, Rossi D. *Curr Opin Genet Dev.* 2000;10:662-67.
36. Harteneck C, Plant TD, Schultz G. *Trends Neurosci.* 2000;23:159-66.
37. Zhao M, Li P, Li X, Zhang L, Winkfein RJ, Chen SRW. *J Biol Chem.* 1999;274:25971-4.
38. Gao L, Balshaw D, Xu L, Tripathy A, Xin C, Meissner G. *Biophys J.* 2000;79:828-40.
39. Chiu J, DeSalle R, Lam HM, Meisel L, Coruzzi G. *Mol Biol Evol.* 1999;16:826-38.
40. Kuwajima G, Futatsugi A, Niinobe M, Nakanishi S, Mikoshiba K. *Neuron.* 1992;9:1133-42.
41. Giannini G, Conti A, Mammarella S, Scrobogna M, Sorrentino V. *J Cell Biol.* 1995;128:893-904.
42. Hamada T, Sakube Y, Ahnn J, Kim DH, Kagawa H. *J Mol Biol.* 2002;324:123-35.
43. Kim YK, Valdivia HH, Maryon EB, Anderson P, Coronado R. *Biophys J.* 1992;63:1379-84.
44. Nicholas WL. *The biology of free living nematodes.* Oxford, UK: Clarendon Press; 1984.
45. Maryon EB, Saari B, Anderson P. *J Cell Sci.* 1998;111:2885-95.
46. Garcia LR, Mehta P, Sternberg PW. *Cell.* 2001;107:777-88.
47. Adachi R, Kagawa H. *Mol Gen Genomics.* 2003;269:797-806.
48. Sullivan KM, Scott K, Zuker CS, Rubin GM. *Proc Natl Acad Sci U S A.* 2000;97:5942-47.
49. O'Brien J, Meissner G, Block BA. *Biophys J.* 1993;65:2418-27.
50. Ivanenko A, McKemy DD, Kenyon JL, Airey JA, Sutko JL. *J. Biol. Chem.* 1995;270:4220-4223.
51. Takeshima H, Ikemoto T, Nishi M, Nishiyama N, Shimuta M, Sugitani Y, Kuno J, Saito I, Saito H, Endo M, Iino M, Noda T. *J Biol Chem.* 1996;271:19649-52.

52. Fujii J, Otsu K, Zorzato F, de Leon S, Khana V, Weiler J, O'Brien P, MacLennan D. *Science.* 1991;253:448-451.
53. Priori SG, Napolitano C, Tiso N, Memmi M, Vignati G, Bloise R, Sorrentino VV, Danieli GA. *Circulation.* 2001;103:196-200.
54. Laitinen PJ, Brown KM, Piippo K, Swan H, Devaney JM, Brahmbhatt B, Donarum EA, Marino M, Tiso N, Viitasalo M, Toivonen L, Stephan DA, Kontula K. *Circulation.* 2001;103:485-90.
55. Franzini-Armstrong C. *J Cell Biol.* 1970;47:488-499.
56. Wagenknecht T, Grassucci R, Frank J, Saito A, Inui M, Fleischer S. *Nature.* 1989;338:167-170.
57. Radermacher M, Rao V, Grassucci R, Frank J, Timerman AP, Fleischer S, Wagenknecht T. *J Cell Biol.* 1994;127:411-423.
58. Serysheva, II, Orlova EV, Chiu W, Sherman MB, Hamilton SL, van Heel M. *Nature Struct. Biol.* 1995;2:18-24.
59. Protasi F, Franzini-Armstrong C, Allen PD. *J Cell Biol.* 1998;140:831-42.
60. Wagenknecht T, Radermacher M. *FEBS Lett.* 1995;369:43-46.
61. Stokes DL, Wagenknecht T. *Eur J Biochem.* 2000;267:5274-9.
62. Block BA, Imagawa T, Campbell KP, Franzini-Armstrong C. *J. Cell Biol.* 1988;107:2587-2600.
63. Bers DM. *Excitation-contraction coupling and cardiac contractile force.* 2nd ed. Dordrecht: Kluwer Academic Publishers; 2001.
64. Jiang Y, Lee A, Chen J, Ruta V, Cadene M, Chait BT, MacKinnon R. *Nature.* 2003;423:33-41.
65. Jiang Y, Ruta V, Chen J, Lee A, MacKinnon R. *Nature.* 2003;423:42-8.
66. Nishi M, Komazaki S, Kurebayashi N, Ogawa Y, Noda T, Iino M, Takeshima H. *J Cell Biol.* 1999;147:1473-80.
67. Du GG, Khanna VK, MacLennan DH. *J Biol Chem.* 2000;275:11778-11783.
68. Lai FA, Misra M, Xu L, Smith HA, Meissner G. *J Biol Chem.* 1989;264:16776-85.
69. Kyte J, Doolittle RF. *J Mol Biol.* 1982;157:105-32.
70. MacLennan DH, Brandl CJ, Korczak B, Green NM. *Nature.* 1985;316:696-700.
71. Brandt NR, Caswell AH, Brandt T, Brew K, Mellgren RL. *J Membr Biol.* 1992;127:35-47.
72. Takeshima H, Nishimura S, Nishi M, Ikeda M, Sugimoto T. *FEBS.* 1993;322:105-110.
73. Bhat MB, Zhao J, Takeshima H, Ma J. *Biophys J.* 1997;73:1329-36.
74. Du GG, Guo X, Khanna VK, MacLennan DH. *J Biol Chem.* 2001;276:31760-71.
75. Du GG, MacLennan DH. *J Biol Chem.* 1998;273:31867-72.
76. Chen SR, Ebisawa K, Li X, Zhang L. *J Biol Chem.* 1998;273:14675-8.
77. Balshaw D, Gao L, Meissner G. *Proc Natl Acad Sci U S A.* 1999;96:3345-7.
78. Wang R, Bolstad J, Kong H, Zhang L, Brown C, Chen SRW. *J Biol Chem.* 2004;279:3635-42.
79. Wang R, Zhang L, Bolstad J, Diao N, Brown C, Ruest L, Welch W, Williams AJ, Chen SRW. *J Biol Chem.* 2003;278:51557-65.
80. Marks AR, Tempst P, Chadwick CC, Riviere L, Fleischer S, Nadal-Ginard B. *J. Biol. Chem.* 1990;265:20719-20722.
81. Chen SR, Airey JA, MacLennan DH. *Journal of Biological Chemistry.* 1993;268:22642-9.
82. Callaway C, Seryshev A, Wang JP, Slavik KJ, Needleman DH, Cantu C, Wu Y, Jayaraman T, Marks AR, Hamilton SL. *J Biol Chem.* 1994;269:15876-84.
83. Grunwald R, Meissner G. *J. Biol. Chem.* 1995;270:11338-11347.
84. Marty I, Villaz M, Arlaud G, Bally I, Ronjat M. *Biochem J.* 1994;298 Pt 3:743-9.
85. Liu Z, Zhang J, Sharma MR, Li P, Chen SR, Wagenknecht T. *Proc Natl Acad Sci U S A.* 2001;98:6104-9.

86. Zhang J, Liu Z, Masumiya H, Wang R, Jiang D, Li F, Wagenknecht T, Chen SR. *J Biol Chem.* 2003;278:14211-8.
87. Liu Z, Zhang J, Li P, Chen SR, Wagenknecht T. *J Biol Chem.* 2002;277:46712-9.
88. Bhat MB, Ma J. *J Biol Chem.* 2002;277:8597-8601.
89. Bhat MB, Ma J. *J Biol Chem.* 2002;277:8597-601.
90. Zorzato F, Yamaguchi N, Xu L, Meissner G, Muller CR, Pouliquin P, Muntoni F, Sewry C, Girard T, Treves S. *Hum Mol Genet.* 2003;12:379-88.
91. Blobel G. *Proc Natl Acad Sci U S A.* 1980;77:1496-500.
92. Persson B, Argos P. *J Mol Biol.* 1994;237:182-92.
93. Mohana Rao JK, Argos P. *Biochim Biophys Acta.* 1986;869:197-214.
94. Galvan DL, Borrego-Diaz E, Perez PJ, Mignery GA. *J Biol Chem.* 1999;274:29483-92.
95. Krogh A, Larsson B, von Heijne G, Sonnhammer EL. *J Mol Biol.* 2001;305:567-80.
96. Berridge MJ, Bootman MD, Roderick HL. *Nat Rev Mol Cell Biol.* 2003;4:517-29.
97. Berridge MJ, Lipp P, Bootman MD. *Nat Rev Mol Cell Biol.* 2000;1:11-21.
98. Frank J. *Annu Rev Biophys Biomol Struct.* 2002;31:303-19.
99. van Heel M, Gowen B, Matadeen R, Orlova EV, Finn R, Pape T, Cohen D, Stark H, Schmidt R, Schatz M, Patwardhan A. *Q Rev Biophys.* 2000;33:307-69.
100. Auer M. *J Mol Med.* 2000;78:191-202.
101. Chiu W, McGough A, Sherman MB, Schmid MF. *Trends Cell Biol.* 1999;9:154-9.
102. Dubochet J, Adrian M, Chang JJ, Homo JC, Lepault J, McDowall AW, Schultz P. *Q Rev Biophys.* 1988;21:129-228.
103. Baker ML, Serysheva, II, Sencer S, Wu Y, Ludtke SJ, Jiang W, Hamilton SL, Chiu W. *Proc Natl Acad Sci U S A.* 2002;99:12155-60.
104. Frank J. *Three-dimensional electron microscopy of macromolecular assemblies.* San Diego, CA: Academic Press; 1996.
105. Sharma MR, Jeyakumar LH, Fleischer S, Wagenknecht T. *J Biol Chem.* 2000;275:9485-91.
106. Orlova EV, Serysheva, II, van Heel M, Hamilton SL, Chiu W. *Nat Struct Biol.* 1996;3:547-52.
107. Serysheva, II, Schatz M, van Heel M, Chiu W, Hamilton SL. *Biophys J.* 1999;77:1936-44.
108. Sharma MR, Jeyakuma LH, Fleischer S, Wagenknecht T. *Biophys J.* 2002;82:644a.
109. Sutko JL, Airey JA, Welch W, Ruest L. *Pharmacol Rev.* 1997;49:53-98.
110. Meissner G. *Front Biosci.* 2002;7:d2072-80.
111. Wagenknecht T, Radermacher M, Grassucci R, Berkowitz J, Xin HB, Fleischer S. *J Biol Chem.* 1997;272:32463-71.
112. Samso M, Trujillo R, Gurrola GB, Valdivia HH, Wagenknecht T. *J Cell Biol.* 1999;146:493-9.
113. Samso M, Wagenknecht T. *J Biol Chem.* 2002;277:1349-53.
114. Liu Z, Zhang J, Wang R, Chen SR, Wagenknecht T. *J Mol Biol.* 2004;338:533-545.
115. Sorrentino V, Volpe P. *Trends Pharmacol Sci.* 1993;14:98-103.
116. Serysheva, II, Ludtke SJ, Baker MR, Chiu W, Hamilton SL. *Proc Natl Acad Sci U S A.* 2002;99:10370-5.
117. Trujillo R, Shaikh TR, Liu Z, Wagenknecht T. *Biophys J.* 2004;86:79a.
118. Wriggers W, Milligan RA, McCammon JA. *J Struct Biol.* 1999;125:185-95.
119. Volkmann N, Hanein D. *J Struct Biol.* 1999;125:176-84.
120. Flucher BE, Franzini-Armstrong C. *Proc Natl Acad Sci U S A.* 1996;93:8101-6.
121. Takeshima H, Komazaki S, Nishi M, Iino M, Kangawa K. *Mol Cell.* 2000;6:11-22.
122. Jorgensen AO, Campbell KP. *J Cell Biol.* 1984;98:1597-602.

123. Jones LR, Zhang L, Sanborn K, Jorgensen AO, Kelley J. *J Biol Chem.* 1995;270:30787-30796.
124. Guo W, Jorgensen AO, Jones LR, Campbell KP. *J Biol Chem.* 1996;271:458-465.
125. Takekura H, Takeshima H, Nishimura S, Takahashi M, Tanabe T, Flockerzi V, Hofmann F, Franzini-Armstrong C. *J Muscle Res Cell Motil.* 1995;16:465-480.
126. Yin CC, Lai FA. *Nat Cell Biol.* 2000;2:669-71.
127. Takekura H, Nishi M, Noda T, Takeshima H, Franzini-Armstrong C. *Proc Natl Acad Sci U S A.* 1995;92:3381-5.
128. Flucher BE, Andrews SB, Fleischer S, Marks AR, Caswell A, Powell JA. *J Cell Biol.* 1993;123:1161-74.
129. Powell JA, Petherbridge L, Flucher BE. *J Cell Biol.* 1996;134:375-87.
130. Takekura H, Franzini-Armstrong C. *Dev Dyn.* 1999;214:372-80.
131. Protasi F, Takekura H, Wang Y, Chen SR, Meissner G, Allen PD, Franzini-Armstrong C. *Biophys J.* 2000;79:2494-508.
132. Wolf M, Eberhart A, Glossmann H, Striessnig J, Grigorieff N. *J Mol Biol.* 2003;332:171-82.
133. Nakai J, Dirksen RT, Nguyen HT, Pessah IN, Beam KG, Allen PD. *Nature.* 1996;380:72-5.
134. Sutko JL, Airey JA. *Physiol Rev.* 1996;76:1027-71.
135. Murayama T, Ogawa Y. *Trends Cardiovasc Med.* 2002;12:305-11.
136. Ward CW, Protasi F, Castillo D, Wang Y, Chen SR, Pessah IN, Allen PD, Schneider MF. *Biophys J.* 2001;81:3216-30.
137. Buck ED, Nguyen HT, Pessah IN, Allen PD. *J Biol Chem.* 1997;272:7360-7.
138. Felder E, Franzini-Armstrong C. *Proc Natl Acad Sci U S A.* 2002;99:1695-700.
139. Dirksen RT, Beam KG. *J Gen Physiol.* 1999;114:393-403.
140. Proenza C, O'Brien J, Nakai J, Mukherjee S, Allen PD, Beam KG. *J Biol Chem.* 2002;277:6530-5.
141. Cleemann L, Morad M. *J Physiol.* 1991;432:283-312.
142. Carl SL, Felix K, Caswell AH, Brandt NR, Ball WJ, Jr., Vaghy PL, Meissner G, Ferguson DG. *J. Cell Biol.* 1995;129:672-82.
143. Sun XH, Protasi F, Takahashi M, Takeshima H, Ferguson DG, Franzini-Armstrong C. *J. Cell Biol.* 1995;129:659-71.
144. Protasi F, Sun XH, Franzini-Armstrong C. *Dev Biol.* 1996;173:265-278.
145. Protasi F, Paolini C, Nakai J, Beam KG, Franzini-Armstrong C, Allen PD. *Biophys J.* 2002;83:3230-44.
146. Paolini C, Fessenden JD, Pessah I, Franzini-Armstrong C. *Biophys J.* 2002;82:78a.
147. Williams AJ, West DJ, Sitsapesan R. *Q Rev Biophys.* 2001;34:61-104.
148. Marks AR. *Physiol Rev.* 1996;76:631-49.
149. Anyatonwu GI, Buck ED, Ehrlich BE. *J Biol Chem.* 2003;278:45528-38.
150. Wang JP, Needleman DH, Seryshev AB, Aghdasi B, Slavik KJ, Liu SQ, Pedersen SE, Hamilton SL. *J Biol Chem.* 1996;271:8387-93.
151. Lynch PJ, Tong J, Lehane M, Mallet A, Giblin L, Heffron JJ, Vaughan P, Zafra G, MacLennan DH, McCarthy TV. *Proc Natl Acad Sci U S A.* 1999;96:4164-69.
152. MacKinnon R. *FEBS Lett.* 2003;555:62-5.
153. Jiang Y, Lee A, Chen J, Cadene M, Chait BT, MacKinnon R. *Nature.* 2002;417:523-6.
154. Morais-Cabral JH, Zhou Y, MacKinnon R. *Nature.* 2001;414:37-42.
155. Zhou Y, Morais-Cabral JH, Kaufman A, MacKinnon R. *Nature.* 2001;414:43-8.
156. Shah PK, Sowdhamini R. *Protein Eng.* 2001;14:867-74.
157. Mead F, Williams AJ. *Biophys J.* 2002;82:1953-63.

158. Mead FC, Sullivan D, Williams AJ. *J Membr Biol.* 1998;163:225-34.

159. Lee JM, Rho SH, Shin DW, Cho C, Park WJ, Eom SH, Ma J, Kim do H. *J Biol Chem.* 2004;279:6994-7000.

160. Welch W, Rheault S, West DJ, Williams AJ. *Biophys J.* 2004;86:402a.

161. Miller C. *Curr Opin Chem Biol.* 2000;4:148-51.

162. Witcher DR, McPherson PS, Kahl SD, Lewis T, Bentley P, Mullinnix MJ, Windass JD, Campbell KP. *J Biol Chem.* 1994;269:13076-13079.

163. Chu A, Diaz-Munoz M, Hawkes MJ, Brush K, Hamilton SL. *Mol Pharmacol.* 1990;37:735-41.

164. Tanna B, Welch W, Ruest L, Sutko JL, Williams AJ. *J Gen Physiol.* 1998;112:55-69.

165. Tanna B, Welch W, Ruest L, Sutko JL, Williams AJ. *J Gen Physiol.* 2000;116:1-9.

166. Tanna B, Welch W, Ruest L, Sutko JL, Williams AJ. *J Gen Physiol.* 2003;121:551-61.

167. Chen SRW, Li P, Zhao M, Li X, Zhang L. *Biophys J.* 2002;82:2436-47.

168. Lamb GD. *Clin Exp Pharmacol Physiol.* 2000;27:216-24.

169. Melzer W, Herrmann-Frank A, Luttgau HC. *Biochim Biophys Acta.* 1995;1241:59-116.

170. Giannini G, Sorrentino V. *Med Res Rev.* 1995;15:313-23.

171. Dirksen RT, Avila G. *Trends Cardiovasc Med.* 2002;12:189-97.

172. Mickelson JR, Louis CF. *Physiol Rev.* 1996;76:537-92.

173. Loke J, MacLennan DH. *Am J Med.* 1998;104:470-86.

174. Jurkat-Rott K, McCarthy T, Lehmann-Horn F. *Muscle Nerve.* 2000;23:4-17.

175. Tong J, Oyamada H, Demaurex N, Grinstein S, McCarthy TV, MacLennan DH. *J Biol Chem.* 1997;272:26332-39.

176. Yang T, Ta TA, Pessah IN, Allen PD. *J Biol Chem.* 2003;278:25722-30.

177. Avila G, O'Connell KM, Dirksen RT. *J Gen Physiol.* 2003;121:277-86.

178. Tiso N, Stephan DA, Nava A, Bagattin A, Devaney JM, Stanchi F, Larderet G, Brahmbhatt B, Brown K, Bauce B, Muriago M, Basso C, Thiene G, Danieli GA, Rampazzo A. *Hum Mol Genet.* 2001;10:189-94.

179. Ikemoto N, Yamamoto T. *Trends Cardiovasc Med.* 2000;10:310-6.

180. Ikemoto N, Yamamoto T. *Front Biosci.* 2002;7:d671-83.

181. Yamamoto T, El-Hayek R, Ikemoto N. *J Biol Chem.* 2000;275:11618-25.

182. Lamb GD, Posterino GS, Yamamoto T, Ikemoto N. *Am J Physiol Cell Physiol.* 2001;281:C207-14.

183. Shtifman A, Ward CW, Yamamoto T, Wang J, Olbinski B, Valdivia HH, Ikemoto N, Schneider MF. *J Gen Physiol.* 2002;119:15-32.

184. Yamamoto T, Ikemoto N. *Biochemistry.* 2002;41:1492-501.

185. Kobayashi H, Ikemoto N. *Biophys J.* 2004;86:397a.

186. El-Hayek R, Saiki Y, Yamamoto T, Ikemoto N. *J Biol Chem.* 1999;274:33341-7.

187. Paul-Pletzer K, Yamamoto T, Bhat MB, Ma J, Ikemoto N, Jimenez LS, Morimoto H, Williams PG, Parness J. *J Biol Chem.* 2002;277:34918-23.

188. Yamamoto T, Ikemoto N. *Biochem Biophys Res Commun.* 2002;291:1102-8.

189. Yano M, Kobayashi S, Kohno M, Doi M, Tokuhisa T, Okuda S, Suetsugu M, Hisaoka T, Obayashi M, Ohkusa T, Matsuzaki M. *Circulation.* 2003;107:477-84.

190. Rios E, Pizarro G. *Physiol Rev.* 1991;71:849-908.

191. Beurg M, Sukhareva M, Ahern CA, Conklin MW, Perez-Reyes E, Powers PA, Gregg RG, Coronado R. *Biophys J.* 1999;76:1744-56.

192. Nakai J, Sekiguchi N, Rando TA, Allen PD, Beam KG. *J Biol Chem.* 1998;273:13403-13406.

193. Leong P, MacLennan DH. *J Biol Chem.* 1998;273:29958-64.
194. Yamazawa T, Takeshima H, Shimuta M, Iino M. *J Biol Chem.* 1997;272:8161-4.
195. Murayama T, Oba T, Katayama E, Oyamada H, Oguchi K, Kobayashi M, Otsuka K, Ogawa Y. *J Biol Chem.* 1999;274:17297-308.
196. Perez CF, Mukherjee S, Allen PD. *J Biol Chem.* 2003;278:39644-52.
197. Yamamoto T, Rodriguez J, Ikemoto N. *J Biol Chem.* 2002;277:993-1001.
198. Yamamoto T, Ikemoto N. *J Biol Chem.* 2002;277:984-92.
199. Gallant EM, Gronert GA, Taylor SR. *Neurosci Lett.* 1982;28:181-6.
200. Fabiato A. *J Gen Physiol.* 1985;85:247-289.
201. Gyorke S, Gyorke I, Lukyanenko V, Terentyev D, Viatchenko-Karpinski S, Wiesner TF. *Front Biosci.* 2002;7:d1454-63.
202. Terentyev D, Viatchenko-Karpinski S, Valdivia HH, Escobar AL, Gyorke S. *Circ Res.* 2002;91:414-20.
203. Lahat H, Pras E, Olender T, Avidan N, Ben-Asher E, Man O, Levy-Nissenbaum E, Khoury A, Lorber A, Goldman B, Lancet D, Eldar M. *Am J Hum Genet.* 2001;69:1378-84.
204. Postma AV, Denjoy I, Hoorntje TM, Lupoglazoff JM, Da Costa A, Sebillon P, Mannens MM, Wilde AA, Guicheney P. *Circ Res.* 2002;91:e21-26.
205. Terentyev D, Viatchenko-Karpinski S, Gyorke I, Volpe P, Williams SC, Gyorke S. *Proc Natl Acad Sci U S A.* 2003;100:11759-64.
206. Viatchenko-Karpinski S, Terentyev D, Gyorke I, Terentyeva R, Volpe P, Priori SG, Napolitano C, Nori A, Williams SC, Gyorke S. *Circ Res.* 2004;94:471-7.
207. Fabiato A. *Adv Exp Med Biol.* 1992;311:245-62.
208. Bassani JW, Yuan W, Bers DM. *Am. J. Phys.* 1995;268:C1313-9.
209. Lukyanenko V, Gyorke I, Gyorke S. *Pflugers Arch.* 1996;432:1047-54.
210. Meissner G. *Annu Rev Physiol.* 1994;56:485-508.
211. Fill M, Copello JA. *Physiol Rev.* 2002;82:893-922.
212. Gyorke I, Gyorke S. *Biophys J.* 1998;75:2801-10.
213. Sitsapesan R, Williams AJ. *J Membr Biol.* 1994;137:215-26.
214. Xu L, Meissner G. *Biophys J.* 1998;75:2302-12.
215. Ching LL, Williams AJ, Sitsapesan R. *Circ Res.* 2000;87:201-6.
216. Gyorke I, Hester N, Jones LR, Gyorke S. *Biophys J.* 2004;86:2121-28.
217. Chen W, Steenbergen C, Levy LA, Vance J, London RE, Murphy E. *J Biol Chem.* 1996;271:7398-403.
218. Shannon TR, Guo T, Bers DM. *Circ Res.* 2003;93:40-45.
219. Yasui K, Palade P, Gyorke S. *Biophys J.* 1994;67:457-60.
220. Sham JS, Song LS, Chen Y, Deng LH, Stern MD, Lakatta EG, Cheng H. *Proc Natl Acad Sci U S A.* 1998;95:15096-101.
221. DelPrincipe F, Egger M, Niggli E. *Nat Cell Biol.* 1999;1:323-29.
222. Sobie EA, Dilly KW, Dos Santos Cruz J, Lederer WJ, Jafri MS. *Biophys J.* 2002;83:59-78.
223. Cheng H, Lederer MR, Lederer WJ, Cannell MB. *Am J Physiol.* 1996;270:C148-59.
224. Lukyanenko V, Viatchenko-Karpinski S, Smirnov A, Wiesner TF, Gyorke S. *Biophys J.* 2001;81:785-98.
225. Shannon TR, Ginsburg KS, Bers DM. *Circ Res.* 2002;91:594-600.
226. Lukyanenko V, Gyorke I, Wiesner TF, Gyorke S. *Circ Res.* 2001;89:614-22.
227. Zhang L, Kelley J, Schmeisser G, Kobayashi YM, Jones LR. *J Biol Chem.* 1997;272:23389-97.

228. Franzini-Armstrong C, Protasi F. *Physiol Rev*. 1997;77:699-729.
229. Beard NA, Sakowska MM, Dulhunty AF, Laver DR. *Biophys J*. 2002;82:310-20.
230. Coumel P, Fidelle J, Lucet V. *Br Heart J*. 1978;40:28-37.
231. January CT, Fozzard HA. *Pharmacol Rev*. 1988;40:219-27.
232. Lederer WJ, Tsien RW. *J Physiol (Lond)*. 1976;263:73-100.
233. Park H, Wu S, Dunker AK, Kang C. *J Biol Chem*. 2003;278:16176-82.
234. Nabauer M, Morad M. *Am J Physiol*. 1990;258:C189-93.
235. Chu A, Fill M, Stefani E, Entman ML. *J Membr Biol*. 1993;135:49-59.
236. Copello JA, Barg S, Onoue H, Fleischer S. *Biophys J*. 1997;73:141-56.
237. Laver DR, Roden LD, Ahern GP, Eager KR, Junankar PR, Dulhunty AF. *J Membr Biol*. 1995;147:7-22.
238. Rousseau E, Meissner G. *Am J Physiol*. 1989;256:H328-337.
239. Blatter LA, Huser J, Ríos E. *Proc Natl Acad Sci U S A*. 1997;94:4176-81.
240. Cheng H, Lederer WJ, Cannell MB. *Science*. 1993;262:740-44.
241. Percival AL, Williams AJ, Kenyon JL, Grinsell MM, Airey JA, Sutko JL. *Biophys J*. 1994;67:1834-50.
242. Gyorke S, Fill M. *Science*. 1993;260:807-9.
243. Gyorke S, Velez P, Suarez-Isla B, Fill M. *Biophys J*. 1994;66:1879-86.
244. Laver DR, Curtis BA. *Biophys J*. 1996;71:732-41.
245. Schiefer A, Meissner G, Isenberg G. *J Physiol*. 1995;489:337-48.
246. Sitsapesan R, Montgomery RA, Williams AJ. *Circ Res*. 1995;77:765-72.
247. Valdivia HH, Kaplan JH, Ellis-Davies GC, Lederer WJ. *Science*. 1995;267:1997-2000.
248. Velez P, Gyorke S, Escobar AL, Vergara J, Fill M. *Biophys J*. 1997;72:691-7.
249. Stern MD. *Biophys J*. 1992;63:497-517.
250. Escobar AL, Velez P, Kim AM, Cifuentes F, Fill M, Vergara JL. *Pflugers Arch*. 1997;434:615-31.
251. Lipp P, Niggli E. *J. Physiol*. 1996;492:31-8.
252. Parker I, Zang WJ, Wier WG. *J Physiol*. 1996;497:31-38.
253. Wier WG, Egan TM, Lopez-Lopez JR, Balke CW. *J Physiol*. 1994;474:463-71.
254. Sitsapesan R, Williams AJ. *J Membr Biol*. 1995;146:133-44.
255. Smith JS, Coronado R, Meissner G. *J. Gen. Physiol*. 1986;88:573-588.
256. Smith JS, Coronado R, Meissner G. *Nature*. 1985;316:446-9.
257. Smith JS, Imagawa T, Ma J, Fill M, Campbell KP, Coronado R. *J Gen Physiol*. 1988;92:1-26.
258. Suarez-Isla BA, Orozco C, Heller PF, Froehlich JP. *Proc Natl Acad Sci U S A*. 1986;83:7741-5.
259. Copello JA, Qi Y, Jeyakumar LH, Ogunbunmi E, Fleischer S. *Cell Calcium*. 2001;30:269-84.
260. Smith JS, Imagawa T, Ma J, Fill M, Campbell KP, Coronado R. *J. Gen. Physiol*. 1988; 2:1-26.
261. Tripathy A, Meissner G. *Biophys J*. 1996;70:2600-15.
262. Copello JA, Porta M, Diaz-Sylvester PL, Nani A, Escobar A, Fleischer S, Fill M. *Biophys J*. 2003;84:17A.
263. Garcia J, Schneider MF. *J Physiol*. 1995;485:437-45.
264. Rios E, Stern MD. *Annu Rev Biophys Biomol Struct*. 1997;26:47-82.
265. Schneider MF. *Annu Rev Physiol*. 1994;56:463-84.
266. Stern MD. *Biophys J*. 1996;70:2100-9.
267. Lukyanenko V, Gyorke S. *J Physiol*. 1999;521:575-85.
268. Armisen R, Sierralta J, Velez P, Naranjo D, Suarez-Isla BA. *Am J Physiol*. 1996;271:C144-53.

269. Fill M, Zahradnikova A, Villalba-Galea CA, Zahradnik I, Escobar AL, Gyorke S. *J Gen Physiol.* 2000;116:873-82.
270. Sachs F, Qin F, Palade P. *Science.* 1995;267:2010-1.
271. Zahradnikova A, Zahradnik I. *Biophys J.* 1995;69:1780-8.
272. Xu L, Mann G, Meissner G. *Circ Res.* 1996;79:1100-9.
273. Laver DR, Lamb GD. *Biophys J.* 1998;74:2352-64.
274. Cannell MB, Cheng H, Lederer WJ. *Science.* 1995;268:1045-49.
275. Cheng H, Cannell MB, Lederer WJ. *Circ Res.* 1995;76:236-41.
276. Cheng H, Cannell MB, Lederer WJ. *Pflugers Arch.* 1994;428:415-17.
277. Cheng H, Lederer MR, Xiao RP, Gomez AM, Zhou YY, Ziman B, Spurgeon H, Lakatta EG, Lederer WJ. *Cell Calcium.* 1996;20:129-40.
278. Shacklock PS, Wier WG, Balke CW. *J Physiol (Lond).* 1995;487:601-8.
279. Franzini-Armstrong C, Protasi F, Ramesh V. *Biophys J.* 1999;77:1528-39.
280. Franzini-Armstrong C, Protasi F, Ramesh V. *Ann N Y Acad Sci.* 1998;853:20-30.
281. Cannell MB, Cheng H, Lederer WJ. *Biophys J.* 1994;67:1942-56.
282. Minta A, Kao JPY, Tsien RY. *J Biol Chem.* 1989;264:8171-78.
283. Santana LF, Cheng H, Gomez AM, Cannell MB, Lederer WJ. *Circ Res.* 1996;78:166-71.
284. Smith GD, Keizer JE, Stern MD, Lederer WJ, Cheng H. *Biophys J.* 1998;75:15-32.
285. Bers DM. *Sci STKE.* 2003;2003:PE13.
286. Guatimosim S, Dilly K, Santana LF, Saleet Jafri M, Sobie EA, Lederer WJ. *J Mol Cell Cardiol.* 2002;34:941-50.
287. Stern MD, Cheng H. *Cell Calcium.* 2004;35:591-601.
288. Wang SQ, Wei C, Zhao G, Brochet DX, Shen J, Song LS, Wang W, Yang D, Cheng H. *Circ Res.* 2004;94:1011-22.
289. Cheng H, Wang SQ. *Front Biosci.* 2002;7:d1867-78.
290. Niggli E, Egger M. *Front Biosci.* 2002;7:d1288-97.
291. Niggli E. *Annu Rev Physiol.* 1999;61:311-35.
292. Wier WG, Balke CW. *Circ Res.* 1999;85:770-6.
293. Wier WG, ter Keurs HE, Marban E, Gao WD, Balke CW. *Circ Res.* 1997;81:462-69.
294. Wehrens XH, Lehnart SE, Huang F, Vest JA, Reiken SR, Mohler PJ, Sun J, Guatimosim S, Song LS, Rosemblit N, D'Armiento JM, Napolitano C, Memmi M, Priori SG, Lederer WJ, Marks AR. *Cell.* 2003;113:829-40.
295. Ginsburg KS, Bers DM. *J Physiol.* 2004;556:463-80.
296. Maier LS, Zhang T, Chen L, DeSantiago J, Brown JH, Bers DM. *Circ Res.* 2003;92:904-11.
297. Li Y, Kranias EG, Mignery GA, Bers DM. *Circ Res.* 2002;90:309-16.
298. Wehrens XH, Lehnart SE, Reiken SR, Marks AR. *Circ Res.* 2004;94:e61-70.
299. Wehrens XH, Lehnart SE, Reiken SR, Deng SX, Vest JA, Cervantes D, Coromilas J, Landry DW, Marks AR. *Science.* 2004;304:292-96.
300. Pogwizd SM, Bers DM. *Trends Cardiovasc Med.* 2004;14:61-66.
301. Pogwizd SM, Schlotthauer K, Li L, Yuan W, Bers DM. *Circ Res.* 2001;88:1159-67.
302. Pogwizd SM, Qi M, Yuan W, Samarel AM, Bers DM. *Circ Res.* 1999;85:1009-19.
303. Weber CR, Ginsburg KS, Bers DM. *Circ Res.* 2003;92:950-52.
304. Esposito G, Santana LF, Dilly K, Cruz JD, Mao L, Lederer WJ, Rockman HA. *Am J Physiol Heart Circ Physiol.* 2000;279:H3101-12.

305. Gomez AM, Valdivia HH, Cheng H, Lederer MR, Santana LF, Cannell MB, McCune SA, Altschuld RA, Lederer WJ. *Science.* 1997;276:800-6.
306. Hasenfuss G, Schillinger W, Lehnart SE, Preuss M, Pieske B, Maier LS, Prestle J, Minami K, Just H. *Circulation.* 1999;99:641-48.
307. del Monte F, Williams E, Lebeche D, Schmidt U, Rosenzweig A, Gwathmey JK, Lewandowski ED, Hajjar RJ. *Circulation.* 2001;104:1424-29.
308. Balijepalli RC, Lokuta AJ, Maertz NA, Buck JM, Haworth RA, Valdivia HH, Kamp TJ. *Cardiovasc Res.* 2003;59:67-77.
309. Gomez AM, Guatimosim S, Dilly KW, Vassort G, Lederer WJ. *Circulation.* 2001;104:688-93.
310. Pieske B, Houser SR, Hasenfuss G, Bers DM. *Cardiovasc Res.* 2003;57:871-2.
311. Pogwizd SM, Sipido KR, Verdonck F, Bers DM. *Cardiovasc Res.* 2003;57:887-96.
312. Litwin SE, Li J, Bridge JH. *Biophys J.* 1998;75:359-71.
313. Lamb GD, Laver DR, Stephenson DG. *J Gen Physiol.* 2000;116:883-90.
314. Gyorke S. *J Gen Physiol.* 1999;114:163-66.
315. Marx SO, Gaburjakova J, Gaburjakova M, Henrikson C, Ondrias K, Marks AR. *Circ Res.* 2001;88:1151-58.
316. Marx SO, Ondrias K, Marks AR. *Science.* 1998;281:818-21.
317. Shannon TR, Ginsburg KS, Bers DM. *Biophys J.* 2000;78:334-43.
318. Trafford AW, Diaz ME, O'Neill SC, Eisner DA. *Front Biosci.* 2002;7:d843-52.
319. Bers DM. *J Mol Cell Cardiol.* 2004;In press.
320. Marks AR, Marx SO, Reiken S. *Trends Cardiovasc Med.* 2002;12:166-70.
321. Trafford AW, Diaz ME, Eisner DA. *Circ Res.* 2001;88:195-201.
322. Brittsan AG, Ginsburg KS, Chu G, Yatani A, Wolska BM, Schmidt AG, Asahi M, MacLennan DH, Bers DM, Kranias EG. *Circ Res.* 2003;92:769-76.
323. Wolska BM, Stojanovic MO, Luo W, Kranias EG, Solaro RJ. *Am J Physiol.* 1996;271:C391-7.
324. Davare MA, Avdonin V, Hall DD, Peden EM, Burette A, Weinberg RJ, Horne MC, Hoshi T, Hell JW. *Science.* 2001;293:98-101.
325. Stange M, Xu L, Balshaw D, Yamaguchi N, Meissner G. *J Biol Chem.* 2003;278:51693-702.
326. Xiao B, Sutherland C, Walsh MP, Chen SR. *Circ Res.* 2004.
327. Hussain M, Drago GA, Coyler J, Orchard CH. *Am J Physiol.* 1997;273:H695-H706.
328. Viatchenko-Karpinski S, Gyorke S. *J Physiol.* 2001;533:837-48.
329. Song LS, Wang SQ, Xiao RP, Spurgeon H, Lakatta EG, Cheng H. *Circ Res.* 2001;88:794-801.
330. Yamaguchi N, Xu L, Pasek DA, Evans KE, Meissner G. *J Biol Chem.* 2003;278:23480-6.
331. Balshaw DM, Xu L, Yamaguchi N, Pasek DA, Meissner G. *J Biol Chem.* 2001;276:20144-53.
332. Xu L, Meissner G. *Biophys J.* 2004;86:797-804.
333. Braun AP, Schulman H. *Annu Rev Physiol.* 1995;57:417-45.
334. Colbran RJ, Soderling TR. *Curr Top Cell Regul.* 1990;31:181-221.
335. Bronstein JM, Farber DB, Wasterlain CG. *Brain Res Brain Res Rev.* 1993;18:135-47.
336. Edman CF, Schulman H. *Biochim Biophys Acta.* 1994;1221:89-101.
337. Tobimatsu T, Fujisawa H. *J Biol Chem.* 1989;264:17907-12.
338. Zhang T, Maier LS, Dalton ND, Miyamoto S, Ross J, Jr., Bers DM, Brown JH. *Circ Res.* 2003;92:912-9.
339. Meyer T, Hanson PI, Stryer L, Schulman H. *Science.* 1992;256:1199-202.
340. Schworer CM, Colbran RJ, Soderling TR. *J Biol Chem.* 1986;261:8581-4.
341. Miller SG, Kennedy MB. *Cell.* 1986;44:861-70.

342. Lai Y, Nairn AC, Greengard P. *Proc Natl Acad Sci U S A*. 1986;83:4253-7.
343. Lou LL, Lloyd SJ, Schulman H. *Proc Natl Acad Sci U S A*. 1986;83:9497-501.
344. Zucchi R, Ronca-Testoni S. *Pharmacol Rev*. 1997;49:1-51.
345. Witcher DR, Kovacs RJ, Schulman H, Cefali DC, Jones LR. *J. Biol. Chem.* 1991;266:11144-52.
346. Hain J, Onoue H, Mayrleitner M, Fleischer S, Schindler H. *J Biol Chem*. 1995;270:2074-81.
347. Takasago T, Imagawa T, Furukawa K, Ogurusu T, Shigekawa M. *J Biochem (Tokyo)*. 1991;109:163-70.
348. Wang J, Best PM. *Nature*. 1992;359:739-41.
349. Rodriguez P, Bhogal MS, Colyer J. *J Biol Chem*. 2003;278:38593-600.
350. Lokuta AJ, Rogers TB, Lederer WJ, Valdivia HH. *J. Phys.* 1995;487:609-22.
351. Li L, Satoh H, Ginsburg KS, Bers DM. *J Physiol*. 1997;501:17-31.
352. Maier LS, Zhang T, Seidler T, Kohlhaas M, Ziolo MT, Zibrova D, Chen L, Brown JH, Bers DM. *Circulation*. 2003;108:IV-54.
353. Guo T, Zhang T, Brown JH, Bers DM. *Biophys J*. 2004;86:241a.
354. Wu Y, Colbran RJ, Anderson ME. *Proc Natl Acad Sci U S A*. 2001;98:2877-81.
355. Hagemann D, Kuschel M, Kuramochi T, Zhu W, Cheng H, Xiao RP. *J Biol Chem*. 2000;275:22532-6.
356. DeSantiago J, Maier LS, Bers DM. *J Mol Cell Cardiol*. 2002;34:975-84.
357. duBell WH, Lederer WJ, Rogers TB. *J. Physiol.* 1996;493:793-800.
358. duBell WH, Gigena MS, Guatimosim S, Long X, Lederer WJ, Rogers TB. *Am J Physiol Heart Circ Physiol*. 2002;282:H38-48.
359. Terentyev D, Viatchenko-Karpinski S, Gyorke I, Terentyeva R, Gyorke S. *J Physiol*. 2003;552:109-18.
360. Tada M, Kirchberger MA, Repke DI, Katz AM. *J Biol Chem*. 1974;249:6174-80.
361. Trafford AW, Diaz ME, Negretti N, Eisner DA. *Circ Res*. 1997;81:477-84.
362. Adachi-Akahane S, Cleemann L, Morad M. *J Gen Physiol*. 1996;108:435-54.
363. Sipido KR, Callewaert G, Carmeliet E. *Circ Res*. 1995;76:102-9.
364. Grantham CJ, Cannell MB. *Circ Res*. 1996;79:194-200.
365. Spencer CI, Berlin JR. *J Physiol*. 1995;488:267-79.
366. Trafford AW, Diaz ME, Sibbring GC, Eisner DA. *J Physiol (Lond)*. 2000;522:259-70.
367. Lukyanenko V, Subramanian S, Gyorke I, Wiesner TF, Gyorke S. *J Physiol*. 1999;518:173-86.
368. Stern MD, Capogrossi MC, Lakatta EG. *Cell Calcium*. 1988;9:247-56.
369. O'Neill SC, Eisner DA. *J Physiol*. 1990;430:519-36.
370. Adams W, Trafford AW, Eisner DA. *Pflugers Arch*. 1998;436:776-81.
371. Overend CL, O'Neill SC, Eisner DA. *J Physiol*. 1998;507:759-69.
372. Choi HS, Trafford AW, Orchard CH, Eisner DA. *J Physiol*. 2000;529:661-68.
373. Fabiato A. *J Gen Physiol*. 1985;85:291-320.
374. Eisner DA, Choi HS, Diaz ME, O'Neill SC, Trafford AW. *Circ Res*. 2000;87:1087-94.
375. Shiferaw Y, Watanabe MA, Garfinkel A, Weiss JN, Karma A. *Biophys J*. 2003;85:3666-86.
376. Euler DE. *Cardiovasc Res*. 1999;42:583-90.
377. Lab MJ, Lee JA. *Circ Res*. 1990;66:585-95.
378. Dumitrescu C, Narayan P, Efimov IR, Cheng Y, Radin MJ, McCune SA, Altschuld RA. *Am J Physiol Heart Circ Physiol*. 2002;282:H1320-6.
379. Ryan JM, Schieve JF, Hull HB, Oser BM. *Circulation*. 1955;12:60-3.

380. Kodama M, Kato K, Hirono S, Okura Y, Hanawa H, Ito M, Fuse K, Shiono T, Watanabe K, Aizawa Y. *J Card Fail.* 2001;7:138-45.
381. Orchard CH, McCall E, Kirby MS, Boyett MR. *Circ Res.* 1991;68:69-76.
382. Qian YW, Clusin WT, Lin SF, Han J, Sung RJ. *Circulation.* 2001;104:2082-7.
383. Huser J, Wang YG, Sheehan KA, Cifuentes F, Lipsius SL, Blatter LA. *J Physiol.* 2000;524:795-806.
384. Diaz ME, Eisner DA, O'Neill SC. *Circ Res.* 2002;91:585-93.
385. Trafford AW, O'Neill SC, Eisner DA. *Pflugers Arch.* 1993;425:181-3.
386. Diaz ME, O'Neill SC, Eisner DA. *Circ Res.* 2004;94:650-56.
387. Moosmang S, Schulla V, Welling A, Feil R, Feil S, Wegener JW, Hofmann F, Klugbauer N. *EMBO J.* 2003;22:6027-34.
388. Tribe RM. *J Physiol.* 2002;538:673.
389. Wellman GC, Nelson MT. *Cell Calcium.* 2003;34:211-29.
390. Somlyo AP, Somlyo AV. *Nature.* 1994;372:231-6.
391. Somlyo AP, Wu X, Walker LA, Somlyo AV. *Rev Physiol Biochem Pharmacol.* 1999;134:201-34.
392. Somlyo AP, Somlyo AV. *Acta Physiol Scand.* 1998;164:437-48.
393. Knot HJ, Nelson MT. *J Physiol.* 1998;508:199-209.
394. Nelson MT, Cheng H, Rubart M, Santana LF, Bonev AD, Knot HJ, Lederer WJ. *Science.* 1995;270:633-637.
395. Heppner TJ, Bonev AD, Santana LF, Nelson MT. *Am J Physiol Heart Circ Physiol.* 2002;283:H2169-76.
396. Ruehlmann DO, Lee CH, Poburko D, van Breemen C. *Circ Res.* 2000;86:E72-9.
397. Jaggar JH, Nelson MT. *Am J Physiol Cell Physiol.* 2000;279:C1528-39.
398. Boittin FX, Macrez N, Halet G, Mironneau J. *Am J Physiol.* 1999;277:C139-51.
399. Lee CH, Poburko D, Sahota P, Sandhu J, Ruehlmann DO, van Breemen C. *J Physiol.* 2001;534:641-50.
400. Peng H, Matchkov V, Ivarsen A, Aalkjaer C, Nilsson H. *Circ Res.* 2001;88:810-815.
401. Cartin L, Lounsbury KM, Nelson MT. *Circ Res.* 2000;86:760-67.
402. Gomez MF, Stevenson AS, Bonev AD, Hill-Eubanks DC, Nelson MT. *J Biol Chem.* 2002;277:37756-37764.
403. Flynn ER, Bradley KN, Muir TC, McCarron JG. *J Biol Chem.* 2001;276:36411-18.
404. Janiak R, Wilson SM, Montague S, Hume JR. *Am J Physiol Cell Physiol.* 2001;280:C22-33.
405. Bolton TR, Lim PS. *J. Physiol.* 1989;409:385-401.
406. Young SH, Ennes HS, McRoberts JA, Chaban VV, Dea SK, Mayer EA. *Am J Physiol.* 1999;276:G1204-12.
407. Endo M, Iino M, Kobayashi T, Yamamoto T. *Prog Clin Biol Res.* 1990;327:193-204.
408. Iino M, Kobayashi T, Endo M. *Biochem. Biophys. Res. Commun.* 1988;152:417.
409. Xu L, Lai FA, Cohn A, Etter E, Guerrero A, Fay FS, Meissner G. *Proc Natl Acad Sci U S A.* 1994;91:3294-98.
410. Herrmann-Frank A, Darling E, Meissner G. *Pflugers Archiv.* 1991;418:353-359.
411. Li PL, Tang WX, Valdivia HH, Zou AP, Campbell WB. *Am J Physiol Heart Circ Physiol.* 2001;280:H208-15.
412. Ledbetter MW, Preiner JK, Louis CF, Mickelson JR. *J Biol Chem.* 1994;269:31544-51.
413. Guerrero-Hernandez A, Gomez-Viquez L, Guerrero-Serna G, Rueda A. *Front Biosci.* 2002;7:d1676-88.

414. Kotlikoff MI. *Prog Biophys Mol Biol.* 2003;83:171-91.
415. Lesh RE, Nixon GF, Fleischer S, Airey JA, Somlyo AP, Somlyo AV. *Circ Res.* 1998;82:175-85.
416. Jaggar JH, Wellman GC, Heppner TJ, Porter VA, Perez GJ, Gollasch M, Kleppisch T, Rubart M, Stevenson AS, Lederer WJ, Knot HJ, Bonev AD, Nelson MT. *Acta Physiol Scand.* 1998;164:577-87.
417. Ohi Y, Yamamura H, Nagano N, Ohya S, Muraki K, Watanabe M, Imaizumi Y. *J Physiol.* 2001;534:313-26.
418. Gollasch M, Wellman GC, Knot HJ, Jaggar JH, Damon DH, Bonev AD, Nelson MT. *Circ Res.* 1998;83:1104-14.
419. Mironneau J, Macrez N, Morel JL, Sorrentino V, Mironneau C. *J Physiol.* 2002;538:707-16.
420. Knot HJ. *Circ Res.* 2001;89:941-3.
421. Lohn M, Jessner W, Furstenau M, Wellner M, Sorrentino V, Haller H, Luft FC, Gollasch M. *Circ Res.* 2001;89:1051-7.
422. Takeshima H, Yamazawa T, Ikemoto T, Takekura H, Nishi M, Noda T, Iino M. *EMBO J.* 1995;14:2999-3006.
423. Takeshima H, Komazaki S, Hirose K, Nishi M, Noda T, Iino M. *EMBO J.* 1998;17:3309-16.
424. Coussin F, Macrez N, Morel JL, Mironneau J. *J Biol Chem.* 2000;275:9596-603.
425. Mironneau J, Coussin F, Jeyakumar LH, Fleischer S, Mironneau C, Macrez N. *J Biol Chem.* 2001;276:11257-64.
426. Ito K, Takakura S, Sato K, Sutko JL. *Circ Res.* 1986;58:730-4.
427. Ito K, Ikemoto T, Takakura S. *Am J Physiol.* 1991;261:H1464-70.
428. Itoh T, Kuriyama H, Suzuki H. *J Physiol.* 1981;321:513-35.
429. Benham CD, Bolton TB. *J Physiol.* 1986;381:385-406.
430. Bolton TB, Imaizumi Y. *Cell Calcium.* 1996;20:141-52.
431. Hisada T, Kurachi Y, Sugimoto T. *Pflugers Arch.* 1990;416:151-61.
432. Ohya Y, Kitamura K, Kuriyama H. *Am J Physiol.* 1987;252:C401-10.
433. Saunders HM, Farley JM. *J Pharmacol Exp Ther.* 1991;257:1114-20.
434. Nelson MT, Quayle JM. *Am. J. Physiol.* 1995;268:C799-C822.
435. Hume JR, Leblanc N. *J Physiol.* 1989;413:49-73.
436. Porter VA, Bonev AD, Knot HJ, Heppner TJ, Stevenson AS, Kleppisch T, Lederer WJ, Nelson MT. *Am J Physiol.* 1998;274:C1346-55.
437. Perez GJ, Bonev AD, Nelson MT. *Am J Physiol Cell Physiol.* 2001;281:C1769-75.
438. Thastrup O, Dawson AP, Scharff O, Foder B, Cullen PJ, Drobak BK, Bjerrum PJ, Christensen SB, Hanley MR. *Agents Actions.* 1989;27:17-23.
439. Ganitkevich VY, Isenberg G. *J Physiol.* 1996;490:305-18.
440. Mironneau J, Arnaudeau S, Macrez-Lepretre N, Boittin FX. *Cell Calcium.* 1996;20:153-60.
441. Gordienko DV, Bolton TB. *J Physiol.* 2002;542:743-62.
442. Herrera GM, Heppner TJ, Nelson MT. *Am J Physiol Cell Physiol.* 2001;280:C481-90.
443. Ji G, Barsotti RJ, Feldman ME, Kotlikoff MI. *J Gen Physiol.* 2002;119:533-44.
444. Ji G, Feldman ME, Greene KS, Sorrentino V, Xin HB, Kotlikoff MI. *J Gen Physiol.* 2004;123:377-86.
445. Gordienko DV, Bolton TB, Cannell MB. *J Physiol.* 1998;507 (Pt 3):707-20.
446. Kirber MT, Etter EF, Bellve KA, Lifshitz LM, Tuft RA, Fay FS, Walsh JV, Fogarty KE. *J Physiol.* 2001;531:315-27.
447. ZhuGe R, Tuft RA, Fogarty KE, Bellve K, Fay FS, Walsh JV. *J Gen Physiol.* 1999;113:215-28.

448. Wellman GC, Cartin L, Eckman DM, Stevenson AS, Saundry CM, Lederer WJ, Nelson MT. *Am J Physiol Heart Circ Physiol.* 2001;281:H2559-67.
449. Collier ML, Ji G, Wang Y, Kotlikoff MI. *J Gen Physiol.* 2000;115:653-62.
450. Itoh T, Ueno H, Kuriyama H. *Experientia.* 1985;41:989-96.
451. Somlyo A. *Circ Res.* 1985;57:497-507.
452. Matsumoto H, Baron CB, Coburn RF. *Am J Physiol.* 1995;268:C458-65.
453. Itoh T, Seki N, Suzuki S, Ito S, Kajikuri J, Kuriyama H. *J Physiol.* 1992;451:307-28.
454. Ganitkevich V, Isenberg G. *J Physiol.* 1993;470:35-44.
455. Ganitkevich V, Isenberg G. *J Physiol.* 1995;484:287-306.
456. Iino M. *J Gen Physiol.* 1989;94:363-83.
457. Imaizumi Y, Torii Y, Ohi Y, Nagano N, Atsuki K, Yamamura H, Muraki K, Watanabe M, Bolton TB. *J Physiol.* 1998;510:705-19.
458. Kirber MT, Guerrero-Hernandez A, Bowman DS, Fogarty KE, Tuft RA, Singer JJ, Fay FS. *J Physiol.* 2000;524:3-17.
459. Wang SQ, Song LS, Lakatta EG, Cheng H. *Nature.* 2001;410:592-96.
460. Bayliss WM. *J. Physiol.* 1902;28:220-231.
461. Nelson MT. *J Physiol.* 1998;507 (Pt 3):629.
462. Nelson MT, Standen NB, Brayden JE, Worley JF, 3rd. *Nature.* 1988;336:382-5.
463. Jaggar JH. *Am J Physiol Cell Physiol.* 2001;281:C439-48.
464. Knot HJ, Standen NB, Nelson MT. *J Physiol (Lond).* 1998;508:211-21.
465. Guia A, Wan X, Courtemanche M, Leblanc N. *Circ Res.* 1999;84:1032-42.
466. ZhuGe R, Sims SM, Tuft RA, Fogarty KE, Walsh JV, Jr. *J Physiol.* 1998;513:711-18.
467. Herrera GM, Nelson MT. *J Physiol.* 2002;541:483-92.
468. Liu G, Shi J, Yang L, Cao L, Park SM, Cui J, Marx SO. *EMBO J.* 2004;23:2196-205.
469. Perez GJ, Bonev AD, Patlak JB, Nelson MT. *J Gen Physiol.* 1999;113:229-38.
470. Brenner R, Perez GJ, Bonev AD, Eckman DM, Kosek JC, Wiler SW, Patterson AJ, Nelson MT, Aldrich RW. *Nature.* 2000;407:870-876.
471. Bonev AD, Jaggar JH, Rubart M, Nelson MT. *Am J Physiol.* 1997;273:C2090-95.
472. Bito H, Deisseroth K, Tsien RW. *Cell.* 1996;87:1203-14.
473. Deisseroth K, Heist EK, Tsien RW. *Nature.* 1998;392:198-202.
474. Sorrentino V. *Front Biosci.* 2003;8:d176-82.
475. Ogawa Y, Murayama T, Kurebayashi N. *Front Biosci.* 2002;7:d1184-94.
476. Bertocchini F, Ovitt CE, Conti A, Barone V, Scholer HR, Bottinelli R, Reggiani C, Sorrentino V. *Embo J.* 1997;16:6956-63.
477. Balschun D, Wolfer DP, Bertocchini F, Barone V, Conti A, Zuschratter W, Missiaen L, Lipp HP, Frey JU, Sorrentino V. *EMBO J.* 1999;18:5264-73.
478. Futatsugi A, Kato K, Ogura H, Li ST, Nagata E, Kuwajima G, Tanaka K, Itohara S, Mikoshiba K. *Neuron.* 1999;24:701-13.
479. Xiao B, Masumiya H, Jiang D, Wang R, Sei Y, Zhang L, Murayama T, Ogawa Y, Lai FA, Wagenknecht T, Chen SR. *J Biol Chem.* 2002;277:41778-85.
480. Murayama T, Ogawa Y. *J Biol Chem.* 1996;271:5079-84.
481. Flucher BE, Conti A, Takeshima H, Sorrentino V. *J Cell Biol.* 1999;146:621-29.
482. Fessenden JD, Wang Y, Moore RA, Chen SR, Allen PD, Pessah IN. *Biophys J.* 2000;79:2509-25.
483. Jeyakumar LH, Copello JA, O'Malley AM, Wu GM, Grassucci R, Wagenknecht T, Fleischer S. *J Biol Chem.* 1998;273:16011-20.

484. Pessah IN, Kim KH, Feng W. *Front Biosci.* 2002;7:a72-9.
485. Murayama T, Ogawa Y. *J Biol Chem.* 2001;276:2953-60.
486. Murayama T, Ogawa Y. *Am J Physiol Cell Physiol.* 2004;287:C36-45.
487. Lee EH, Lopez JR, Li J, Protasi F, Pessah IN, Kim DH, Allen PD. *Am J Physiol Cell Physiol.* 2004;286:C179-89.
488. Rios E, Brum G. *Front Biosci.* 2002;7:d1195-211.
489. Ogawa Y, Murayama T, Kurebayashi N. *Mol Cell Biochem.* 1999;190:191-201.
490. Rossi R, Bottinelli R, Sorrentino V, Reggiani C. *Am J Physiol Cell Physiol.* 2001;281:C585-94.
491. Conklin MW, Ahern CA, Vallejo P, Sorrentino V, Takeshima H, Coronado R. *Biophys J.* 2000;78:1777-85.
492. Perez CF, Voss A, Pessah IN, Allen PD. *Biophys J.* 2003;84:2655-63.
493. Rossi D, Simeoni I, Micheli M, Bootman M, Lipp P, Allen PD, Sorrentino V. *J Cell Sci.* 2002;115:2497-504.
494. Yang D, Pan Z, Takeshima H, Wu C, Nagaraj RY, Ma J, Cheng H. *J Biol Chem.* 2001;276:40210-4.
495. Takekura H, Flucher BE, Franzini-Armstrong C. *Dev Biol.* 2001;239:204-14.
496. Takeshima H. *Ann N Y Acad Sci.* 1993;707:165-77.
497. Sakube Y, Ando H, Kagawa H. *J Mol Biol.* 1997;267:849-64.
498. Fleig A, Takeshima H, Penner R. *J Physiol.* 1996;496:339-45.
499. Yamazawa T, Takeshima H, Sakurai T, Endo M, Iino M. *EMBO J.* 1996;15:6172-7.
500. Moore RA, Nguyen H, Galgaran J, Pessah IN, Allen PD. *J Cell Biol.* 1998;140:843-51.
501. Adachi-Akahane S, Cleemann L, Morad M. *Am J Physiol.* 1999;276:H1178-89.
502. Uehara A, Yasukochi M, Imanaga I, Nishi M, Takeshima H. *Cell Calcium.* 2002;31:89-96.
503. Ikemoto T, Komazaki S, Takeshima H, Nishi M, Noda T, Iino M, Endo M. *J Physiol (Lond).* 1997;501:305-12.
504. Clancy JS, Takeshima H, Hamilton SL, Reid MB. *Am J Physiol.* 1999;277:R1205-9.
505. Kouzu Y, Moriya T, Takeshima H, Yoshioka T, Shibata S. *Brain Res Mol Brain Res.* 2000;76:142-50.
506. Shimuta M, Yoshikawa M, Fukaya M, Watanabe M, Takeshima H, Manabe T. *Mol Cell Neurosci.* 2001;17:921-30.
507. Komazaki S, Ikemoto T, Takeshima H, Iino M, Endo M, Nakamura H. *Cell Tissue Res.* 1998;294:467-73.
508. Nishi M, Komazaki S, Iino M, Kangawa K, Takeshima H. *FEBS Lett.* 1998;432:191-6.
509. Nishi M, Mizushima A, Nakagawara K, Takeshima H. *Biochem Biophys Res Commun.* 2000;273:920-7.
510. Nishi M, Sakagami H, Komazaki S, Kondo H, Takeshima H. *Brain Res Mol Brain Res.* 2003;118:102-10.
511. Yoshida M, Sugimoto A, Ohshima Y, Takeshima H. *Biochem Biophys Res Commun.* 2001;289:234-9.
512. Komazaki S, Ito K, Takeshima H, Nakamura H. *FEBS Lett.* 2002;524:225-9.
513. Ito K, Komazaki S, Sasamoto K, Yoshida M, Nishi M, Kitamura K, Takeshima H. *J Cell Biol.* 2001;154:1059-67.
514. Komazaki S, Nishi M, Takeshima H. *FEBS Lett.* 2003;542:69-73.
515. Nishi M, Hashimoto K, Kuriyama K, Komazaki S, Kano M, Shibata S, Takeshima H. *Biochem Biophys Res Commun.* 2002;292:318-24.

516. Fabiato A. *Am J Physiol.* 1983;245:C1-C14.
517. Endo M, Tanaka M, Ogawa Y. *Nature.* 1970;228:34-36.
518. Coronado R, Morrissette J, Sukhareva M, Vaughan DM. *Am J Physiol.* 1994;266:C1485-504.
519. Diaz-Munoz M, Hamilton S, Kaetzel M, Hazarika P, Dedman J. *J. Biol. Chem.* 1990;265:15894-15899.
520. Knudson CM, Stang KK, Jorgenson AO, Campbell KP. *J. Biol. Chem.* 1993;268:12646-12645.
521. Lokuta AJ, Meyers MB, Sander PR, Fishman GI, Valdivia HH. *J. Biol. Chem.* 1997;272:25333-8.
522. Brillantes AB, Ondrias K, Scott A, Kobrinsky E, Ondriasova E, Moschella MC, Jayaraman T, Landers M, Ehrlich BE, Marks AR. *Cell.* 1994;77:513-23.
523. Currie S, Loughrey CM, Craig MA, Smith GL. *Biochem J.* 2004;377:357-66.
524. Wehrens XH, Marks AR. *Nat Rev Drug Discov.* 2004;In press.
525. Zaccolo M, Pozzan T. *Science.* 2002;295:1711-5.
526. Berridge MJ. *Cell Calcium.* 1996;20:95-6.
527. DeSouza N, Reiken S, Ondrias K, Yang YM, Matkovich S, Marks AR. *J Biol Chem.* 2002;277:39397-39400.
528. Marx SO, Kurokawa J, Reiken S, Motoike H, D'Armiento J, Marks AR, Kass RS. *Science.* 2002;295:496-9.
529. Hulme JT, Lin TW, Westenbroek RE, Scheuer T, Catterall WA. *Proc Natl Acad Sci U S A.* 2003;100:13093-8.
530. Allen P, Ouimet C, Greengard P. *Proc. Natl. Acad. Sci. USA.* 1997;94:9956-9961.
531. Jayaraman T, Brillantes AM, Timerman AP, Erdjument-Bromage H, Fleischer S, Tempst P, Marks AR. *J Biol Chem.* 1992;267:9474-77.
532. Timerman AP, Ogunbumni E, Freund E, Wiederrecht G, Marks AR, Fleischer S. *Journal of Biological Chemistry.* 1993;268:22992-9.
533. Timerman AP, Onoue H, Xin HB, Barg S, Copello J, Wiederrecht G, Fleischer S. *J Biol Chem.* 1996;271:20385-91.
534. Van Acker K, Bultynck G, Rossi D, Sorrentino V, Boens N, Missiaen L, De Smedt H, Parys JB, Callewaert G. *J Cell Sci.* 2004;117:1129-37.
535. Jeyakumar LH, Ballester L, Cheng DS, McIntyre JO, Chang P, Olivey HE, Rollins-Smith L, Barnett JV, Murray K, Xin HB, Fleischer S. *Biochem Biophys Res Commun.* 2001;281:979-986.
536. Gaburjakova M, Gaburjakova J, Reiken S, Huang F, Marx SO, Rosemblit N, Marks AR. *J Biol Chem.* 2001;276:16931-5.
537. Bultynck G, Rossi D, Callewaert G, Missiaen L, Sorrentino V, Parys JB, De Smedt H. *J Biol Chem.* 2001;276:47715-24.
538. Masumiya H, Wang R, Zhang J, Xiao B, Chen SR. *J Biol Chem.* 2003;278:3786-92.
539. Porter Moore C, Zhang JZ, Hamilton SL. *J Biol Chem.* 1999;274:36831-4.
540. Moore CP, Rodney G, Zhang JZ, Santacruz-Toloza L, Strasburg G, Hamilton SL. *Biochemistry.* 1999;38:8532-7.
541. Zhang H, Zhang JZ, Danila CI, Hamilton SL. *J Biol Chem.* 2003;278:8348-55.
542. Meyers MB, Pickel VM, Sheu SS, Sharma VK, Scotto KW, Fishman GI. *J Biol Chem.* 1995;270:26411-8.
543. Meyers MB, Puri TS, Chien AJ, Gao T, Hsu PH, Hosey MM, Fishman GI. *J Biol Chem.* 1998;273:18930-5.
544. Collins J, Tarcsafalvi A, Ikemoto N. *Biochem Biophys Res Commun.* 1990;167:189-193.
545. Culligan K, Banville N, Dowling P, Ohlendieck K. *J Appl Physiol.* 2002;92:435-45.

546. Ohkura M, Furukawa K, Fujimori H, Kuruma A, Kawano S, Hiraoka M, Kuniyasu A, Nakayama H, Ohizumi Y. *Biochemistry.* 1998;37:12987-93.
547. Szegedi C, Sarkozi S, Herzog A, Jona I, Varsanyi M. *Biochem J.* 1999;337:19-22.
548. Beard NA, Laver DR, Dulhunty AF. *Prog Biophys Mol Biol.* 2004;85:33-69.
549. Hain J, Nath S, Mayrleitner M, Fleischer S, Schindler H. *Biophys J.* 1994;67:1823-33.
550. Marks AR. *J Mol Cell Cardiol.* 2001;33:615-24.
551. Wehrens XH, Marks AR. *Trends Biochem Sci.* 2003;28:671-8.
552. Lakatta EG. *Cell Calcium.* 2004;35:629-42.
553. Zhou YY, Song LS, Lakatta EG, Xiao RP, Cheng H. *J Physiol.* 1999;521:351-61.
554. Witcher DR, Strifler BA, Jones LR. *J. Biol. Chem.* 1992;267:4963-7.
555. Reiken S, Lacampagne A, Zhou H, Kherani A, Lehnart SE, Ward C, Huang F, Gaburjakova M, Gaburjakova J, Rosemblit N, Warren MS, He KL, Yi GH, Wang J, Burkhoff D, Vassort G, Marks AR. *J Cell Biol.* 2003;160:919-28.
556. Sonnleitner A, Fleischer S, Schindler H. *Cell Calcium.* 1997;21:283-90.
557. Yoshida A, Takahashi M, Imagawa T, Shigekawa M, Takisawa H, Nakamura T. *J Biochem (Tokyo).* 1992;111:186-90.
558. Bers DM. *Front Biosci.* 2002;7:d1697-711.
559. Kaftan E, Marks AR, Ehrlich BE. *Circ Res.* 1996;78:990-97.
560. Jiang MT, Lokuta AJ, Farrell EF, Wolff MR, Haworth RA, Valdivia HH. *Circ Res.* 2002;91:1015-22.
561. Marks AR. *Front Biosci.* 2002;7:D970-77.
562. McCall E, Li L, Satoh H, Shannon TR, Blatter LA, Bers DM. *Circ Res.* 1996;79:1110-21.
563. Ahern GP, Junankar PR, Dulhunty AF. *FEBS Letters.* 1994;352:369-74.
564. Ahern GP, Junankar PR, Dulhunty AF. *Biophys J.* 1997;72:146-62.
565. Wang SQ, Stern MD, Rios E, Cheng H. *Proc Natl Acad Sci U S A.* 2004;101:3979-84.
566. Maier LS, Bers DM. *J Mol Cell Cardiol.* 2002;34:919-39.
567. Bowditch HP. *Arbeit aus der Physiologischen Anstalt zu Leipzig.* 1871;6:139-176.
568. Dulhunty AF, Laver D, Curtis SM, Pace S, Haarmann C, Gallant EM. *Biophys J.* 2001;81:3240-52.
569. Zhao S, Brandt NR, Caswell AH, Lee EY. *Biochemistry.* 1998;37:18102-9.
570. Neumann J, Boknik P, Herzig S, Schmitz W, Scholz H, Gupta RC, Watanabe AM. *Am J Physiol.* 1993;265:H257-66.
571. Carr AN, Schmidt AG, Suzuki Y, del Monte F, Sato Y, Lanner C, Breeden K, Jing SL, Allen PB, Greengard P, Yatani A, Hoit BD, Grupp IL, Hajjar RJ, DePaoli-Roach AA, Kranias EG. *Mol Cell Biol.* 2002;22:4124-35.
572. Santana LF, Chase EG, Votaw VS, Nelson MT, Greven R. *J Physiol.* 2002;544:57-69.
573. Lehnart SE, Wehrens XHT, Laitinen PJ, Reiken SR, Deng SX, Chen Z, Landry DW, Kontula K, Swan H, Marks AR. *Circulation.* 2004:r113-19.
574. Laver DR, Baynes TM, Dulhunty AF. *J Membr Biol.* 1997;156:213-29.
575. Meissner G, Rios E, Tripathy A, Pasek DA. *J Biol Chem.* 1997;272:1628-38.
576. Kawano S. *Receptors Channels.* 1998;5:405-16.
577. Hayek SM, Zhu X, Bhat MB, Zhao J, Takeshima H, Valdivia HH, Ma J. *Biochem J.* 2000;351:57-65.
578. Li P, Chen SR. *J Gen Physiol.* 2001;118:33-44.
579. Lacampagne A, Klein MG, Schneider MF. *J Gen Physiol.* 1998;111:207-24.

580. Laver DR, Owen VJ, Junankar PR, Taske NL, Dulhunty AF, Lamb GD. *Biophys J.* 1997;73:1913-24.
581. MacKrill JJ. *Biochem J.* 1999;337:345-61.
582. Bahler M, Rhoads A. *FEBS Lett.* 2002;513:107-13.
583. Hoeflich KP, Ikura M. *Cell.* 2002;108:739-42.
584. Vetter SW, Leclerc E. *Eur J Biochem.* 2003;270:404-14.
585. Zamponi GW. *Neuron.* 2003;39:879-81.
586. Babu YS, Bugg CE, Cook WJ. *J Mol Biol.* 1988;204:191-204.
587. Zhang M, Tanaka T, Ikura M. *Nat Struct Biol.* 1995;2:758-67.
588. Ikura M, Clore GM, Gronenborn AM, Zhu G, Klee CB, Bax A. *Science.* 1992;256:632-8.
589. Rhoads AR, Friedberg F. *Faseb J.* 1997;11:331-40.
590. Wu X, Reid RE. *Biochemistry.* 1997;36:3608-16.
591. Black DJ, Tikunova SB, Johnson JD, Davis JP. *Biochemistry.* 2000;39:13831-7.
592. Meissner G. *Biochemistry.* 1986;25:244-51.
593. Tripathy A, Xu L, Mann G, Meissner G. *Biophys J.* 1995;69:106-19.
594. Rodney GG, Williams BY, Strasburg GM, Beckingham K, Hamilton SL. *Biochemistry.* 2000;39:7807-12.
595. Beckingham K. *J Biol Chem.* 1991;266:6027-30.
596. Martin SR, Maune JF, Beckingham K, Bayley PM. *Eur J Biochem.* 1992;205:1107-14.
597. Mukherjea P, Maune JF, Beckingham K. *Protein Sci.* 1996;5:468-77.
598. Rodney GG, Krol J, Williams B, Beckingham K, Hamilton SL. *Biochemistry.* 2001;40:12430-5.
599. Pate P, Mochca-Morales J, Wu Y, Zhang JZ, Rodney GG, Serysheva, II, Williams BY, Anderson ME, Hamilton SL. *J Biol Chem.* 2000;275:39786-92.
600. Xiong LW, Newman RA, Rodney GG, Thomas O, Zhang JZ, Persechini A, Shea MA, Hamilton SL. *J Biol Chem.* 2002;277:40862-70.
601. Yamaguchi N, Xin C, Meissner G. *J Biol Chem.* 2001;276:22579-85.
602. Moore CP, Zhang JZ, Hamilton SL. *J Biol Chem.* 1999;274:36831-34.
603. Zhang JZ, Wu Y, Williams BY, Rodney G, Mandel F, Strasburg GM, Hamilton SL. *Am J Physiol.* 1999;276:C46-53.
604. Xia R, Stangler T, Abramson JJ. *J Biol Chem.* 2000;275:36556-61.
605. Hidalgo C, Aracena P, Sanchez G, Donoso P. *Biol Res.* 2002;35:183-93.
606. Wu Y, Aghdasi B, Dou SJ, Zhang JZ, Liu SQ, Hamilton SL. *J Biol Chem.* 1997;272:25051-61.
607. Zaidi NF, Lagenaur CF, Abramson JJ, Pessah I, Salama G. *J Biol Chem.* 1989;264:21725-36.
608. Liu G, Abramson JJ, Zable AC, Pessah IN. *Mol Pharmacol.* 1994;45:189-200.
609. Feng W, Liu G, Allen PD, Pessah IN. *J Biol Chem.* 2000;275:35902-7.
610. Hamilton SL, Reid MB. *Antioxid Redox Signal.* 2000;2:41-5.
611. Xu L, Eu JP, Meissner G, Stamler JS. *Science.* 1998;279:234-37.
612. Eu JP, Sun J, Xu L, Stamler JS, Meissner G. *Cell.* 2000;102:499-509.
613. Aracena P, Sanchez G, Donoso P, Hamilton SL, Hidalgo C. *J Biol Chem.* 2003;278:42927-35.
614. Marengo JJ, Hidalgo C, Bull R. *Biophys J.* 1998;74:1263-77.
615. Oba T, Murayama T, Ogawa Y. *Am J Physiol Cell Physiol.* 2002;282:C684-92.
616. Sun J, Xin C, Eu JP, Stamler JS, Meissner G. *Proc Natl Acad Sci U S A.* 2001;98:11158-62.
617. Sun J, Xu L, Eu JP, Stamler JS, Meissner G. *J Biol Chem.* 2003;278:8184-9.
618. Zuhlke RD, Reuter H. *Proc Natl Acad Sci U S A.* 1998;95:3287-94.

619. Pitt GS, Zuhlke RD, Hudmon A, Schulman H, Reuter H, Tsien RW. *J Biol Chem.* 2001;276:30794-802.
620. Sencer S, Papineni RV, Halling DB, Pate P, Krol J, Zhang JZ, Hamilton SL. *J Biol Chem.* 2001;276:38237-41.
621. O'Connell KM, Yamaguchi N, Meissner G, Dirksen RT. *J Gen Physiol.* 2002;120:337-47.
622. Lewis GP. *Mediators of inflammation.* Bristol, UK: Wright; 1986.
623. Lane SJ, Lee TH. *J Allergy Clin Immunol.* 1996;98:S67-S71.
624. Gallin JI, Snuyderman R. *Inflammation: Basic principals and clinical correlates.* Philadephia, PA: Lippincott Williams & Wilkins; 1999.
625. Trowbridge HO, Emling R. *Inflammation: A review of the process.* Chicago, IL: Quintessence Books; 1997.
626. Pricop L, Salmon JE. *Antioxid Redox Signal.* 2002;4:85-95.
627. Thollon C, Iliou JP, Cambarrat C, Robin F, Vilaine JP. *Cardiovasc Res.* 1995;30:648-55.
628. Dvorak AM. *Prog Histochem Cytochem.* 1998;33:169-320.
629. Perez RL, Rivera-Marrero CA, Roman J. *Semin Respir Infect.* 2003;18:23-32.
630. Schins RP. *Inhal Toxicol.* 2002;14:57-78.
631. Shiels IA, Taylor SM, Fairlie DP. *Med Hypotheses.* 2000;54:193-7.
632. Hyvelin JM, Martin C, Roux E, Marthan R, Savineau JP. *Am J Respir Crit Care Med.* 2000;162:687-94.
633. Partida-Sanchez S, Cockayne DA, Monard S, Jacobson EL, Oppenheimer N, Garvy B, Kusser K, Goodrich S, Howard M, Harmsen A, Randall TD, Lund FE. *Nat Med.* 2001;7:1209-16.
634. Hosoi E, Nishizaki C, Gallagher KL, Wyre HW, Matsuo Y, Sei Y. *J Immunol.* 2001;167:4887-94.
635. Moonga BS, Li S, Iqbal J, Davidson R, Shankar VS, Bevis PJ, Inzerillo A, Abe E, Huang CL, Zaidi M. *Am J Physiol Renal Physiol.* 2002;282:F921-32.
636. Rang HP, Urban L. *Br J Anaesth.* 1995;75:145-56.
637. Marone G, Casolaro V, Cirillo R, Stellato C, Genovese A. *Clin Immunol Immunopathol.* 1989;50:S24-40.
638. Barrett KE. *World J Gastroenterol.* 2004;10:617-9.
639. Schwartz LB. *Curr Opin Immunol.* 1994;6:91-7.
640. Metcalf D. *Ciba Found Symp.* 1997;204:40-50.
641. De Backer MD, Loonen I, Verhasselt P, Neefs JM, Luyten WH. *Biochem J.* 1998;335:663-70.
642. Brown N, Robers L. Histamine, bradykinin, and their antagonists. In: Hardman J, Limbird L, Gilman A, eds. *Goodman and Gilman's pharmacological basis of therapeutics.* USA: McGraw-Hill; 2001.
643. Gokina NI, Bevan JA. *Am J Physiol Heart Circ Physiol.* 2000;278:H2105-14.
644. Maton PN, Burton ME. *Drugs.* 1999;57:855-70.
645. Wang LD, Gantz I, Butler K, Hoeltzel M, Del Valle J. *Biochem Biophys Res Commun.* 2000;276:539-45.
646. del Rio E, McLaughlin M, Downes CP, Nicholls DG. *Eur J Neurosci.* 1999;11:3015-22.
647. Rueda A, Garcia L, Soria-Jasso LE, Arias-Montano JA, Guerrero-Hernandez A. *Cell Calcium.* 2002;31:161-73.
648. Nathan C, Xie QW. *Cell.* 1994;78:915-8.
649. Kaminski HJ, Andrade FH. *Neuromuscul Disord.* 2001;11:517-24.
650. Beckman J. Physiological and pathological chemistry of nitric oxide. In: Lancaster J, ed. *Nitric oxide principals and action.* San Diego, CA: Academic Press; 1996:1-82.

651. Stuehr DJ, Marletta MA. *Proc Natl Acad Sci U S A*. 1985;82:7738-42.
652. Moncada S, Palmer RM, Higgs EA. *Pharmacol Rev*. 1991;43:109-42.
653. Langrehr JM, Hoffman RA, Lancaster JR, Jr., Simmons RL. *Transplantation*. 1993;55:1205-12.
654. Bogdan C, Rollinghoff M, Diefenbach A. *Curr Opin Immunol*. 2000;12:64-76.
655. Garcia-Cardena G, Martasek P, Masters BS, Skidd PM, Couet J, Li S, Lisanti MP, Sessa WC. *J Biol Chem*. 1997;272:25437-40.
656. Kobzik L, Stringer B, Balligand JL, Reid MB, Stamler JS. *Biochem Biophys Res Commun*. 1995;211:375-81.
657. Bidri M, Feger F, Varadaradjalou S, Ben Hamouda N, Guillosson JJ, Arock M. *Int Immunopharmacol*. 2001;1:1543-58.
658. Coleman JW. *Clin Exp Immunol*. 2002;129:4-10.
659. Kobzik L, Reid MB, Bredt DS, Stamler JS. *Nature*. 1994;372:546-8.
660. Meszaros LG, Minarovic I, Zahradnikova A. *FEBS Lett*. 1996;380:49-52.
661. Zahradnikova A, Minarovic I, Venema RC, Meszaros LG. *Cell Calcium*. 1997;22:447-54.
662. Bao JX, Kandel ER, Hawkins RD. *Science*. 1997;275:969-73.
663. Hawkins RD, Son H, Arancio O. *Prog Brain Res*. 1998;118:155-72.
664. Jin I, Hawkins RD. *J Neurosci*. 2003;23:7288-97.
665. Lang E, Novak A, Reeh PW, Handwerker HO. *J Neurophysiol*. 1990;63:887-901.
666. Fock S, Mense S. *Brain Res*. 1976;105:459-69.
667. Nishi K, Sakanashi M, Takenaka F. *Pflugers Arch*. 1977;372:53-61.
668. Kanaka R, Schaible HG, Schmidt RF. *Brain Res*. 1985;327:81-90.
669. Longhurst JC, Kaufman MP, Ordway GA, Musch TI. *Am J Physiol*. 1984;247:R552-9.
670. Stewart JM. In: Henson PM, Murphy RC, eds. *Mediators of the inflammatory process*. Amsterdam, Netherlands: Elsevier; 1989:189-217.
671. Marceau F, Hess JF, Bachvarov DR. *Pharmacol Rev*. 1998;50:357-86.
672. Hall J, Morton I. The pharmacology and immunopharmacology of kinin receptors. In: Farmer S, ed. *The handbook of immunopharmacology: The kinin system*. London, United Kingdom: Acedemic Press; 1997:9-43.
673. Kaplan A, Joseph K, Shibayama Y, Nakazawa Y, Ghebrehiwet B, Reddigari S, Silverberg M. Bradykinin formation: Plasma and tissue pathways and cellular interactions. In: Gallin JI, Snyderman R, eds. *Inflammation: Basic principals and clinical correlates*. Philadelphia: Lippincott Williams & Wilkins; 1999:311-347.
674. Bhoola KD, Figueroa CD, Worthy K. *Pharmacol Rev*. 1992;44:1-80.
675. Schremmer-Danninger E, Offner A, Siebeck M, Roscher AA. *Biochem Biophys Res Commun*. 1998;243:246-52.
676. Foucart S, Grondin L, Couture R, Nadeau R. *Can J Physiol Pharmacol*. 1997;75:639-45.
677. Watson SP, Arkinstall L. Bradykinin. In: *The G protein-linked receptor factsbook*. London: Academic Press; 1994:67-77.
678. McGuirk SM, Dolphin AC. *Neuroscience*. 1992;49:117-28.
679. Ronde P, Dougherty JJ, Nichols RA. *J Physiol*. 2000;529:307-19.
680. Shuttleworth TJ. *J Biol Chem*. 1996;271:21720-5.
681. Mignen O, Shuttleworth TJ. *J Biol Chem*. 2000;275:9114-9.
682. Striggow F, Ehrlich BE. *Biochem Biophys Res Commun*. 1997;237:413-18.
683. Miller DK, Gillard JW, Vickers PJ, Sadowski S, Leveille C, Mancini JA, Charleson P, Dixon RA, Ford-Hutchinson AW, Fortin R, *et al*. *Nature*. 1990;343:278-81.

684. Dixon RA, Diehl RE, Opas E, Rands E, Vickers PJ, Evans JF, Gillard JW, Miller DK. *Nature.* 1990;343:282-4.

685. Matsumoto T, Funk CD, Radmark O, Hoog JO, Jornvall H, Samuelsson B. *Proc Natl Acad Sci U S A.* 1988;85:26-30.

686. Shimizu T, Radmark O, Samuelsson B. *Proc Natl Acad Sci U S A.* 1984;81:689-93.

687. Funk CD, Radmark O, Fu JY, Matsumoto T, Jornvall H, Shimizu T, Samuelsson B. *Proc Natl Acad Sci U S A.* 1987;84:6677-81.

688. Samuelsson B, Dahlen SE, Lindgren JA, Rouzer CA, Serhan CN. *Science.* 1987;237:1171-6.

689. Dahlen SE, Hedqvist P, Hammarstrom S, Samuelsson B. *Nature.* 1980;288:484-6.

690. Back M. *Life Sci.* 2002;71:611-22.

691. Kannan S. *Med Hypotheses.* 2002;59:261-5.

692. Bouchelouche K, Andersen L, Nordling J, Horn T, Bouchelouche P. *J Urol.* 2003;170:638-44.

693. Eun SY, Jung SJ, Park YK, Kwak J, Kim SJ, Kim J. *Biochem Biophys Res Commun.* 2001;285:1114-20.

694. Hwang SW, Cho H, Kwak J, Lee SY, Kang CJ, Jung J, Cho S, Min KH, Suh YG, Kim D, Oh U. *Proc Natl Acad Sci U S A.* 2000;97:6155-60.

695. Mehta K, Cheema S. *Leuk Lymphoma.* 1999;32:441-9.

696. Deshpande DA, Walseth TF, Panettieri RA, Kannan MS. *FASEB J.* 2003;17:452-54.

697. Howard M, Grimaldi JC, Bazan JF, Lund FE, Santos-Argumedo L, Parkhouse RM, Walseth TF, Lee HC. *Science.* 1993;262:1056-9.

698. Galione A, Lee HC, Busa WB. *Science.* 1991;253:1143-46.

699. Ozawa T. *Int J Mol Med.* 2001;7:21-25.

700. Lambert RK, Wiggs BR, Kuwano K, Hogg JC, Pare PD. *J Appl Physiol.* 1993;74:2771-81.

701. Ohlstein EH, Horohonich S, Hay DW. *J Pharmacol Exp Ther.* 1989;250:548-55.

702. Parameswaran K, Janssen LJ, O'Byrne PM. *Chest.* 2002;121:621-4.

703. Janssen LJ, Premji M, Lu-Chao H, Cox G, Keshavjee S. *Am J Physiol Lung Cell Mol Physiol.* 2000;278:L899-905.

704. Lee HC, Aarhus R, Graeff R, Gurnack ME, Walseth TF. *Nature.* 1994;370:307-9.

705. Guse AH. *Cell Signal.* 1999;11:309-16.

706. Dalpiaz A, Spisani S, Biondi C, Fabbri E, Nalli M, Ferretti ME. *Curr Drug Targets Immune Endocr Metabol Disord.* 2003;3:33-42.

707. Jenden DJ, Fairhurst AS. *Pharmacol Rev.* 1969;21:1-25.

708. Jones LR, Besch HR, Jr., Sutko JL, Willerson JT. *J Pharmacol Exp Ther.* 1979;209:48-55.

709. Bidasee KR, Besch HR, Jr. *J Biol Chem.* 1998;273:12176-86.

710. Tinker A, Sutko JL, Ruest L, Deslongchamps P, Welch W, Airey JA, Gerzon K, Bidasee KR, Besch HR, Jr., Williams AJ. *Biophys J.* 1996;70:2110-19.

711. Humerickhouse RA, Bidasee KR, Gerzon K, Emmick JT, Kwon S, Sutko JL, Ruest L, Besch HR. *J Biol Chem.* 1994;269:30243-53.

712. Buck E, Zimanyi I, Abramson JJ, Pessah IN. *J Biol Chem.* 1992;267:23560-67.

713. Gonzalez A, Kirsch WG, Shirokova N, Pizarro G, Brum G, Pessah IN, Stern MD, Cheng H, Rios E. *Proc Natl Acad Sci U S A.* 2000;97:4380-5.

714. Hui C, Besch HR, Jr., Bidasee KR. *Biophys J.* 2004;88:In press.

715. Callaway C, Slavik K, Wang D, Needleman T, Jayaraman T, Marks AR, Hamilton SL. *Biophys J.* 1994;66:A225.

716. Bidasee KR, Xu L, Meissner G, Besch HR, Jr. *J Biol Chem.* 2003;278:14237-48.

717. Humerickhouse RA, Besch HR, Jr., Gerzon K, Ruest L, Sutko JL, Emmick JT. *Mol Pharmacol.* 1993;44:412-21.
718. Dulhunty AF, Curtis SM, Watson S, Cengia L, Casarotto MG. *J Biol Chem.* 2004;279:11853-62.
719. Hill AP, Kingston O, Sitsapesan R. *Mol Pharmacol.* 2004;65:1258-68.
720. Tripathy A, Bidasee KR, Meissner G, Besch HR, Jr. *Biophys J.* 2000;78:A125.
721. Welch W, Ahmad S, Airey JA, Gerzon K, Humerickhouse RA, Besch HR, Jr., Ruest L, Deslongchamps P, Sutko JL. *Biochemistry.* 1994;33:6074-85.
722. Jefferies PR, Gengo PJ, Watson MJ, Casida JE. *J Med Chem.* 1996;39:2339-46.
723. Jefferies PR, Blumenkopf TA, Gengo PJ, Cole LC, Casida JE. *J Med Chem.* 1996;39:2331-8.
724. Welch W, Sutko JL, Mitchell KE, Airey J, Ruest L. *Biochemistry.* 1996;35:7165-73.
725. Bidasee KR, Xu L, Meissner G, Besch HR, Jr., Nallani K. *Biophys J.* 2002;82:113A.
726. Williams AJ. *Front Biosci.* 2002;7:d1223-30.
727. Blayney LM, Zissimopoulos S, Ralph E, Abbot E, Matthews L, Lai FA. *J Biol Chem.* 2004;279:14639-48.
728. Kohno M, Yano M, Kobayashi S, Doi M, Oda T, Tokuhisa T, Okuda S, Ohkusa T, Matsuzaki M. *Am J Physiol Heart Circ Physiol.* 2003;284:H1035-42.
729. Hille B. *Ion channels of excitable membranes.* 3rd ed. Sunderland: Sinauer Associates; 2001.
730. Possani LD, Becerril B, Tytgat J, Delepierre M. High affinity scorpion toxins for studying potassium and sodium channels. In: Lopatin A, Nichols CG, eds. *Methods in Pharmacology and Toxicology.* Totowa, NJ: Humana Press; 2001.
731. DeBin JA, Maggio JE, Strichartz GR. *Am J Physiol.* 1993;264:C361-9.
732. Gao YD, Garcia ML. *Proteins.* 2003;52:146-54.
733. Valdivia HH, Fuentes O, el-Hayek R, Morrissette J, Coronado R. *J Biol Chem.* 1991;266:19135-38.
734. Valdivia HH, Kirby MS, Lederer WJ, Coronado R. *Proc. Natl. Acad. Sci.* 1992;89:12185-12189.
735. Zamudio FZ, Conde R, Arevalo C, Becerril B, Martin BM, Valdivia HH, Possani LD. *J Biol Chem.* 1997;272:11886-94.
736. el-Hayek R, Lokuta AJ, Arevalo C, Valdivia HH. *J Biol Chem.* 1995;270:28696-28704.
737. Ji YH, Liu Y, Yu K, Ohishi T, Hoshino M, Mochizuki T, Yanaihara N. *Chin Sci Bull.* 1997;42:952-956.
738. Fajloun Z, Kharrat R, Chen L, Lecomte C, Di Luccio E, Bichet D, El Ayeb M, Rochat H, Allen PD, Pessah IN, De Waard M, Sabatier JM. *FEBS Lett.* 2000;469:179-85.
739. Zhu X, Zamudio FZ, Olbinski BA, Possani LD, Valdivia HH. *J Biol Chem.* 2004;279:26588-96.
740. Zamudio FZ, Gurrola GB, Arevalo C, Sreekumar R, Walker JW, Valdivia HH, Possani LD. *FEBS Lett.* 1997;405:385-89.
741. Menez A, Bontems F, Roumestand C, Gilquin B, Toma F. *Proc Royal Soc Edinburg.* 1992;99B:83-103.
742. Darbon H. *J Soc Biol.* 1999;193:445-50.
743. Narasimhan L, Singh J, Humblet C, Guruprasad K, Blundell T. *Nat Struct Biol.* 1994;1:850-2.
744. Pallaghy PK, Nielsen KJ, Craik DJ, Norton RS. *Protein Sci.* 1994;3:1833-9.
745. Lee CW, Lee EH, Takeuchi K, Takahashi H, Shimada I, Sato K, Shin SY, Kim do H, Kim JI. *Biochem J.* 2004;377:385-94.
746. Mosbah A, Kharrat R, Fajloun Z, Renisio JG, Blanc E, Sabatier JM, El Ayeb M, Darbon H. *Proteins.* 2000;40:436-42.
747. el-Hayek R, Antoniu B, Wang J, Hamilton SL, Ikemoto N. *J. Biol.Chem.* 1995;270:22116-8.

748. Gurrola GB, Arevalo C, Sreekumar R, Lokuta AJ, Walker JW, Valdivia HH. *J Biol Chem.* 1999;274:7879-86.
749. Esteve E, Smida-Rezgui S, Sarkozi S, Szegedi C, Regaya I, Chen L, Altafaj X, Rochat H, Allen P, Pessah IN, Marty I, Sabatier JM, Jona I, De Waard M, Ronjat M. *J Biol Chem.* 2003;278:37822-31.
750. Casarotto MG, Green D, Pace SM, Curtis SM, Dulhunty AF. *Biophys J.* 2001;80:2715-26.
751. Casarotto MG, Gibson F, Pace SM, Curtis SM, Mulcair M, Dulhunty AF. *J Biol Chem.* 2000;275:11631-37.
752. Green D, Pace S, Curtis SM, Sakowska M, Lamb GD, Dulhunty AF, Casarotto MG. *Biochem J.* 2003;370:517-27.
753. Bannister ML, Williams AJ, Sitsapesan R. *Biochem Biophys Res Commun.* 2004;314:667-74.
754. Tripathy A, Resch W, Xu L, Valdivia HH, Meissner G. *J Gen Physiol.* 1998;111:679-90.
755. Simeoni I, Rossi D, Zhu X, Garcia J, Valdivia HH, Sorrentino V. *FEBS Lett.* 2001;508:5-10.
756. Shtifman A, Ward CW, Wang J, Valdivia HH, Schneider MF. *Biophys J.* 2000;79:814-27.
757. Chen L, Esteve E, Sabatier JM, Ronjat M, De Waard M, Allen PD, Pessah IN. *J Biol Chem.* 2003;278:16095-106.
758. Richard JP, Melikov K, Vives E, Ramos C, Verbeure B, Gait MJ, Chernomordik LV, Lebleu B. *J Biol Chem.* 2003;278:585-90.
759. Lindgren M, Hallbrink M, Prochiantz A, Langel U. *Trends Pharmacol Sci.* 2000;21:99-103.
760. Mabrouk K, Van Rietschoten J, Vives E, Darbon H, Rochat H, Sabatier JM. *FEBS Lett.* 1991;289:13-7.
761. Beutner G, Sharma VK, Giovannucci DR, Yule DI, Sheu SS. *J Biol Chem.* 2001;10:10.
762. Abramson JJ, Salama G. *J Bioenerg Biomembr.* 1989;21:283-94.
763. Aghdasi B, Reid MB, Hamilton SL. *J Biol Chem.* 1997;272:25462-67.
764. Eu JP, Hare JM, Hess DT, Skaf M, Sun J, Cardenas-Navina I, Sun QA, Dewhirst M, Meissner G, Stamler JS. *Proc Natl Acad Sci U S A.* 2003;100:15229-34.
765. Hwang C, Sinskey AJ, Lodish HF. *Science.* 1992;257:1496-502.
766. Csala M, Fulceri R, Mandl J, Benedetti A, Banhegyi G. *Biochem Biophys Res Commun.* 2001;287:696-700.
767. Reid MB. *News Physiol Sci.* 1996;11:114-121.
768. Zima AV, Copello JA, Blatter LA. *J Physiol.* 2004;555:727-41.
769. Kawakami M, Okabe E. *Mol Pharmacol.* 1998;53:497-503.
770. Xia R, Webb JA, Gnall LL, Cutler K, Abramson JJ. *Am J Physiol Cell Physiol.* 2003;285:C215-21.
771. Zima AV, Copello JA, Blatter LA. *FEBS Lett.* 2003;547:32-6.
772. Cherednichenko G, Zima AV, Feng W, Schaefer S, Blatter LA, Pessah IN. *Circ Res.* 2004;94:478-86.
773. Park JW, Chun YS, Kim MS, Park YC, Kwak SJ, Park SC. *Int J Cardiol.* 1998;65:139-47.
774. Stamler JS, Meissner G. *Physiol Rev.* 2001;81:209-237.
775. Xu KY, Huso DL, Dawson TM, Bredt DS, Becker LC. *Proc Natl Acad Sci U S A.* 1999;96:657-62.
776. Barouch LA, Harrison RW, Skaf MW, Rosas GO, Cappola TP, Kobeissi ZA, Hobai IA, Lemmon CA, Burnett AL, O'Rourke B, Rodriguez ER, Huang PL, Lima JA, Berkowitz DE, Hare JM. *Nature.* 2002;416:337-9.
777. Kelly RA, Balligand JL, Smith TW. *Circ Res.* 1996;79:363-80.

778. Stamler JS, Lamas S, Fang FC. *Cell.* 2001;106:675-83.
779. Sun J, Xu L, Eu JP, Stamler JS, Meissner G. *J Biol Chem.* 2001;276:15625-30.
780. Wang P, Zweier JL. *J Biol Chem.* 1996;271:29223-30.
781. Stoyanovsky D, Murphy T, Anno PR, Kim YM, Salama G. *Cell Calcium.* 1997;21:19-29.
782. Hart JD, Dulhunty AF. *J Membr Biol.* 2000;173:227-36.
783. Suko J, Drobny H, Hellmann G. *Biochim Biophys Acta.* 1999;1451:271-87.
784. Ziolo MT, Katoh H, Bers DM. *Am J Physiol Heart Circ Physiol.* 2001;281:H2295-303.
785. Petroff MG, Kim SH, Pepe S, Dessy C, Marban E, Balligand JL, Sollott SJ. *Nat Cell Biol.* 2001;3:867-73.
786. mellitus Ecotdacod. *Diabetes Spectrum.* 2004;17:51-59.
787. Prout TE. *Md Med J.* 1990;39:933-7.
788. Turok DK, Ratcliffe SD, Baxley EG. *Am Fam Physician.* 2003;68:1767-72.
789. Mahgoub MA, Abd-Elfattah AS. *Mol Cell Biochem.* 1998;180:59-64.
790. Chatham JC, Forder JR, McNeill JH. *The diabetic heart.* Boston, MA: Kluwer Academic Press; 1996.
791. Chen S, Evans T, Mukherjee K, Karmazyn M, Chakrabarti S. *J Mol Cell Cardiol.* 2000;32:1621-9.
792. Sellers DJ, Chess-Williams R. *J Auton Pharmacol.* 2001;21:15-21.
793. Dincer UD, Bidasee KR, Guner S, Tay A, Ozcelikay AT, Altan VM. *Diabetes.* 2001;50:455-61.
794. Dhalla NS, Liu X, Panagia V, Takeda N. *Cardiovasc Res.* 1998;40:239-47.
795. Viberti G. *J Hypertens Suppl.* 2003;21 Suppl 1:S3-6.
796. Service FJ, O'Brien PC. *Diabetologia.* 2001;44:1215-20.
797. Arnold JM, Yusuf S, Young J, Mathew J, Johnstone D, Avezum A, Lonn E, Pogue J, Bosch J. *Circulation.* 2003;107:1284-90.
798. Okin PM, Devereux RB, Nieminen MS, Jern S, Oikarinen L, Viitasalo M, Toivonen L, Kjeldsen SE, Julius S, Dahlof B. *J Am Coll Cardiol.* 2001;38:514-20.
799. Keane WF, Lyle PA. *Am J Kidney Dis.* 2003;41:S22-5.
800. Athyros VG, Papageorgiou AA, Mercouris BR, Athyrou VV, Symeonidis AN, Basayannis EO, Demitriadis DS, Kontopoulos AG. *Curr Med Res Opin.* 2002;18:220-8.
801. Furberg CD, Psaty BM, Pahor M, Alderman MH. *Ann Intern Med.* 2001;135:1074-8.
802. Bell DS. *Ethn Dis.* 2002;12:S1-12-8.
803. Gaede P, Vedel P, Larsen N, Jensen GV, Parving HH, Pedersen O. *N Engl J Med.* 2003;348:383-93.
804. Yu Z, McNeill JH. *Can J Physiol Pharmacol.* 1991;69:1268-76.
805. Yu Z, Tibbits GF, McNeill JH. *Am J Physiol.* 1994;266:H2082-9.
806. Guner S, Arioglu E, Tay A, Tasdelen A, Aslamaci S, Bidasee KR, Dincer UD. *Mol Cell Biochem.* 2004;In press.
807. Razeghi P, Young ME, Cockrill TC, Frazier OH, Taegtmeyer H. *Circulation.* 2002;106:407-11.
808. Netticadan T, Temsah RM, Kent A, Elimban V, Dhalla NS. *Diabetes.* 2001;50:2133-8.
809. Teshima Y, Takahashi N, Saikawa T, Hara M, Yasunaga S, Hidaka S, Sakata T. *J Mol Cell Cardiol.* 2000;32:655-64.
810. Zhong Y, Ahmed S, Grupp IL, Matlib MA. *Am J Physiol Heart Circ Physiol.* 2001;281:H1137-47.
811. Bidasee KR, Dincer UD, Besch HR, Jr. *Mol Pharmacol.* 2001;60:1356-64.
812. Eisner DA, Diaz ME, O'Neill SC, Trafford AW. *J Mol Cell Cardiol.* 2000;32:1377-78.
813. Bidasee KR, Nallani K, Henry B, Dincer UD, Besch HR, Jr. *Mol Cell Biochem.* 2003;249:113-23.

814. Bidasee KR, Nallani K, Yu Y, Cocklin RR, Zhang Y, Wang M, Dincer UD, Besch HR, Jr. *Diabetes*. 2003;52:1825-36.

815. Fessenden JD, Chen L, Wang Y, Paolini C, Franzini-Armstrong C, Allen PD, Pessah IN. *Proc Natl Acad Sci U S A*. 2001;98:2865-70.

816. Eager KR, Roden LD, Dulhunty AF. *Am J Physiol*. 1997;272:C1908-18.

817. Droge W. *Physiol Rev*. 2002;82:47-95.

818. Bidasee KR, Nallani K, Besch HR, Jr., Dincer UD. *J Pharmacol Exp Ther*. 2003;305:989-98.

819. Ulrich P, Cerami A. *Recent Prog Horm Res*. 2001;56:1-21.

820. Gronert GA. Malignant hyperthermia. In: Engel AG, Franzini-Armstrong C, eds. *Myology*. New York: McGraw-Fill; 1994:1661-1678.

821. Ellis FR. *Br J Anaesth*. 1984;56:1181-82.

822. Larach MG. *Anesth Analg*. 1989;69:511-15.

823. Ording H, Brancadoro V, Cozzolino S, Ellis FR, Glauber V, Gonano EF, Halsall PJ, Hartung E, Heffron JJ, Heytens L, Kozak-Ribbens G, Kress H, Krivosic-Horber R, Lehmann-Horn F, Mortier W, Nivoche Y, Ranklev-Twetman E, Sigurdsson S, Snoeck M, Stieglitz P, Tegazzin V, Urwyler A, Wappler F. *Acta Anaesthesiol Scand*. 1997;41:955-66.

824. Allen GC, Larach MG, Kunselman AR. *Anesthesiology*. 1998;88:579-88.

825. Shuaib A, Paasuke RT, Brownell KW. *Medicine (Baltimore)*. 1987;66:389-96.

826. McCarthy TV, Healy JM, Heffron JJ, Lehane M, Deufel T, Lehmann-Horn F, Farrall M, Johnson K. *Nature*. 1990;343:562-4.

827. MacLennan DH, Duff C, Zorzato F, Fujii J, Phillips M, Korneluk RG, Frodis W, Britt BA, Worton RG. *Nature*. 1990;343:559-61.

828. Gillard EF, Otsu K, Fujii J, Duff C, de Leon S, Khanna VK, Britt BA, Worton RG, MacLennan DH. *Genomics*. 1992;13:1247-54.

829. Quane KA, Healy JM, Keating KE, Manning BM, Couch FJ, Palmucci LM, Doriguzzi C, Fagerlund TH, Berg K, Ording H, Bendixen D, Mortier W, Linz U, Muller CR, McCarthy TV. *Nat Genet*. 1993;5:51-55.

830. Zhang Y, Chen HS, Khanna VK, De Leon S, Phillips MS, Schappert K, Britt BA, Brownell KW, MacLennan DH. *Nat Genet*. 1993;5:46-49.

831. Roberts MC, Mickelson JR, Patterson EE, Nelson TE, Armstrong PJ, Brunson DB, Hogan K. *Anesthesiology*. 2001;95:716-25.

832. Levitt RC, Olckers A, Meyers S, Fletcher JE, Rosenberg H, Isaacs H, Meyers DA. *Genomics*. 1992;14:562-6.

833. Iles DE, Lehmann-Horn F, Scherer SW, Tsui LC, Olde Weghuis D, Suijkerbuijk RF, Heytens L, Mikala G, Schwartz A, Ellis FR, *et al*. *Hum Mol Genet*. 1994;3:969-75.

834. Sudbrak R, Procaccio V, Klausnitzer M, Curran JL, Monsieurs K, van Broeckhoven C, Ellis R, Heyetens L, Hartung EJ, Kozak-Ribbens G. *Am J Hum Genet*. 1995;56:684-91.

835. Robinson RL, Monnier N, Wolz W, Jung M, Reis A, Nuernberg G, Curran JL, Monsieurs K, Stieglitz P, Heytens L, Fricker R, van Broeckhoven C, Deufel T, Hopkins PM, Lunardi J, Mueller CR. *Hum Mol Genet*. 1997;6:953-61.

836. Monnier N, Procaccio V, Stieglitz P, Lunardi J. *Am J Hum Genet*. 1997;60:1316-25.

837. Robinson RL, Anetseder MJ, Brancadoro V, van Broekhoven C, Carsana A, Censier K, Fortunato G, Girard T, Heytens L, Hopkins PM, Jurkat-Rott K, Klinger W, Kozak-Ribbens G, Krivosic R, Monnier N, Nivoche Y, Olthoff D, Rueffert H, Sorrentino V, Tegazzin V, Mueller CR. *Eur J Hum Genet*. 2003;11:342-8.

838. Sambuughin N, Sei Y, Gallagher KL, Wyre HW, Madsen D, Nelson TE, Fletcher JE, Rosenberg H, Muldoon SM. *Anesthesiology.* 2001;95:594-99.

839. Girard T, Urwyler A, Censier K, Mueller CR, Zorzato F, Treves S. *Hum Mutat.* 2001;18:357-8.

840. Brandt A, Schleithoff L, Jurkat-Rott K, Klingler W, Baur C, Lehmann-Horn F. *Hum Mol Genet.* 1999;8:2055-62.

841. Monnier N, Krivosic-Horber R, Payen JF, Kozak-Ribbens G, Nivoche Y, Adnet P, Reyford H, Lunardi J. *Anesthesiology.* 2002;97:1067-74.

842. Urwyler A, Deufel T, McCarthy T, West S. *Br J Anaesth.* 2001;86:283-7.

843. Sei Y, Sambuughin N, Muldoon S. *Anesthesiology.* 2004;100:464-5.

844. Wappler F, Fiege M, Steinfath M, Agarwal K, Scholz J, Singh S, Matschke J, Schulte Am Esch J. *Anesthesiology.* 2001;94:95-100.

845. Davis MR, Haan E, Jungbluth H, Sewry C, North K, Muntoni F, Kuntzer T, Lamont P, Bankier A, Tomlinson P, Sanchez A, Walsh P, Nagarajan L, Oley C, Colley A, Gedeon A, Quinlivan R, Dixon J, James D, Muller CR, Laing NG. *Neuromuscul Disord.* 2003;13:151-7.

846. Robinson R, Hopkins P, Carsana A, Gilly H, Halsall J, Heytens L, Islander G, Jurkat-Rott K, Muller C, Shaw MA. *Hum Genet.* 2003;112:217-8.

847. Jungbluth H, Muller CR, Halliger-Keller B, Brockington M, Brown SC, Feng L, Chattopadhyay A, Mercuri E, Manzur AY, Ferreiro A, Laing NG, Davis MR, Roper HP, Dubowitz V, Bydder G, Sewry CA, Muntoni F. *Neurology.* 2002;59:284-87.

848. Monnier N, Romero NB, Lerale J, Landrieu P, Nivoche Y, Fardeau M, Lunardi J. *Hum Mol Genet.* 2001;10:2581-92.

849. Ferreiro A, Monnier N, Romero NB, Leroy JP, Bonnemann C, Haenggeli CA, Straub V, Voss WD, Nivoche Y, Jungbluth H, Lemainque A, Voit T, Lunardi J, Fardeau M, Guicheney P. *Ann Neurol.* 2002;51:750-59.

850. Monnier N, Ferreiro A, Marty I, Labarre-Vila A, Mezin P, Lunardi J. *Hum Mol Genet.* 2003;12:1171-78.

851. Romero NB, Monnier N, Viollet L, Cortey A, Chevallay M, Leroy JP, Lunardi J, Fardeau M. *Brain.* 2003;126:2341-9.

852. Dirksen RT. *Front Biosci.* 2002;7:d659-70.

853. Cannon SC. *Neuromuscul Disord.* 2002;12:533-43.

854. Jurkat-Rott K, Lerche H, Lehmann-Horn F. *J Neurol.* 2002;249:1493-502.

855. Taratuto AL. *Curr Opin Neurol.* 2002;15:553-61.

856. Lueck JD, Goonasekera SA, Dirksen RT. *Basic Applied Myology.* 2004;In Press.

857. Manzur AY, Sewry CA, Ziprin J, Dubowitz V, Muntoni F. *Neuromuscul Disord.* 1998;8:467-73.

858. Monnier N, Romero NB, Lerale J, Nivoche Y, Qi D, MacLennan DH, Fardeau M, Lunardi J. *Hum Mol Genet.* 2000;9:2599-608.

859. Jungbluth H, Sewry CA, Muntoni F. *Eur J Paediatr Neurol.* 2003;7:23-30.

860. Scacheri PC, Hoffman EP, Fratkin JD, Semino-Mora C, Senchak A, Davis MR, Laing NG, Vedanarayanan V, Subramony SH. *Neurology.* 2000;55:1689-96.

861. Gallant EM, Lentz LR. *Am J Physiol.* 1992;262:C422-6.

862. Gallant EM, Jordan RC. *Muscle Nerve.* 1996;19:68-73.

863. Dietze B, Henke J, Eichinger HM, Lehmann-Horn F, Melzer W. *J Physiol.* 2000;526:507-14.

864. Tong J, McCarthy TV, MacLennan DH. *J Biol Chem.* 1999;274:693-702.

865. Avila G, Dirksen RT. *J Gen Physiol.* 2001;118:277-90.

866. Tilgen N, Zorzato F, Halliger-Keller B, Muntoni F, Sewry C, Palmucci LM, Schneider C, Hauser E, Lehmann-Horn F, Muller CR, Treves S. *Hum Mol Genet.* 2001;10:2879-87.
867. Avila G, O'Brien JJ, Dirksen RT. *Proc Natl Acad Sci U S A.* 2001;98:4215-20.
868. Rossi D, Sorrentino V. *Cell Calcium.* 2002;32:307-19.
869. Harrison GG. *Br J Anaesth.* 1988;60:279-86.
870. Krause T, Gerbershagen MU, Fiege M, Weisshorn R, Wappler F. *Anaesthesia.* 2004;59:364-73.
871. Ellis KO, Castellion AW, Honkomp LJ, Wessels FL, Carpenter JE, Halliday RP. *J Pharm Sci.* 1973;62:948-51.
872. Snyder HR, Jr., Davis CS, Bickerton RK, Halliday RP. *J Med Chem.* 1967;10:807-10.
873. Elovic E. *Phys Med Rehabil Clin N Am.* 2001;12:793-816.
874. Reddy VG. *Middle East J Anesthesiol.* 2002;16:419-42.
875. Kim DH, Sreter FA, Ohnishi ST, Ryan JF, Roberts J, Allen PD, Meszaros LG, Antoniu B, Ikemoto N. *Biochim Biophys Acta.* 1984;775:320-27.
876. Nelson TE. *J Clin Invest.* 1983;72:862-70.
877. Britt BA. *Malignant hyperthermia.* Boston: Martinus Nijhoff; 1987.
878. Ellis KO, Carpenter JF. *Arch Phys Med Rehabil.* 1974;55:362-69.
879. Ellis KO, Bryant SH. *Naunyn Schmiedebergs Arch Pharmacol.* 1972;274:107-9.
880. Ellis KO, Carpenter JF. *Naunyn Schmiedebergs Arch Pharmacol.* 1972;275:83-94.
881. Ellis KO, Wessels FL. *Naunyn Schmiedebergs Arch Pharmacol.* 1978;301:237-40.
882. Denborough M. *Lancet.* 1998;352:1131-36.
883. Wappler F. *Eur J Anaesthesiol.* 2001;18:632-52.
884. MacLennan DH. *Eur J Biochem.* 2000;267:5291-7.
885. Protasi F. *Front Biosci.* 2002;7:d650-58.
886. McCarthy TV, Quane KA, Lynch PJ. *Hum Mutat.* 2000;15:410-17.
887. Fill M, Coronado R, Mickelson JR, Vilven J, Ma JJ, Jacobson BA, Louis CF. *Biophys J.* 1990;57:471-75.
888. Gallant EM, Curtis S, Pace SM, Dulhunty AF. *Biophys J.* 2001;80:1769-82.
889. Nelson TE. *Anesthesiology.* 1992;76:588-95.
890. Allen PD, Lopez JR, Sanchez V, Ryan JF, Sreter FA. *Anesthesiology.* 1992;76:132-38.
891. Van Winkle WB. *Science.* 1976;193:1130-31.
892. Koshita M, Yamamoto M, Hotta K. *J Biochem.* 1982;92:1103-8.
893. Nelson TE. *FEBS Lett.* 1984;167:123-30.
894. Ohnishi ST, Taylor S, Gronert GA. *FEBS Lett.* 1983;161:103-7.
895. White MD, Collins JG, Denborough MA. *Biochem J.* 1983;212:399-405.
896. Dehpour AR, Mofakham S, Mahmoudian M. *Biochem Pharmacol.* 1982;31:965-68.
897. Sengupta C, Meyer UA, Carafoli E. *FEBS Lett.* 1980;117:37-38.
898. Parness J, Palnitkar SS. *J Biol Chem.* 1995;270:18465-72.
899. Palnitkar SS, Mickelson JR, Louis CF, Parness J. *Biochem J.* 1997;326:847-52.
900. Fruen BR, Mickelson JR, Louis CF. *J Biol Chem.* 1997;272:26965-71.
901. Zhao F, Li P, Chen SR, Louis CF, Fruen BR. *J Biol Chem.* 2001;276:13810-16.
902. Palnitkar SS, Bin B, Jimenez LS, Morimoto H, Williams PG, Paul-Pletzer K, Parness J. *J Med Chem.* 1999;42:1872-80.
903. Paul-Pletzer K, Palnitkar SS, Jimenez LS, Morimoto H, Parness J. *Biochemistry.* 2001;40:531-42.
904. El Hayek SM, Zhao J, Bhat M, Xu X, Nagaraj R, Pan Z, Takeshima H, Ma J. *FEBS Lett.* 1999;461:157-64.

905. Kobayashi S, Yamamoto T, Parness J, Ikemoto N. *Biochem J.* 2004;380:561-69.
906. Nelson TE, Lin M, Zapata-Sudo G, Sudo RT. *Anesthesiology.* 1996;84:1368-79.
907. Szentesi P, Collet C, Sarkozi S, Szegedi C, Jona I, Jacquemond V, Kovacs L, Csernoch L. *J Gen Physiol.* 2001;118:355-75.
908. Ohta T, Ito S, Ohga A. *Eur J Pharmacol.* 1990;178:11-19.
909. Butkow N, Wheatley AM, Lippe IT, Marcus RH, Rosendorff C. *Basic Res Cardiol.* 1990;85:297-306.
910. Meissner A, Min JY, Haake N, Hirt S, Simon R. *Eur J Heart Fail.* 1999;1:177-86.
911. Mitchell MB, Winter CB, Banerjee A, Harken AH. *J Surg Res.* 1993;54:411-17.
912. Yu G, Zucchi R, Ronca-Testoni S, Ronca G. *Basic Res Cardiol.* 2000;95:137-43.
913. Zucchi R, Ronca F, Ronca-Testoni S. *Pharmacol Ther.* 2001;89:47-65.
914. Min JY, Meissner A, Feng X, Wang J, Malek S, Wang JF, Simon R, Morgan JP. *Eur J Pharmacol.* 2003;471:41-47.
915. Horton JW, White DJ, Maass D, Sanders B, Thompson M, Giroir B. *J Surg Res.* 1999;87:39-50.
916. Thompson M, Kliewer A, Maass D, Becker L, White DJ, Bryant D, Arteaga G, Horton J, Giroir BP. *Pediatr Res.* 2000;47:669-76.
917. Westhoff JH, Hwang SY, Scott DR, Ozawa F, Volpe P, Inokuchi K, Koulen P. *Cell Calcium.* 2003;34:261-69.
918. Choi BR, Burton F, Salama G. *J Physiol.* 2002;543:615-31.
919. Pogwizd SM, Bers DM. *Ann N Y Acad Sci.* 2002;976:454-65.
920. Shorofsky SR, Balke CW. *Am J Med.* 2001;110:127-40.
921. Allen PD. *Circ Res.* 2002;91:181-82.
922. George CH, Higgs GV, Lai FA. *Circ Res.* 2003;93:531-40.
923. Marks AR, Reiken S, Marx SO. *Circulation.* 2002;105:272-75.
924. Marks AR. *Circulation.* 2002;106:8-10.
925. Eisenhofer G, Friberg P, Rundqvist B, Quyyumi AA, Lambert G, Kaye DM, Kopin IJ, Goldstein DS, Esler MD. *Circulation.* 1996;93:1667-76.
926. Thomas JA, Marks BH. *Am J Cardiol.* 1978;41:233-43.
927. Antos CL, Frey N, Marx SO, Reiken S, Gaburjakova M, Richardson JA, Marks AR, Olson EN. *Circ Res.* 2001;89:997-1004.
928. Morgan JP, Erny RE, Allen PD, Grossman W, Gwathmey JK. *Circulation.* 1990;81:III21-32.
929. Arai M, Matsui H, Periasamy M. *Circ Res.* 1994;74:555-64.
930. Gwathmey JK, Copelas L, MacKinnon R, Schoen FJ, Feldman MD, Grossman W, Morgan JP. *Circ Res.* 1987;61:70-76.
931. Beuckelmann DJ, Nabauer M, Erdmann E. *Circulation.* 1992;85:1046-55.
932. Hasenfuss G, Mulieri LA, Leavitt BJ, Allen PD, Holubarsch C, Just H, Alpert NR. *Basic Res Cardiol.* 1992;87 Suppl 1:107-16.
933. Pieske B, Maier LS, Bers DM, Hasenfuss G. *Circ Res.* 1999;85:38-46.
934. Hobai IA, O'Rourke B. *Circulation.* 2001;103:1577-84.
935. Pogwizd SM, Bers DM. *J Cardiovasc Electrophysiol.* 2002;13:88-91.
936. Schwinger RH, Munch G, Bolck B, Karczewski P, Krause EG, Erdmann E. *J Mol Cell Cardiol.* 1999;31:479-91.
937. Meyer M, Schillinger W, Pieske B, Holubarsch C, Heilmann C, Posival H, Kuwajima G, Mikoshiba K, Just H, Hasenfuss G. *Circulation.* 1995;92:778-84.
938. Shannon TR, Pogwizd SM, Bers DM. *Circ Res.* 2003;93:592-94.

939. Kapiloff MS, Jackson N, Airhart N. *J Cell Sci.* 2001;114:3167-76.
940. Reiken S, Gaburjakova M, Gaburjakova J, He Kl KL, Prieto A, Becker E, Yi Gh GH, Wang J, Burkhoff D, Marks AR. *Circulation.* 2001;104:2843-48.
941. Yano M, Ono K, Ohkusa T, Suetsugu M, Kohno M, Hisaoka T, Kobayashi S, Hisamatsu Y, Yamamoto T, Noguchi N, Takasawa S, Okamoto H, Matsuzaki M. *Circulation.* 2000;102:2131-36.
942. Wu Y, MacMillan LB, McNeill RB, Colbran RJ, Anderson ME. *Am J Physiol.* 1999;276:H2168-78.
943. Bers DM, Li L, Satoh H, McCall E. *Ann N Y Acad Sci.* 1998;853:157-77.
944. Studer R, Reinecke H, Bilger J, Eschenhagen T, Bohm M, Hasenfuss G, Just H, Holtz J, Drexler H. *Circ Res.* 1994;75:443-53.
945. Weber CR, Piacentino V, 3rd, Ginsburg KS, Houser SR, Bers DM. *Circ Res.* 2002;90:182-89.
946. Piacentino V, 3rd, Margulies KB, Houser SR. *Ann N Y Acad Sci.* 2002;976:476-7.
947. Piacentino V, 3rd, Weber CR, Chen X, Weisser-Thomas J, Margulies KB, Bers DM, Houser SR. *Circ Res.* 2003;92:651-8.
948. Dhalla NS, Dixon IM, Rupp H, Barwinsky J. *Basic Res Cardiol.* 1991;86 Suppl 3:13-23.
949. Houser SR, Freeman AR, Jaeger JM, Breisch EA, Coulson RL, Carey R, Spann JF. *Am J Physiol.* 1981;240:H168-76.
950. Koumi S, Backer CL, Arentzen CE. *Circulation.* 1995;92:164-74.
951. Beuckelmann DJ, Nabauer M, Erdmann E. *Circulation Research.* 1993;73:379-385.
952. Tomaselli GF, Beuckelmann DJ, Calkins HG, Berger RD, Kessler PD, Lawrence JH, Kass D, Feldman AM, Marban E. *Circulation.* 1994;90:2534-9.
953. Matsuda H, Noma A, Kurachi Y, Irisawa H. *Circ Res.* 1982;51:142-51.
954. Clusin WT. *Nature.* 1983;301:248-50.
955. Giles W, Shimoni Y. *J Physiol.* 1989;417:465-81.
956. Collier ML, Levesque PC, Kenyon JL, Hume JR. *Circ Res.* 1996;78:936-44.
957. Schlotthauer K, Bers DM. *Circ Res.* 2000;87:774-80.
958. Sipido KR, Volders PG, de Groot SH, Verdonck F, Van de Werf F, Wellens HJ, Vos MA. *Circulation.* 2000;102:2137-44.
959. Armoundas AA, Hobai IA, Tomaselli GF, Winslow RL, O'Rourke B. *Circ Res.* 2003;93:46-53.
960. Pogwizd SM, Corr PB. *Circ Res.* 1987;61:352-71.
961. Billington CK, Joseph SK, Swan C, Scott MG, Jobson TM, Hall IP. *Am J Physiol.* 1999;276:L412-9.
962. Swan H, Piippo K, Viitasalo M, Heikkila P, Paavonen T, Kainulainen K, Kere J, Keto P, Kontula K, Toivonen L. *J Am Coll Cardiol.* 1999;34:2035-42.
963. Priori SG, Napolitano C, Memmi M, Colombi B, Drago F, Gasparini M, DeSimone L, Coltorti F, Bloise R, Keegan R, Cruz Filho FE, Vignati G, Benatar A, DeLogu A. *Circulation.* 2002;106:69-74.
964. Ono K, Yano M, Ohkusa T, Kohno M, Hisaoka T, Tanigawa T, Kobayashi S, Matsuzaki M. *Cardiovasc Res.* 2000;48:323-31.
965. Mohler PJ, Schott JJ, Gramolini AO, Dilly KW, Guatimosim S, duBell WH, Song LS, Haurogne K, Kyndt F, Ali ME, Rogers TB, Lederer WJ, Escande D, Le Marec H, Bennett V. *Nature.* 2003;421:634-9.
966. Schott JJ, Charpentier F, Peltier S, Foley P, Drouin E, Bouhour JB, Donnelly P, Vergnaud G, Bachner L, Moisan JP. *Am J Hum Genet.* 1995;57:1114-22.

967. Ahern GP, Junankar PR, Dulhunty AF. *Neuroscience Letters*. 1997;225:81-4.

968. Berlin JR, Bassani JW, Bers DM. *Biophysical Journal*. 1994;67:1775-87.

969. Reiken S, Wehrens XH, Vest JA, Barbone A, Klotz S, Mancini D, Burkhoff D, Marks AR. *Circulation*. 2003;107:2459-66.

970. Doi M, Yano M, Kobayashi S, Kohno M, Tokuhisa T, Okuda S, Suetsugu M, Hisamatsu Y, Ohkusa T, Matsuzaki M. *Circulation*. 2002;105:1374-9.

971. Echt DS, Liebson PR, Mitchell LB, Peters RW, Obias-Manno D, Barker AH, Arensberg D, Baker A, Friedman L, Greene HL, *et al. N Engl J Med*. 1991;324:781-8.

972. Marban E. *Nature*. 2002;415:213-8.

973. Prestle J, Janssen PM, Janssen AP, Zeitz O, Lehnart SE, Bruce L, Smith GL, Hasenfuss G. *Circ Res*. 2001;88:188-94.

974. De la Bastie D, Levitsky D, Rappaport L, Mercardier J, Marotte F, Winewsky C, Brovkovich V, Schwartz K, Lompre A. *Circ. Res*. 1990;66:554-564.

975. Cory CR, McCutcheon LJ, O'Grady M, Pang AW, Geiger JD, O'Brien PJ. *Am. J. Physiol.* 1993;264:H926-H937.

976. Linck B, Boknik P, Eschenhagen T, Muller FU, Neumann J, Nose M, Jones LR, Schmitz W, Scholz H. *Cardiovasc Res*. 1996;31:625-32.

977. Litwin SE, Vatner DE, Morgan JP. *Am J Physiol*. 1995;269:H1553-63.

978. Yamamoto T, Yano M, Kohno M, Hisaoka T, Ono K, Tanigawa T, Saiki Y, Hisamatsu Y, Ohkusa T, Matsuzaki M. *Cardiovasc Res*. 1999;44:146-55.

979. Marks AR. *Am J Physiol*. 1997;272:H597-605.

980. Lam E, Martin MM, Timerman AP, Sabers C, Fleischer S, Lukas T, Abraham RT, O'Keefe SJ, O'Neill EA, Wiederrecht GJ. *J Biol Chem*. 1995;270:26511-22.

981. Sewell TJ, Lam E, Martin MM, Leszyk J, Weidner J, Calaycay J, Griffin P, Williams H, Hung S, Cryan J. *J Biol Chem*. 1994;269:21094-102.

982. Chidsey CA, Harrison DC, Braunwald E. *N Engl J Med*. 1962;267:650-58.

983. Bristow MR. *Circulation*. 2000;101:558-69.

984. Kaneko N. *Drug Dev Res*. 1994;33:429-438.

985. Bruckschlegel G, Holmer SR, Jandeleit K, Grimm D, Muders F, Kromer EP, Riegger GA, Schunkert H. *Hypertension*. 1995;25:250-9.

986. Zierhut W, Studer R, Laurent D, Kastner S, Allegrini P, Whitebread S, Cumin F, Baum HP, de Gasparo M, Drexler H. *Cardiovasc Res*. 1996;31:758-68.

987. Okuda S, Yano M, Doi M, Oda T, Tokuhisa T, Kohno M, Kobayashi S, Yamamoto T, Ohkusa T, Matsuzaki M. *Circulation*. 2004;109:911-9.

988. Oosterhuis HJGH. Clinical aspects. In: DeBates MH, Oosterhuis HJGH, eds. *Myasthenia gravis*. Florida: CRC Press; 1993.

989. Lindstrom JM, Seybold ME, Lennen VA, Whittingham S, Duane DD. *Neurology*. 1998;51:933-939.

990. Drachman DB. *N Engl J Med*. 1994;330:1797-810.

991. Aarli JA. *Arch Neurol*. 1999;56:25-7.

992. Bedlack RS, Sanders DB. *Postgrad Med*. 2000;107:211-4, 220-2.

993. Beekman R, Kuks JB, Oosterhuis HJ. *J Neurol*. 1997;244:112-8.

994. Vincent A, Willcox N. *Pathol Res Pract*. 1999;195:535-40.

995. Wekerle H, Muller-Hermelink HK. The thymus in myasthenia gravis. In: Muller-Hermelink HK, Berry CL, Grundmann E, eds. *The human thymus: histopathology and pathology*. Berlin, Heidelberg: Springer-Verlag; 1986.
996. Myking AO, Skeie GO, Varhaug JE, Andersen KS, Gilhus NE, Aarli JA. *Eur J Neurol.* 1998;5:401-405.
997. Romi F, Skeie GO, Aarli JA, Gilhus NE. *J Neurol.* 2000;247:369-75.
998. Mygland A, Tysnes OB, Matre R, Aarli JA, Gilhus NE. *Autoimmunity.* 1994;17:327-31.
999. Benacquista BL, Sharma MR, Samso M, Zorzato F, Treves S, Wagenknecht T. *Biophys J.* 2000;78:1349-58.
1000. Skeie GO, Mygland A, Treves S, Gilhus NE, Aarli JA, Zorzato F. *Muscle Nerve.* 2003;27:81-9.
1001. Skeie GO, Lunde PK, Sejersted OM, Mygland A, Aarli JA, Gilhus NE. *Muscle Nerve.* 1998;21:329-35.
1002. Romi F, Skeie GO, Vedeler C, Aarli JA, Zorzato F, Gilhus NE. *J Neuroimmunol.* 2000;111:169-76.
1003. Gilhus NE, Aarli JA, Christensson B, Matre R. *J Neuroimmunol.* 1984;7:55-64.
1004. Marx A, Osborn M, Tzartos S, Geuder KI, Schalke B, Nix W, Kirchner T, Muller-Hermelink HK. *Dev Immunol.* 1992;2:77-84.
1005. Mygland A, Kuwajima G, Mikoshiba K, Tysnes OB, Aarli JA, Gilhus NE. *J Neuroimmunol.* 1995;62:79-83.
1006. Romi F, Bo L, Skeie GO, Myking A, Aarli JA, Gilhus NE. *J Neuroimmunol.* 2002;128:82-9.
1007. Vanderlugt CJ, Miller SD. *Curr Opin Immunol.* 1996;8:831-6.
1008. Mygland A, Tysnes OB, Aarli JA, Matre R, Gilhus NE. *J Autoimmun.* 1993;6:507-15.
1009. Yanase K, Smith RM, Puccetti A, Jarett L, Madaio MP. *J Clin Invest.* 1997;100:25-31.
1010. Teillaud JL. *Pathol Biol (Paris).* 1999;47:771-5.
1011. Iwasa K, Komai K, Takamori M. *Muscle Nerve.* 1998;21:1655-60.
1012. Somnier FE, Skeie GO, Aarli JA, Trojaborg W. *Eur J Neurol.* 1999;6:555-63.
1013. Mygland A, Aarli JA, Matre R, Gilhus NE. *J Neurol Neurosurg Psych.* 1994;57:843-46.
1014. Skeie GO, Bartoccioni E, Evoli A, Aarli J, Gilhus NE. *Eur J Neurol.* 1996;3:136-140.
1015. Agius MA, Richman DP, Fairclough RH, Aarli J, Gilhus NE, Romi F. *Ann N Y Acad Sci.* 2003;998:453-6.
1016. Aarli JA. *Eur J Neurol.* 1997;4:203-209.
1017. Dropcho EJ. *Ann N Y Acad Sci.* 1998;841:246-61.
1018. Romi F. Muscle autoantibodies in myasthenia gravis: clinical, immunological, and therapeutic implications. In: *Dept. of Neurology*. Bergen: University of Bergen; 2001.
1019. Romi F, Skeie GO, Aarli JA, Gilhus NE. *Arch Neurol.* 2000;57:1596-600.
1020. Venuta F, Rendina EA, De Giacomo T, Della Rocca G, Antonini G, Ciccone AM, Ricci C, Coloni GF. *Eur J Cardiothorac Surg.* 1999;15:621-24.
1021. Romi F, Gilhus NE, Varhaug JE, Myking A, Aarli JA. *Eur Neurol.* 2003;49:210-7.
1022. Frist WH, Thirumalai S, Doehring CB, Merrill WH, Stewart JR, Fenichel GM, Bender HW, Jr. *Ann Thorac Surg.* 1994;57:334-8.
1023. Romi F, Gilhus NE, Varhaug JE, Myking A, Skeie GO, Aarli JA. *Eur J Neurol.* 2002;9:55-61.
1024. Evoli A, Minisci C, Di Schino C, Marsili F, Punzi C, Batocchi AP, Tonali PA, Doglietto GB, Granone P, Trodella L, Cassano A, Lauriola L. *Neurology.* 2002;59:1844-50.

INDEX

E

I